Resounding praise for

THE THYROID CONNECTION

by Amy Myers

"Dr. Myers's plan is one of the most accessible, inspiring, and effective programs I have ever encountered. Anyone with a diagnosed, misdiagnosed, or even undiagnosed thyroid disorder will benefit from reading *The Thyroid Connection.*"

—Robb Wolf, author of *The Paleo Solution*

"People who feel overweight, sluggish, or depressed can find solace and advice in this holistic look at disorders of the thyroid, the hormone-secreting gland that effects metabolism."

—Karen Springen, *Booklist*

"Who doesn't want to eat delicious foods, have more energy, and feel their absolute best? You don't have to upend your life to see amazing results—you just have to read *The Thyroid Connection.*"

—Mark Hyman, MD, author of *Food Fix*

"Thyroid disease is incredibly prevalent and affects every organ system in the human body. In *The Thyroid Connection,* Dr. Amy Myers skillfully and eloquently guides us to the understanding that our lifestyle choices play major roles in determining thyroid health and function. Her message is empowering for those with thyroid issues as well as those who want to maintain thyroid health and resistance to disease. This book belongs on the reference shelf for anyone wishing to remain healthy!"

—David Perlmutter, MD, author of *Grain Brain* and *Brain Maker*

"In *The Thyroid Connection*, Dr. Amy Myers dismantles myths and exposes the truth about thyroid dysfunctions—some of the most misunderstood disorders plaguing millions of Americans."

—Frank Lipman, MD, author of *The New Health Rules*

"As a sufferer of thyroid dysfunction herself, Dr. Myers writes with a compassion and understanding that is not only comforting, but hugely inspiring."

—Terry Wahls, MD, author of *The Wahls Protocol*

The
THYROID
CONNECTION

Also by Amy Myers, MD

The Autoimmune Solution: Prevent and Reverse the Full Spectrum of Inflammatory Symptoms and Diseases

The
THYROID
CONNECTION

Why You Feel Tired, Brain-Fogged, and Overweight— and How to Get Your Life Back

AMY MYERS, MD

LITTLE, BROWN SPARK
New York   Boston   London

To all of us who have been failed by
conventional medicine

Little, Brown Spark
Hachette Book Group
1290 Avenue of the Americas, New York, NY 10104
littlebrownspark.com

Originally published in hardcover by Little, Brown and Company, September 2016
First Little, Brown Spark paperback edition, March 2021

Little, Brown Spark is an imprint of Little, Brown and Company, a division of Hachette Book Group, Inc. The Little, Brown Spark name and logo are trademarks of Hachette Book Group, Inc.

The publisher is not responsible for websites (or their content) that are not owned by the publisher.

The Hachette Speakers Bureau provides a wide range of authors for speaking events. To find out more, go to hachettespeakersbureau.com or call (866) 376-6591.

Drawings by Ali Fine

ISBN 978-0-316-27286-5 (hc) / 978-0-316-27285-8 (pb)
LCCN 2016939895

Printing 1, 2021

LSC-C

Printed in the United States of America

Contents

The
THYROID
CONNECTION

Introduction

Hey there.

You may be reading this book because you think you've got a thyroid problem or you *know* you've got one. Either way, you probably have the sinking feeling that your doctor is missing something, because he or she keeps insisting that you're fine, whereas *you* know that "fine" is the last thing you are.

Maybe you've been gaining weight even though you're sticking like glue to your weight-loss plan. Or maybe you've been eating and exercising just the way you always have—good, bad, or indifferent—but you used to have a stable weight and now the pounds are mounting up.

Or perhaps you have the opposite problem—your weight is suddenly dropping, quickly, even though you're eating way more than usual and seem to be hungry even after finishing a huge meal. Maybe you're struggling with a racing heart or sudden palpitations. Perhaps you're in a continual state of dread, a low-grade anxiety that has you constantly on edge.

Maybe you're having way too many senior moments—and you're only in your twenties. Or maybe you are in your sixties, but you *know* your brain should be working better than it is.

Perhaps you're tired all the time. Or listless. Or depressed. Maybe your hormones are all over the place. Or you can't get pregnant, even though you've been trying for a while. Or your sex drive seems to have gone permanently AWOL. Perhaps you've got some other upsetting symptom— indigestion, constipation, diarrhea. Maybe your anxiety has begun to erupt into devastating panic attacks that seem to happen for no reason.

Or perhaps your problem is achy joints, trembling hands, weakened muscles, flaky skin. Maybe you're always cold. Or maybe—and this one can be the most disturbing of all—your hair is starting to fall out.

Any or all of these symptoms can indicate a thyroid problem—either a thyroid that is *under*performing or one that is *over*performing (while the symptoms might be distinct, there can be a lot of overlap). And if your doctor has assured you that you *don't* have a thyroid problem—that your labs are normal, or that you're already getting the right amount of supplemental thyroid hormone, or that your issues are caused by female hormones (if you're a woman) or low testosterone (if you're a man) or by depression or stress or anxiety or not being disciplined enough about your diet—well, I'm here to tell you that, while some of this might be true, you still might have a thyroid problem.

That's right. Even if your doctor says you *don't* have a thyroid problem, you very well might. It is all too sadly possible that the tests you're getting aren't accurate, that your doctor is misinterpreting the results, that you're being undermedicated, that you're getting the wrong type of medication—or that you're suffering from some combination of all those factors.

Meanwhile, you're feeling lousy, exhausted, old before your time, and—since your doctor won't believe you—possibly crazy. So breathe a big sigh of relief and get ready to feel better. Because in this book, you're going to find out that you were right all along. There *is* something wrong with you. You *do* have thyroid dysfunction, it *can* be treated, and as soon as it is, you're going to feel like a whole new person.

MAKING YOUR OWN THYROID CONNECTION

It's remarkable how many symptoms—large, small, and in between—are connected to your thyroid. In fact, just about every aspect of your body depends on thyroid function; if your thyroid isn't working up to par, you won't be either. Healing and supporting your thyroid is one of the most important ways you can connect to your body, and one of the best ways to achieve optimal health.

In this book, you're going to learn all about your thyroid—how it works, why it can make you feel so miserable, and what you can do to get a more accurate diagnosis. You're going to learn which tests to ask for and what treatment options to explore.

You're also going to discover how to transform your health through the right diet and lifestyle—healing your gut, getting the nutrients your thyroid needs, avoiding inflammatory foods, ridding your body of its toxic burden, treating infections, and practicing effective stress reduction. Toward this end, you'll learn just how much exercise is good for your thyroid, since exercising too much or too intensely can actually disrupt thyroid function.

Best of all, you're going to find out how to get rid of those symptoms. How to clear away the brain fog. How to soothe the anxiety and ease the depression. How to heal those achy joints and raging hormones. How to get your sex life back. How to drop those extra pounds and never regain them. And, yes, how to get your hair growing all thick and healthy—better than you've ever seen it—and have clear glowing skin and boatloads of energy to boot.

That's what I want for you—total vibrant health and nothing less. That's what you can look forward to when your thyroid is working optimally and you're following the diet and lifestyle that supports excellent health. I know you can do it, because that's what thousands of my patients have achieved. If they could get there, you can too.

TAKING CHARGE OF YOUR HEALTH

There are two key aspects to thyroid health.

The most important depends on you. If you follow The Myers Way® Thyroid Connection Plan, my protocol for total thyroid health that I outline in this book, you'll see a dramatic improvement in your health, vitality, and well-being. After ten years of using this protocol both in my practice and for myself, I can promise you that nothing— and I mean *nothing*—makes you feel as good as giving your body what it needs.

The second aspect of thyroid health involves working with your doctor. In this book, you're going to learn everything you need to know to work with your physician so you can be 100 percent sure you are getting the right diagnosis and the most effective treatment. And *wow,* are you going to feel better when you do!

Few things feel as awful as a messed-up thyroid and a doctor who doesn't believe you have a problem. How do I know? Because before I became a thyroid doctor, I was a thyroid patient. I know how miserable your life can be when your thyroid is out of whack. I know how frustrating it is when your doctor doesn't believe you, or when you are told that everything is fine when you *know* that it isn't. I especially know how devastating it can be to think that you've run out of options, to believe that there's nothing you can do but resign yourself to a life of mood swings and weight gain, anxiety and depression, brain fog and fatigue and thinning hair.

I know it because I've lived it. At age thirty-two, I had my own raging thyroid to deal with, a terrifying disorder that made me feel as though my body was not my own and my mind was spinning out of control. And even though I was a second-year medical student and had more understanding of basic anatomy than most people, my own doctor refused to believe me. "Oh," she said, "it's just stress. And you medical students always think you've got every problem you read about in your textbooks."

No. I had a genuinely disordered thyroid, which my doctor initially refused to test. And even after I insisted on a full workup and got my diagnosis, the treatments offered to me by conventional medicine were often worse than the disease. Sad to say, most traditional doctors — not all, but most — do a very, very poor job of treating thyroid dysfunction. They just keep missing the boat.

So let me share with you my own personal thyroid connection, because that's what has inspired me throughout my medical career to listen to my patients, understand what's really going on, and seek out the best possible treatments — the ones that rely on your body's own natural ability to achieve optimal health. Conventional medicine failed me — there's no other way to put it. It's my mission not to let it fail you too.

WHEN YOUR DOCTOR WON'T
BELIEVE YOU...

"You don't have a thyroid problem."

Like millions of other patients before and after me, I heard those dismissive words and my heart sank. I had just started my second year of medical school. I had always been strong and healthy. I knew how to work hard, and I liked nothing better than to rise to a challenge, whether it was my two-year stint in the Peace Corps or that first year of medical school. Even through those long, grueling months of my mother's battle with cancer and her early death, I had found a way to rise to the occasion. And after she died, I had begun work in a research lab where I studied and patented a natural compound that might prevent others from dying as she did.

But now, seemingly out of nowhere, my body was totally out of control. Every day I struggled with anxiety that at times would erupt into full-blown panic attacks, complete with racing pulse, rapid breathing, and a growing feeling of doom. At night, I lay awake, hearing my heart beat double-time in sync with the ticking clock, unable to calm myself into sleep.

I was also losing weight at an alarming rate. If I didn't eat two pieces of Ezekiel toast spread thickly with butter right before bedtime, I would weigh in at two pounds lighter the next morning. And if that sounds like the ideal weight-loss plan, let me tell you, it was anything but. I was gaunt, haggard, and frail, my muscles trembling so badly when I went down the stairs that I had to clutch the railing for dear life. I was always hungry, even after I ate. It got so bad that while I was sitting in our school's giant lecture hall, I couldn't even take proper notes—my hands had developed such a pronounced tremor that my fingers couldn't control the pen.

Anybody's friends would have been worried. My friends were medical students who observed my symptoms firsthand. "Amy, go see a doctor," they insisted. So I went—only to have her tell me that I had "medical-student syndrome": believing that I had every symptom we were learning about in school.

No, I insisted. I knew my body. Something terrible was going on.

"Maybe it's just stress," the doctor suggested, already preparing to move on to her next patient. "After all, the second year of medical school is one of the hardest."

Stress? I had helped care for my dying mother and made it through her funeral. I had spent more than two years in the Peace Corps in a Paraguayan village so small, it wasn't even on a map, with no running water and an eight-hour journey to the nearest telephone. I had successfully completed my first year of medical school. *That* was all stress — and my body had never responded with weight loss, insomnia, panic, and tremors; nothing even close.

It wasn't easy to listen to my own self-knowledge rather than the authoritative pronouncements of my doctor, especially when I was so ill I could barely function. But I've always been a feisty Louisiana woman — that's how my mother raised me — and I just couldn't go along with a diagnosis that I *knew* was so off base.

"Please," I insisted, "I need a complete workup." Somehow I managed to stand my ground, and, reluctantly, she ordered a complete battery of blood tests.

One week later I was spending the weekend at my aunt's house on the Gulf Coast when I got a phone call from this very same doctor. I don't think she actually apologized. But she did tell me that I had a serious disorder of my thyroid.

As you'll see later in this book, there are two ways your thyroid can go out of whack. The most common is *hypothyroidism,* when your thyroid *under*performs. Hypothyroid conditions may or may not be autoimmune. The autoimmune version is known as Hashimoto's thyroiditis and is actually the most common form of underactive thyroid.

Or you can have *hyperthyroidism,* when your thyroid *over*performs. That less common condition is what I had, and it also may or may not be autoimmune. I had the autoimmune kind, known as Graves' disease.

When you've got an autoimmune disease of any type your body is basically attacking itself. The vast majority of thyroid disorders are autoimmune in nature — your immune system begins attacking your thyroid. To get at the root of the problem, you need to address both the thyroid gland *and* the immune system, but sadly, most conventional doctors just ignore the immune system and treat only the thyroid. I would later discover that this is a very incomplete way to treat both Hashimoto's and Graves'.

Later, too, I would learn that I could have treated my condition through a combination of diet, high-quality supplements, and lifestyle changes—the protocol that has become The Myers Way Thyroid Connection Plan. But I didn't know then what I know now, so when I was referred to an endocrinologist—a physician who specializes in hormonal disorders, including thyroid dysfunction—I was sort of stuck with what he told me.

"You've got three choices," he said. "One, take a medication known as propylthiouracil, or PTU, which will shut down your thyroid and stop it from overperforming. Two, use radioactive iodine"—I-131—"to blow up your thyroid." (Like Hiroshima, I thought with a shudder.) "Or, three, have a surgeon remove all or part of your thyroid."

In fact, none of those choices sat well with me. My parents had been into holistic health and Chinese medicine. I grew up eating home-cooked meals made of organic whole foods. Mom grew organic tomatoes and sprouts and fed us home-baked whole-wheat bread and homemade plain yogurt. Until I left home, I didn't know that rice came in any color but brown. At fourteen, I became a vegetarian. Even when I entered medical school, I planned to be a holistic doctor of some kind—someone who relied on the healing properties of good food and viewed the body as a whole—although at the time, I had no idea how to pursue that goal.

Of course, now I know that dairy, gluten, grains, legumes, and nightshades (tomatoes, peppers, eggplants, potatoes) can trigger *inflammation*—an immune system response that is at the heart of autoimmune conditions, thyroid dysfunction, and many other chronic health problems. I also know that my body needs the nutrients in wild, organic animal protein to support both immune and thyroid health as well as other bodily functions. Ironically, my vegetarianism and Mom's "healthy foods" were part of what was making me sick.

But that was something I'd learn later on. Meanwhile, I was rightly suspicious of those three conventional choices. Harsh medication with devastating side effects? Assaulting my thyroid with radioactive poison? Surgery? None of them sounded like how I wanted to treat my body.

So I tried to go another way, working with a doctor of Chinese medicine who had her own herbs and dietary protocols. She loaded me up with fermented foods, sprouted grains, disgusting powders and teas and tinctures. Fermented foods can be good for your health, but not when your system is as distressed as mine was. And all the rest of it just made me feel worse.

So back I went to the endocrinologist, and at this point, my symptoms were really bad. The insomnia was insane — I was lucky to get three hours of sleep a night. My heart was racing so fast that it felt as though it were beating out of my chest — and yes, I was taking beta-blockers, a prescription medication to slow my heart rate, which contributed to the brain fog. I had the sinking feeling that whatever symptom I brought in, the doctor was going to medicate it. Then I'd be dealing with my thyroid dysfunction *and* all the side effects. Thanks to all those sleepless nights, I was having a hard time showing up for class, and I couldn't afford to fail medical school. So, grudgingly, I began a long, draining, and dispiriting series of conventional medical treatments.

First I tried the PTU, because that seemed like the least invasive choice. Maybe it was, but it was still pretty brutal. The medicine dried out my mouth and nose to an agonizing extent, and to top it all off, the meds turned my *over*active thyroid into an *under*active one. Say hello to a whole new set of symptoms: fatigue, constantly feeling cold, dried-out skin, and hair that started to fall out in clumps.

After a few weeks of feeling terrible, I returned to the endocrinologist. He was more worried by my chronic fatigue than my other symptoms and ran some blood tests. Later that day, he told me that the PTU was beginning to destroy my liver in a condition known as toxic hepatitis. That was a one-in-a-million risk, but it had happened to me, and if I didn't get off the medication right away, I might eventually die of full-blown liver failure. I was ordered to get into bed and stay there until my liver recovered — which could be weeks or even months.

Okay, instead of three conventional choices, I was down to only two: surgery or the destruction of my thyroid via radioactive iodine. As little as the nuclear option appealed to me, surgery seemed an even more frightening prospect. I had become so debilitated and demoralized that if something had gone wrong under the knife, I seriously questioned my ability to fight my way back to life. I spent day after day searching for alternative treatments but found none. So I chose to *ablate*—or destroy—my thyroid with radioactive iodine.

If you go this route, your thyroid gland, while it is being destroyed, can dump large amounts of thyroid hormone into your bloodstream. Eventually, you won't have a thyroid at all, and you'll have to take supplemental thyroid hormone for life. But before I could get to that point, those sudden, massive surges of hormone sent me into even more severe panic attacks made all the more upsetting because they could strike at any time. I had to add Xanax to my personal pharmacy because I literally never knew where I would freak out next—at the dog park? The supermarket? In church? I began to avoid leaving my house for any reason whatsoever; the fear of having to struggle through a public panic attack was just too great.

Then, as if I were caught in a medical pinball machine, my system ricocheted back in the other direction—low thyroid. Once again I was exhausted and constantly cold. I quickly gained ten pounds, and, yep, I was back to losing hair. To make matters even worse, I developed irritable bowel syndrome.

Since my thyroid had been intentionally destroyed, I now needed to take supplemental thyroid hormone, so my doctor put me on Synthroid. But my symptoms continued. And here's the thing: even though I felt like death warmed over, *my thyroid labs were normal.*

So once again, I was begging a doctor to believe me. I'd run through my symptoms and say how awful I felt, and my doctor would look at my lab reports and shake his head. Talk about adding insult to injury.

BUT *I* BELIEVE YOU

Now, I know my story is more extreme than most. But whether your story is just like mine or somewhat different, you are likely suffering from the same root cause: a dysfunctional thyroid, perhaps also a disordered immune system, and a body that is struggling with a damaged gut, a toxic burden, an underlying infection, or an overload of stress. Like me, you are probably dealing with a doctor who either doesn't believe you or simply doesn't have the right approach—to thyroid *or* diet and lifestyle—to make you feel better.

I'm so sorry you are going through this! You deserve to feel terrific. The information in this book can get you there.

How can I be so sure? Because I have treated thousands of thyroid patients over the past ten years, and believe me, I've heard it all. I've treated people whose symptoms were so subtle and whose labs seemed so normal, they could barely believe they had thyroid dysfunction—except for the periodic brain fog, the slow drain of energy, the mild depression, and the weight that just wouldn't go away. I've treated women who couldn't get pregnant and men who felt as though their sex drive had completely disappeared. And I've worked with patients who, like me, had Graves' disease and helped them completely reverse their symptoms, get off medication, and return their thyroid hormones back to normal levels without the use of any of the harsh medications or extreme treatments that I was offered.

Each of these stories has its own unique details, and certainly yours does too. But here's what they all have in common: a person whose life is being diminished because his or her thyroid just isn't working the way it's supposed to.

Here's another thing these stories have in common: a doctor who is failing to effectively diagnose and treat thyroid dysfunction. And, wow, do I understand how frustrating *that* is—frustrating, debilitating, devastating. My patients tell me how dismissive and unhelpful their previous doctors have been, how these physicians insist that the real problem is depression, or sex hormones, or stress, or anxiety, or even that the issues are "all in your head." How insulting is that?

It's outrageous, but it's true: the way conventional medicine approaches the thyroid virtually guarantees that many—perhaps even most—cases will be misdiagnosed or mistreated, frequently both. Most conventional doctors don't run nearly enough tests. They don't interpret the tests properly. They don't offer enough treatment options. And they don't back up their treatments with a diet and lifestyle that can help restore thyroid health.

Which is why I was beyond relieved to finally discover another way — a better way — than conventional medicine. It's called *functional medicine,* and it transformed my life.

FINDING A BETTER WAY

I first discovered functional medicine at an integrative health symposium, and it was like a bright light turned on to illuminate the darkness. I sat in the auditorium listening to a physician lay out the true root causes of chronic illness, and I thought, *Yes.* This *is the explanation I've been looking for.*

For the first time, I understood the role that diet, gut health, toxins, infections, and stress had played in my health. I found out that foods I'd always believed to be healthy were undermining my gut, my immune system, and my thyroid, especially the gluten, grains, and legumes that had been the mainstay of my diet.

I learned about a condition known as leaky gut, in which the gut wall literally leaks partially digested food into the body, compromising the immune system and assaulting the body with toxins. I discovered many other ways that toxins had compromised my health. I found out that seemingly minor infections were weakening my immune system and that psychological stress was indeed a prime contributor to autoimmune disease.

My life would never be the same. After that conference, I took my health into my own hands. I eliminated the toxic and inflammatory foods from my diet and added in the high-quality supplements needed for optimal thyroid function. I healed my gut, detoxified my system, treated underlying infections, and relieved my stress. Within weeks, I began to feel healthy — for the first time in seven years.

What a difference this new protocol made! My anxiety and panic attacks evaporated. My energy came bounding back. My hair and skin looked terrific. Best of all, I had that glowing sense of well-being that you get only when your body is getting exactly what it needs. Welcome to optimal health!

I stopped seeing the conventional doctors who wanted to ignore the bigger picture and moved my care to a functional medicine physician. I also enrolled in the functional medicine certification program through the Institute for Functional Medicine. I wanted to learn everything I could about this new approach to medicine and health—to become the kind of physician who had helped me achieve such extraordinary results.

If I had known about functional medicine when I first got Graves', I might not have had to suffer through the harsh medications, and I wouldn't have had to destroy my thyroid. I might have been able to treat my overactive thyroid with herbs while eliminating inflammatory foods, healing my gut, and ridding my body of the toxins, infections, and stress that were at the root of my illness. It's remarkable but true that diet and lifestyle can conquer diseases that conventional medicine can scarcely tame. I was sorry I hadn't discovered functional medicine sooner. But at least I could share this tremendous healing with others.

So I eventually left my position as an emergency room physician and opened my own functional medicine practice in Austin, Texas. There I treat a wide variety of patients, with a focus on leaky gut, inflammation, autoimmune conditions, and thyroid dysfunction. I developed The Myers Way, my own personal protocol for healing that has helped thousands of people. I wrote my first book, *The Autoimmune Solution,* which quickly became a *New York Times* bestseller. And now I'm writing this book, because I want you to benefit from everything I've learned.

A WHOLE NEW WORLD

When I first encountered functional medicine, a whole new world opened up. A world where doctors actually *listened* to their patients. A world where each patient was treated as an individual, with a kind of personalized medicine that can make all the difference between dragging yourself along—not really sick, but not really well—and striding through life feeling absolutely terrific. A world where thyroid dysfunction is no longer mislabeled as *depression, anxiety, obesity,* or *hormone problems* but is correctly diagnosed and treated with the right kind of supplemental thyroid hormone or medication plus the diet and lifestyle that your thyroid and immune system need. A world where the body is supported with the right food, exercise, sleep, and stress relief to achieve total, optimal health. Functional medicine has enabled me to help thousands of patients — and, thrillingly, to heal myself.

Now it's your turn. You shouldn't have to go through one more day of having your symptoms misdiagnosed and your condition poorly treated. So I'm going to help you understand what's happening in your body, including what your thyroid, your immune system, and your gut are doing. If you want to find a functional medicine practitioner, I'll provide you with the resources to do that. But if you want to continue with your own conventional doctor, I'll help you work with him or her more effectively so that you can get the tests, diagnosis, and treatment you need and that you deserve.

In this book, you'll learn about which blood tests are typically ordered and what all those numbers mean. You'll find out about other blood tests that you can ask for so that you and your doctor can get a more comprehensive picture of what's really going on. (Yes, the majority of conventional doctors don't ask for enough tests — but most of the labs I'll tell you about are standard blood tests that can be run in any office or by any lab.)

I'll also explain which types of supplemental thyroid hormones are usually prescribed — and what your other options are. Most doctors prescribe a synthetic form of supplemental thyroid hormone known as levothyroxine (popular brand names are Synthroid, Levoxyl, and Tirosint). That form of supplemental hormone has both strengths and weaknesses, and I'll help you understand exactly what they are. You'll also learn about the strengths and weaknesses of desiccated porcine thyroid (popular brand names are Armour, Nature-Throid, and Westhroid) — a natural alternative that works better for some people — as well as about some other options, including specially compounded supplemental thyroid hormone geared precisely to your biology.

In true functional medicine style, I'm going to help you develop a *personalized* health plan to support your thyroid, your immune system, and your gut. In part 5, you'll also find out whether you are suffering from such common gut problems as yeast overgrowth, small intestine bacterial overgrowth (SIBO), and parasites, as well as adrenal dysfunction, and I'll suggest specific remedies for each condition.

Last but not least, I'll provide you with a complete guide to The Myers Way Thyroid Connection Plan: the meal plans, recipes, supplements, and lifestyle recommendations that will jump-start your thyroid function, support your immune system, heal your gut, and make you healthier overall. If your thyroid dysfunction is the result of an autoimmune condition, The Myers Way is even more important for you, since people with one autoimmune condition are three times more likely than the general population to develop a second. Following The Myers Way can help you revitalize your immune system and eliminate your symptoms while preventing additional disorders and diseases.

I don't want you to suffer one more day because your doctor didn't offer the right diagnosis or treatment. I don't want you to have to do what I did—take toxic medication or undergo a permanent medical procedure that cannot be reversed. I don't want you to wonder for one more moment whether your problem is "all in your head" or beat yourself up about not being able to lose weight. Knowledge is power—it's a cliché, but it's true—and in this book, you'll find all the knowledge you need to partner with your doctor and take control of your health. I'm so excited for you, because I know you *can* feel terrific—lean, energized, empowered.

So turn the page and let's get started. A whole new world is waiting.

Part One

THE NEW THYROID EPIDEMIC

CHAPTER 1

The Thyroid Crisis

There's a new epidemic sweeping the country—and your doctor probably doesn't even know about it.

This epidemic might cause you to gain weight that suddenly becomes impossible to lose. Or it could cause you to *lose* weight at an alarming rate, even though you're constantly eating—and constantly hungry.

One version of this epidemic leaves you feeling tired and fatigued, sapped of energy and drained of motivation. Another fills your life with anxiety and dread that frequently erupt into full-blown panic attacks.

Some people with this epidemic suffer from brain fog—loss of clarity and focus, frustrating memory lapses, "senior moments." Others struggle with depression. Hair falling out is another symptom. Aching joints and muscles. A racing heart. Trembling hands. Weakened muscles. Feeling old before your time—even if you're still in your twenties. Difficulty falling asleep. Difficulty *staying* asleep.

This epidemic could increase your chance of having a miscarriage. Or keep you from getting pregnant in the first place. It could kill your sex drive. Or make it difficult to perform sexually whether you're a man (in which case you'd suffer from erectile dysfunction) or a woman (vaginal dryness). It might even put you at increased risk of developing an autoimmune disease.

The worst part is that conventional medicine frequently misses your diagnosis. Your conventional doctor might say, "Your labs are normal. Those symptoms you're feeling? That's just what happens as you get older." Or "Your numbers are within the normal range, so if you don't feel well, it's probably just stress." Or "Your blood work looks good. If you're feeling low, you've got to expect that as you approach menopause."

If your doctor misses your diagnosis, you might be incorrectly pre-scribed an antidepressant or an anti-anxiety medication. You might be given birth control pills to regulate your cycle or hormone replacement therapy to treat your mood swings. Or maybe your doctor just says, "Get some rest, don't work so hard, how about a vacation?"

Even if you have been properly diagnosed, you might not be getting the right treatment. So when you come in still feeling unwell — feeling as though you've turned into another person whom you don't even recognize — your doctor replies, "Hey, whatever you've got, it's not showing up in any of the blood tests I ran — your labs are normal. I'm sorry you're feeling so lousy, but I've done everything I can."

This raging epidemic illness affects at least twenty-seven million Americans and some two hundred million worldwide that we know of — and millions more have never been diagnosed. Although it is most common among women over forty, this epidemic can strike anyone, anywhere — in fact, my colleagues and I are seeing a sharp increase in cases, especially among women in their twenties and thirties.

This epidemic is called *thyroid dysfunction*. And if it's not properly treated, it can destroy your life.

When You Have Too Little Thyroid Hormone...

You often feel cold and might not sweat.
You can become constipated.
You gain weight or cannot lose weight.
You develop brain fog: memory lapses, difficulty concentrating.
You can feel listless and unmotivated.
You struggle with fatigue.
You sleep far more than usual.
You might become depressed or have mood swings.
Your hair falls out.
Your skin feels lifeless and dry.

You suffer from hormone irregularities.

You have been diagnosed with infertility or have had miscarriages.

You may see a goiter in your neck or experience neck swelling.

You feel under par, off, just not yourself.

You have a slow heartbeat.

You have been diagnosed with high cholesterol.

When You Have Too Much Thyroid Hormone...

You often feel warm or have increased perspiration.

You feel anxious, wired, have mood swings.

You struggle with insomnia.

You might develop panic attacks.

Your heart races and you can develop palpitations.

You suffer from loose stools or diarrhea.

You can develop tremors.

You lose weight without trying.

You might develop muscle weakness.

Your eyes might seem to bulge out of their sockets.

You may see a goiter in your neck or experience neck swelling.

You may have irregular periods or infertility.

You may have a rash or thickening of skin on the front of your shins.

Your hair may be falling out.

You may suffer from chronic urticaria or hives.

When you have thyroid dysfunction, you might also have symptoms from *both* lists at the same time or alternating back and forth. You might feel tired *and* wired, exhausted *and* unable to sleep, anxious *and* depressed. I've had patients whose response to an underactive thyroid was to *lose* weight rather than gain it, because their adrenal glands overcompensated for the thyroid issue by overproducing stress hormones. The thyroid signaling system is supercomplex, and there are lots of ways it can misfire. That is why doing a complete thyroid panel of blood tests is so important: to sort through the sometimes confusing symptoms and come up with a reliable diagnosis.

THE THYROID EPIDEMIC

Okay, so here's the thing: *Conventional medicine is failing far too many people.* And nowhere is this failure more evident than with thyroid dysfunction.

The American Thyroid Association says that over the course of a lifetime, at least 12 percent of the U.S. population will suffer from thyroid dysfunction. That's one person in eight. And women are five to eight times more likely than men to be affected. According to the association, up to 60 percent of people with thyroid dysfunction don't even realize they have a problem.

With so many suffering, you'd think conventional medicine would sound the alarm. You'd expect your conventional doctor to be all over thyroid dysfunction — testing you regularly, giving you the right amount and type of medication and/or supplemental thyroid hormone, ensuring that you're getting the right kind of diet and supplements and sleep and stress relief to keep your thyroid in peak condition.

Nope. Not even close. Instead, thyroid dysfunction is one of the most underdiagnosed and improperly treated health conditions. Conventional doctors are failing us in so many ways regarding thyroid dysfunction, it's hard to list them all, but let's give it a try.

- Even when you present with thyroid symptoms, many doctors fail to test for thyroid disorders and misdiagnose the condition, especially if you're younger than forty or you are a man.
- When you *are* tested, you often don't get all the tests you need.
- When you are finally diagnosed and treated, if you are hypothyroid (have an underactive thyroid), you often don't get the right amount or proper form of supplemental thyroid hormone.
- If you are hyperthyroid (have an overactive thyroid), your conventional medical options carry severe, sometimes disabling side effects or irreversible damage and you aren't told about natural herbal treatments that might be equally effective while sparing you the downsides.
- You never learn about the extraordinary effects you can achieve by making certain changes in your diet and lifestyle: consuming the

nutrients your thyroid needs, avoiding foods that trigger *inflammation* (an immune system response that can create numerous problems), healing your gut, getting rid of your toxic overload, treating underlying infections, avoiding overexercising, getting good, restful sleep, and relieving stress.

• You don't find out how to reverse autoimmune conditions and support your immune system — a crucial need, since the vast majority of thyroid dysfunction is due to autoimmunity.

As both a functional medicine physician and a thyroid patient, I hate thinking how badly conventional medicine is failing people with thyroid dysfunction, because I *know* how awful it feels to go through the medical mill. The doctors who tell you it's all in your head. The treatments that are supposed to work but don't, or don't work well enough, or leave you struggling with side effects. The symptoms that get worse and worse and worse, while your doctor brushes them off and insists that you are getting standard-of-care treatment.

All that is bad enough. But what really bothers me is that we've all been sold a bill of goods. We've been told that depression and brain fog and weight gain are an inevitable part of aging — that loss of sex drive and lack of energy and memory lapses are just something you have to learn to live with. We've been fooled into thinking that even in our twenties and thirties, we should expect to feel stressed, burned out, and miserable. The ideal of optimal health and function in every aspect of our bodies — and our lives — is made to seem like some kind of impossible dream, some kind of New Age fantasy instead of an absolutely achievable medical goal that every single one of us should be able to attain.

Well, I'm here to tell you that vibrant, glowing health is *not* a fantasy. My patients achieve it every day, and I know you can too. When you finally get your thyroid back into balance, you won't believe how terrific you feel.

So welcome to *The Thyroid Connection* — the book that's going to turn it all around for you and get you back on track.

WHY IS YOUR THYROID SO IMPORTANT?

When your thyroid function is off, you feel beyond rotten. When it's optimal, you feel terrific: vital, energized, optimistic. How can one small gland have such far-reaching effects? What gives your thyroid so much power?

In fact, your thyroid is absolutely critical to every single cell in your body. Every cell has a receptor for thyroid hormone, which means that no cell can function without it. Thyroid hormone is like the gas in your car's tank—you need a steady stream of it fueling each cell.

But it's not enough to have "some" thyroid hormone. Every cell needs *exactly the right amount*—neither too much nor too little. You thought Goldilocks was fussy? She's nothing compared to how frantic your cells get without the optimal amount of thyroid hormone.

Too little, and your metabolism slows way down. You become cold, depressed, and constipated, with brain fog that fuddles your mind and a listlessness that saps you of energy. You gain weight at the drop of a hat. Your sex hormones might go completely out of whack.

Too much, and your metabolism revs up to warp speed. You become panicky, anxious, and plagued by frequent bowel movements, perhaps even diarrhea. You lose weight even when you eat constantly. Your muscles feel weak and your hands begin to shake.

These are the dramatic extremes. But even when things don't get so out of hand, the wrong amount of thyroid hormone can make your life a misery. It's like a subtle saboteur sapping you of good health and well-being, drop by drop by drop.

Not only your thyroid is involved. The thyroid gland is at the center of a complex network of communication that includes your hypothalamus, your pituitary, your thyroid, and, ultimately, every single one of your cells. This system involves multiple feedback loops providing a constant stream of information—again, so that each of your cells gets exactly the right amount of thyroid hormone. The network is called the *thyroid signaling system,* and it's so detailed and intricate, it puts the Internet to shame.

The thyroid signaling system interacts with all your other hormones, including stress hormones, sex hormones, and all the hormones that enable your brain to process thought and emotion. When your thyroid is off, you don't process stress properly. Your sexual function can be disrupted in many different ways: lowered sex drive, impaired sexual performance, menstrual irregularities, difficulties getting or staying pregnant. Your brain is also affected; thyroid dysfunction has an impact on your levels of anxiety and depression as well as your ability to think, remember, and focus.

Okay. So achieving optimal thyroid function is now your number-one goal. How do you get there?

In most cases, you have to follow two approaches at the same time. You need to practice a healthy diet and lifestyle, The Myers Way Thyroid Connection Plan. You may also need the right type of medical treatment.

THE MYERS WAY THYROID CONNECTION PLAN

- Consume the nutrients your body needs for optimal thyroid function: iodine, protein (to provide you with tyrosine, an amino acid), selenium, zinc, iron, vitamin D, vitamin A, omega-3 fatty acids, and a variety of B vitamins.
- Avoid inflammatory foods, especially gluten and dairy.
- For autoimmune conditions, also avoid all grains and legumes.
- Heal your gut.
- Relieve your body of its toxic burden:
  - Avoid exposure to toxins.
  - Support your body's natural ability to detox.
- Heal any lingering infections you might have, including subtle ones you might not be aware of.
- Relieve stress:
  - Practice stress relief: paced breathing, neurofeedback, float tanks, acupuncture, yoga, meditation, saunas, time in nature, fun and pleasure, whatever reduces your stress. Get the right type of exercise—nothing that is too extreme or intense for your body.
  - Get enough deep restful sleep each night.

Whether your thyroid is *underactive* (*hypo*thyroid) or *overactive* (*hyper*-thyroid), your diet and lifestyle should be basically the same (although my exercise recommendations are somewhat different for each). However, your medical treatment will differ vastly, so let's break it down.

IF YOUR THYROID IS *UNDER*ACTIVE . . .

Let's start by asking *why* your thyroid is underperforming in the first place. There are two basic possibilities: autoimmune or something else.

If you've got an autoimmune disorder...

This is the most common form of thyroid dysfunction: an autoimmune condition in which, over time, your immune system attacks and destroys so much of your thyroid that your thyroid can no longer produce enough hormone to power your cells.

If that's the problem, our goal is to calm your immune system and get it to stop attacking your thyroid. We do this through the diet and lifestyle protocols of The Myers Way.

If we can reverse the dysfunction early enough, we can preserve all or most of your thyroid gland. That's a great outcome, because then your thyroid can still produce all the thyroid hormone you need, and you won't need supplemental hormone.

However, most conventional doctors don't even try to reverse an autoimmune condition—they just don't believe it's possible. They won't suggest an anti-inflammatory diet and lifestyle; they'll just give you supplemental thyroid hormone.

If that's your situation, your thyroid might already have been partially destroyed. That, I'm afraid, is irreversible—we don't yet know how to regenerate thyroid tissue. Depending on how long you've had your autoimmune condition and on what your diet and lifestyle have been, you will probably still need supplemental thyroid hormone. In that case, our goal becomes ensuring that your doctor is giving you exactly the right type and amount. (Don't worry. In part 3, you'll learn exactly what you need to work effectively with your doctor.)

Meanwhile, following The Myers Way Thyroid Connection Plan

will prevent any further damage to your thyroid and keep you from developing another autoimmune condition. Remember, having one autoimmune condition makes you three times more likely to develop another.

If you don't have an autoimmune disorder...

Although most thyroid disorders are autoimmune in nature, some are not. If your thyroid is underperforming but not because of an autoimmune disorder, these are the most common factors at play:

- Your thyroid gland isn't getting the nutrients it needs to produce thyroid hormone.
- Your body isn't getting the nutrients it needs to convert thyroid hormone into the active form that your body can actually use.
- Your body isn't getting the nutrients it needs to enable thyroid hormone to enter your cells.
- Some other imbalance in your stress hormones or sex hormones is disrupting thyroid function.
- Too much of your thyroid hormone is being *bound* to the proteins in your blood, making it unavailable to your cells.

In these cases, too, you'll be making changes to your diet and lifestyle.

If you have never taken supplemental thyroid hormone, The Myers Way Thyroid Connection Plan might be enough to reverse the dysfunction and get you back on track. In some cases, though, you might also need to take supplemental hormone, especially if you're already taking it. In that case, again, our goal is to make sure that your doctor gives you the right dose and type. It's possible that, over time, following The Myers Way will get you into such good shape that you can reduce or even eliminate that supplemental thyroid hormone.

IF YOUR THYROID IS *OVER*ACTIVE...

If you've got an overactive thyroid, we can absolutely get you to a state of optimal health. It just takes longer—sometimes a lot longer—than with an underactive thyroid. As I tell my patients, with an underactive thyroid, it's as though you're trying to coax a reluctant horse out of the gate, whereas with an overactive thyroid, the horse has already burst through and is galloping swiftly away. Coaxing the slow horse out is usually easier than catching the fast one—but in the end, we can still end up with two well-behaved horses!

As with hypothyroidism, hyperthyroidism is usually—but not always—autoimmune in nature. Whether it's autoimmune or not, you'll do well to follow The Myers Way Thyroid Connection Plan, and you'll also take herbs that can help calm your thyroid. It can take several months before your "runaway horse" returns to a calm and optimal state, but once it does, you can enjoy glowing health. At that point, you'll no longer need to take the herbs—but, as in all cases, you should continue to follow The Myers Way, especially if you have an autoimmune condition. You'll also need to keep working with your doctor to check your labs and monitor your progress, especially since an overactive thyroid carries a number of risks, including osteoporosis, heart arrhythmia, and heart failure. Meanwhile, The Myers Way can both help prevent another autoimmune disorder and support your thyroid along with your entire body.

GREAT EXPECTATIONS: JUST HOW GOOD CAN IT GET?

If you have an underperforming thyroid...

Once you're on the right type and dose of supplemental thyroid hormone, *wow,* does your condition improve, especially if you are making the diet and lifestyle changes that support optimal function and health.

The excess weight comes off as if by magic. Your missing energy comes surging back. Your brain fog evaporates. Your hair stops falling out and is thicker and more beautiful than ever before. Your depression and anxiety go away. Your sex drive and sexual function are back to normal. You feel vital, powerful, sharp, and focused, radiating the vibrant health that is your birthright. All you needed was a few simple changes—but it seems like a medical miracle.

If you have an overperforming *thyroid...*

This process is slower, but over time, it is equally dramatic. It might take several months or maybe even longer for your health to improve, but with the right treatment, you can eventually get rid of the panic attacks, the racing heart, and the trembling hands. You'll be able to sleep again, relax again, focus again, enjoy life again. You will feel beyond terrific: calm and energized, vital and relaxed, glowing with deep, reliable health. Your journey might have taken longer, but when you are finally in amazing health, you will enjoy your own medical miracle.

THE TOP SEVEN MYTHS ABOUT THYROID

In part 2 of this book, you'll get a thorough explanation of your thyroid and your immune system. In part 3, you'll learn what most doctors miss and get everything you need to work more effectively with your doctor. And in part 4, you'll find out how The Myers Way Thyroid Connection Plan can help you reverse your symptoms and support your body with a proven protocol for diet and lifestyle.

But I don't want you to have to wait that long to break through the demoralizing myths that surround thyroid dysfunction. I want you to have some good, solid facts at your disposal right now. When your doctor tells you that you don't have a thyroid problem or that you are being properly treated, it can be really hard to believe the opposite. When several doctors all agree that you don't have thyroid dysfunction, it becomes even more difficult to disagree. Conventional wisdom is a powerful beast!

Well, it's time to kill the beast and free yourself from the thyroid myths. Just because a lot of people believe something doesn't make it true — and a lot of doctors believing something doesn't make it any more true. In my first book, *The Autoimmune Solution*, I told the story of Ignaz Semmelweis, the Hungarian doctor who tried for decades to convince his fellow physicians to wash their hands in between attending at childbirths so they didn't transfer germs from one new mother to the next. It took more than fifty years for his newfangled notion to become standard of care, even though his insight seems obvious to us now. I think in fifty years—hopefully, even less—these common thyroid myths are going to seem just as outlandish as not washing your hands. I want you to have that information *now,* though, so here we go:

MYTH 1: Gaining weight, losing energy, and having a lowered sex drive are all normal parts of getting older, and there's just not that much you can do about it.

FACT: These symptoms are often indicators of thyroid dysfunction, and there is quite a bit you can do about it.

Here is where functional medicine is just so much better than conventional medicine. Conventional medicine tends to view decline as inevitable and assumes that with age, the body naturally breaks down.

Well, to some extent that's true, of course—but not nearly to the extent that conventional medicine would have you believe. In fact, if you support the optimal function of your body—if you know what every organ and system needs to function at its best—you can maintain a brisk metabolism, a vigorous sex drive, and a lean, healthy weight, not to mention a strong, steady supply of energy, for your entire life. Yes, you might slow down a bit with each passing decade, but only a bit, because age isn't really the issue. Function is.

The problem is, most people don't know how to support the optimal function of their bodies, and so, indeed, as they get older, function begins to break down. That's not age, though. That's poor diet, leaky gut, too many toxins from a world that is overburdened with heavy metals, industrial chemicals, and factory-farmed foods, underlying infections, not enough exercise or the wrong type of exercise, and too much unrelieved stress. Too many medications add to your body's abuse—including antibiotics, by the way, which disrupt gut function and destroy all the good bacteria while promoting weight gain, among other problems.

The great news, though, is that all this poor function can be corrected through healthier choices—which is particularly exciting for anyone out there with thyroid dysfunction, an autoimmune disorder, or both. You can improve function and eliminate your symptoms, and you can do it at any age. I'll never have the pleasure of meeting most of you, but I can offer the benefit of my experience in the pages of this book.

> MYTH 2: You're in perimenopause or menopause, or you've just had a baby. Brain fog, depression, weight gain, hormonal issues, and generally feeling crummy are par for the course. And the best treatments are birth control pills or hormone replacement therapy.

> FACT: Thyroid dysfunction does frequently kick in as menopause approaches or after you give birth. But the proper treatment can have you feeling sharp and optimistic while maintaining a healthy weight.

One of the things that make me maddest about conventional medicine is how pessimistic conventional doctors seem to be about their patients' prospects. They accept so much less for their patients than I am willing to accept for mine! I want you glowing and energized, lean and strong, mentally sharp while feeling calm and happy. I know you can get there—if your thyroid is getting the support it needs and if the rest of your body is too.

So many symptoms that seem to be caused by female hormones have their root in an unhealthy thyroid. True, the hormonal shifts of pregnancy, birth, and menopause often trigger thyroid dysfunction—although sometimes, it's faulty thyroid function that kicks off a sex hormone crisis. Either way, when I see a patient with female-hormone problems, I make sure to check her thyroid too—and almost inevitably, one type of hormonal problem goes with another. That means that we have to treat both the thyroid and the estrogen-progesterone issues; otherwise, whichever system is left untreated will likely make the other system worse.

So if you're approaching menopause, in menopause, or dealing with postpartum issues, do not assume that you don't *also* have thyroid dysfunction. It's entirely possible that you can resolve your female-hormone problems through thyroid treatment and The Myers Way, without ever taking a birth control pill or estrogen replacement.

Even if you do need bio-identical hormone replacement therapy, it's likely to be incomplete without attention to your thyroid, your diet, and your lifestyle. Take comfort in knowing that solving the thyroid dysfunction and supporting your body's total health is going to make a huge difference to every hormone in your body.

MYTH 3: Diet doesn't affect your thyroid.

FACT: It absolutely does, especially if your thyroid dysfunction has an autoimmune component.

As you'll learn in part 2, one significant aspect of autoimmune conditions is a phenomenon known as *molecular mimicry*. That's what can cause your immune system to get confused between a type of food and a part of your body.

Let's take a step back and consider the problem of food sensitivity. This occurs when your immune system decides that a particular food is dangerous to your body. Gluten—a group of proteins found in wheat, barley, rye, and many other grains—often triggers this type of sensitivity. When your immune system mistakes gluten for a dangerous invader, it mobilizes an attack of killer chemicals every time you consume a gluten-containing food. Bread, pasta, and baked goods are the most common gluten-containing foods, but gluten is also used as a preservative and thickener, so you can find it in a number of prepared and packaged foods and sauces.

This violent reaction to a gluten invasion might give you side effects like a stuffy nose, brain fog, joint pain, fatigue, a skin rash, a headache, indigestion, or some other response to your body's attempts to fight off an enemy. However, because the molecular structure of gluten seems to resemble the structure of a thyroid cell, consuming gluten can also provoke an attack on your thyroid.

That's why, when I have my thyroid patients cut out gluten 100 percent, we see an immediate improvement in their thyroid function and a sharp decrease in their thyroid antibodies (an indication that the immune system is poised to attack the thyroid). Diet absolutely makes a difference to their thyroid function—and if you have auto-immune thyroid dysfunction, it will make a big difference to your overall health and entire immune system too.

In part 4, you'll learn many other ways in which thyroid function is affected by diet. And in part 5, you'll have the chance to put The Myers Way Thyroid Connection Plan into action, so you can see for yourself what a significant difference diet can make.

MYTH 4: The health of your gut has no bearing on your thyroid.

FACT: Gut health is actually one of the most important factors affecting your thyroid.

Although gut health is important for many reasons, it's absolutely vital for treating and preventing autoimmune conditions. After all, nearly 80 percent of your immune system is right on the other side of your gut wall. If your gut wall lacks integrity—if partially digested food and toxins can leak through—your immune system takes the hit. As we'll see in part 2, this can trigger an autoimmune condition and a number of other symptoms as well. My patients with autoimmune diseases—including Hashimoto's and Graves'—immediately do better as their gut begins to heal.

You'll learn more about the importance of your gut in parts 2 and 4. And in part 5, you'll have a chance to find out whether you have one or both of two common gut infections, yeast overgrowth (aka Candida) and small intestine bacteria overgrowth (SIBO). If so, you'll learn how to treat them and prevent them from coming back. You'll also see how quickly The Myers Way Thyroid Connection Plan helps you heal your gut, which vastly improves both your thyroid and your overall health. For now, let me say yet again that this is an aspect of health that conventional medicine tends to ignore. Functional medicine, by contrast, focuses on gut health as central to your overall well-being.

MYTH 5: These days, we're all stressed and sleep-deprived. *That's* the problem—not poor thyroid function.

FACT: Stress and sleep problems cause us so much trouble in part because of the way they disrupt thyroid function.

As you'll see in part 4, I'm going to be all over your sleep habits, and I'm going to push you on the stress issue too. If you don't get enough good, restful sleep each night, your thyroid is going to suffer, and so will your immune system. If you're not finding ways to relieve stress, it'll be twice as bad. Sleep and stress relief are crucial to The Myers Way and to any effective treatment of thyroid and immune dysfunction.

But—and this is very important—you might be struggling with sleep and stress *because* your thyroid is out of whack. When your thyroid isn't working well, your whole body suffers. It's a vicious cycle, a catch-22. As you'll learn in part 2, every single cell in your body relies on thyroid hormone to power it up. While sleep is a wonderful, relaxing experience, creating healthy sleep requires a certain amount of work from your brain. If your brain doesn't have enough thyroid hormone, it might not be able to organize sleep.

Likewise, your thyroid and your adrenal glands—which produce stress hormones—are intimately involved. So if your thyroid is unbalanced, your adrenal function likely will also be in a poor state. You might have fewer reserves to deal with stress, a greater tendency to fly off the handle at little things, or an overall lack of motivation and "oomph." To make matters worse, your stress hormones might overcompensate for low thyroid, keeping you wired up far into the night. So insomnia, irritability, listlessness, and feeling wired are often due to thyroid dysfunction as well as adrenal dysfunction—and getting you the right dose of supplemental thyroid hormone can make a world of difference.

Last but in no way least, sleep problems and stress issues can result from poor diet and lifestyle. If you aren't giving every organ and gland and system what they need to function, if your body is overloaded with toxins, and if you never find a way to relieve your stress, your sleep and your stress levels will suffer, and your thyroid and adrenals right along with them. And then poor thyroid and adrenal function will just make everything worse. It's a vicious cycle—but you have the power to turn it around. Support your thyroid and your adrenals with The Myers Way Thyroid Connection Plan and you'll be amazed by how your sleep and stress issues melt away.

MYTH 6: If you feel depressed, anxious, unmotivated, or listless, that's depression, not thyroid dysfunction.

FACT: Poor thyroid function *creates* depression, anxiety, and lack of motivation—problems that are frequently solved or at least improved through effective thyroid treatment.

Hey, I'll be the first to agree that depression is a complex condition, as are anxiety, brain fog, and the loss of motivation. Many factors can be involved, an intricate mix of the physical and psychological.

Having said that, it's extraordinary how much your body can affect your mood—and even more extraordinary how much of an impact the right dose of supplemental thyroid hormone can have on your ability to process emotions. I've seen it time and time again: patients who are certain that they will be depressed for life—including patients with a family history of depression—notice a complete transformation in how they feel as soon as their thyroid hormones are properly adjusted.

Another significant aspect of depression, anxiety, and brain fog is gut health. After all, 95 percent of your body's serotonin—a crucial natural antidepressant—is made in the gut. When your serotonin levels are low, you feel anxious, depressed, and pessimistic, and you might also struggle with sleep problems. When your serotonin levels are optimal, you feel calm, optimistic, self-confident, and empowered. A key aspect of The Myers Way Thyroid Connection Plan is to heal your gut, and that, too, will go a long way toward healing depression and anxiety while significantly improving mental function.

So if you struggle with depression, anxiety, brain fog, or a general lack of motivation, please, please, *please* consider that your thyroid may play a *significant* role in your condition. Use this book. Work with your doctor. Get the best possible diagnosis and treatment. You might be astonished at how quickly you emerge into a clearer, brighter world.

MYTH 7: When you feel "blah" or lousy, there's often nothing you can do about it.

FACT: If you understand how to support your body's function, you can almost always get from *lousy* to *terrific*.

Although I've saved this myth for last, it's probably the most important one of all, and the one that I most want you to take to heart. So often when you go in to see a conventional doctor and say that you just don't feel good, the doctor shrugs. So many problems don't show up on their radar—your body might be performing within the standard reference range, but you feel rotten anyway. So many problems that *do* show up are nearly impossible for conventional medicine to treat, except possibly with medications that often create problems of their own. Feeling less than terrific is just not considered a genuine problem by most conventional doctors.

But I *do* consider feeling less than terrific a problem—a big problem. I know that if you're not feeling great—energized, vital, clear-thinking, at a healthy weight—then some part of your body's function is off. Maybe your thyroid is out of whack. Or your sex hormones are imbalanced. Maybe your adrenals are not performing as they should. Most likely your gut has lost some integrity and is beginning to leak. These problems affect your neurotransmitters, and your immune system, and your joints, and your muscles, and every single one of your organs. That tiny little problem—"I just don't feel great a lot of the time"—indicates much bigger problems throughout your anatomy.

Maybe you can drag along for many years just not feeling so great. Or maybe, sooner or later, "not great" turns into heart disease, or diabetes, or an autoimmune condition, or another type of chronic disorder.

Hey, when you have thyroid dysfunction, it can make your life a misery. When your thyroid is functioning well, you feel focused, energized, and fully alive. I wrote this book to help you get there, to give you a comprehensive view of how your thyroid works, what might be going wrong, and how to set it right. Some of this you can achieve by working with your doctors. Some of it you can do on your own. Either way, I want you to get the help you need to turn "not great" into "terrific!" I want you to have the support you deserve to make sure your thyroid, your gut, your immune system, and every other part of your anatomy are functioning at their absolute best. That's what keeps you lean, energized, glowing, and optimistic. And that's the optimal health that is your birthright.

CHAPTER 2

You *Can* Be Helped

If, like so many people, you've struggled to get your doctor to believe that something is wrong with you, my heart goes out to you. When you're feeling sick, tired, and scared, there's nothing worse than having a physician—the person whose help you desperately need—tell you that you're fine and there's nothing more that he or she can do to help you. "It's all in your head," "This just happens as you get older," "I've already done everything I can"—these are unconscionable responses, in my opinion, and frankly, they make my blood boil. They are far too common among conventional doctors, and the sad thing is, most patients are stuck believing them.

Well, it ends here. In this chapter, you're going to meet other patients whose doctors told them that help was not available in *conventional* medicine—and who then went on to get help from *functional* medicine. I want you to know that you are not alone, that you *can* be helped, and that any doctor who dismisses you or brushes you off is failing in his or her professional duties.

There's a kind of trauma involved in having one or more doctors ignore your pain—I've seen it in patient after patient, and I've certainly felt it myself. This chapter is about making sense of that trauma. If you've been frustrated with your doctor's response—and especially if you've been frustrated by the responses of several doctors—perhaps you'll see yourself in the patient stories that follow. And after you've read the stories, we'll take a closer look at why and how conventional medicine fails so many thyroid patients.

I also want you to see how powerful certain changes can be: getting the nutrients, vitamins, and minerals that your thyroid needs to make thyroid hormone and that your body needs to correctly respond to that hormone; healing your gut; lowering your levels of inflammation; getting the right kind of exercise for your body, neither too little nor too much; decreasing your exposure to toxins and improving your body's ability to detoxify; healing underlying infection; and countering the stress in your life with enough relaxation to keep your stress hormones at an optimal level. These elements of The Myers Way Thyroid Connection Plan are hardly the stuff of TV dramas, and they are pooh-poohed by many conventional doctors as changes that are "not really going to make much difference."

But in fact, the difference they make can be extremely dramatic, as your symptoms retreat, your energy returns, your anxiety and depression lift, and your entire body enjoys a reliable, steady glow of vitality and well-being.

You'll begin to experience these benefits yourself when you've completed the twenty-eight-day plan. Depending on your condition, you may be feeling 100 percent by that time, or you may need several months to fully achieve optimal health. You might also use herbs to calm your overactive thyroid (if you're hyperthyroid) or work with your doctor to determine the right type and amount of supplemental thyroid hormone (if you're hypothyroid). Either way, as the patients in this chapter discovered, the changes embodied in The Myers Way can transform your health — and your life.

WHAT DOES SUCCESS LOOK LIKE?

Here's the good news: Virtually everyone reading this book can expect to achieve a state of vibrant health and well-being. If you follow The Myers Way Thyroid Connection Plan and, if necessary, work with your doctor (which you'll find out how best to do in part 3), you can eventually become free of the symptoms on pages 20 and 21, energized and vital, with a balanced mood, a healthy weight, and a sense of optimism and calm.

Now, there are many different routes to this goal, depending on a number of factors: whether you are hypo- or hyperthyroid, if it is autoimmune or not, how long you've been having thyroid dysfunction, and whether you've got any other chronic conditions. Those other factors will help determine how long it takes you to feel terrific, and they'll also determine what you need to do going forward.

Because here's the bottom line: Your thyroid is a vital organ—you cannot live without it. If it has been ablated with I-131, surgically removed, or even damaged by chronic inflammation, you will need to take some amount of supplemental thyroid hormone.

In my book *The Autoimmune Solution,* I show you how to reverse autoimmune symptoms and renew your health without any medications or supplemental hormones whatsoever. But the thyroid and the immune system are different in that regard. That's because the immune system is a set of biochemicals, which are more flexible and easier to change. The thyroid is a vital organ, and once a significant part of it is damaged, that damage is permanent. In that case, we need to compensate for the hormone that the thyroid is not producing.

However, the news is still very, very good, because once you've made the diet and lifestyle changes that your body needs and once you've got the supplemental thyroid hormone (*if* you need it), you can feel terrific and enjoy a vibrant, healthy life. Here are all the options for that good outcome:

- If you're hypothyroid and you've caught your thyroid issues early on, you might be able to reverse your condition completely through The Myers Way Thyroid Connection Plan. You may never need supplemental thyroid hormone or any other type of medical treatment and can rely entirely on diet supplements, and lifestyle changes.

- If you have been hypothyroid for several years, the damage to your thyroid might be so significant that it is no longer able to produce enough thyroid hormone for your needs. Following The Myers Way *will* help you to feel healthy and terrific—but only if your doctor also prescribes the right type and amount of supplemental thyroid hormone to compensate for what your own thyroid can no longer produce.

- If you are hyperthyroid and have not yet had I-131 ablation or surgery, you can very likely reverse your condition through The Myers Way Thyroid Connection Plan while also taking several natural herbs to calm your thyroid. This is true whether you are currently taking thyroid-suppressing medication or not. Depending on your condition, you might need several weeks or even months to get off your thyroid-suppressing medication and achieve optimal health. Once you've done it, however, remaining on The Myers Way will typically be all you need—no meds, no herbs, just the right diet and lifestyle.

- If you were hyperthyroid and all or part of your thyroid was ablated or removed, or if your thyroid has become damaged in some other way, you will need to take some form of supplemental thyroid hormone to compensate for what your own thyroid can no longer produce. We can't regenerate your thyroid, but The Myers Way can help reverse your symptoms, and you may also be able to reduce your supplemental thyroid hormone dose.

Going forward, when I say *reverse* in this book, I mean reverse the damage to your body and your immune system, not the damage to your *thyroid*. We can reverse *symptoms* and an *autoimmune response*. We can't reverse thyroid damage—but, luckily, we can compensate for it with the right type and amount of supplemental thyroid hormone.

The Myers Way Thyroid Connection Plan *Can*...

Help eliminate your symptoms

Calm an overactive thyroid

Provide your body with the nutrients it needs for optimal thyroid response

Reduce the obstacles to optimal thyroid response, including overexercise, stress, and the burden of excess toxins

Reduce inflammation in your thyroid and body

Reverse damage to your immune system and get it to function optimally (i.e., reverse your autoimmunity)

The Myers Way Thyroid Connection Plan *Cannot*...

Repair damage to your thyroid itself

Cure your autoimmunity

MARTINA: "YOUR LABS ARE FINE. YOU'RE JUST GETTING OLDER"

Martina had always been a powerful, energetic woman. A lawyer in a small Texas town, she was well known and well liked, so in her late forties, she decided to run for city council.

Martina's husband, a local businessman, fully supported his wife's decision, and her two kids—one a senior in high school, the other a junior at a nearby college—were proud and excited for their mom. Still, the stresses of running her campaign along with maintaining her law practice started to catch up with Martina and she began to have a number of symptoms she hadn't experienced before: fatigue, brain fog, frequently feeling cold, a sudden weight gain of about ten pounds, and, most disturbing of all, hair loss.

Martina had been diagnosed with hypothyroidism after the birth of her second child, and she'd been taking a small dose of supplemental thyroid hormone for the past eighteen years. Martina's thyroid was simply not producing enough thyroid hormone, so she needed supplemental thyroid hormone to make up the rest. So far, so good.

Then Martina began having symptoms. After all those years, something was no longer working. She asked her doctor to recheck her thyroid labs. He did—and told her everything was fine.

"Your labs are fine," her doctor assured Martina. "You're just getting older. It's normal to slow down. Try taking it easy for the next few months."

Martina just wouldn't accept that, at forty-eight, she could no longer live a demanding, ambitious life. She also knew her body — and she *knew* something was off. She wanted a better solution than "just relax."

"You can't argue with your labs," the doctor insisted. "It's all there in black-and-white. But you *are* almost fifty, so maybe it's perimenopause." He prescribed birth control pills for Martina to regulate any sex hormone imbalances.

Instead of making things better, the pills made everything worse. After only a few weeks, Martina was climbing the walls; mood swings, insomnia, and occasional waves of anxiety were added to her existing fatigue and brain fog. She gained another five pounds. And even more hair fell out.

Martina had heard some of my podcasts in which I talked about the importance of listening to the patient. That sounded good to Martina, so she came to me.

"These symptoms are making my life unlivable," she told me. "I can't perform. I can't cope. I wanted my doctor to work with me, but he just brushed me off. As if I was supposed to adjust to fit the treatment, instead of him adjusting the treatment to fit *me*."

Clearly, Martina was suffering, and I was determined to help. So I ran a complete set of labs for her, including a complete thyroid panel — far more detailed than the ones her conventional doctor had ordered.

While we waited for Martina's labs to come back, I recommended that she start on The Myers Way Thyroid Connection Plan, which includes diet and lifestyle changes as well as several supplements that would provide her thyroid with the nutrients it needed to function properly.

I also wanted to get Martina off the birth control pills. I explained that when your system has too much estrogen — especially the synthetic estrogens found in birth control pills and hormone replacement therapy—your body makes more of a protein called *thyroxine-binding globulin,* or TBG. Typically, most of your thyroid hormone binds to the proteins in your blood, leaving a portion of it free to enter your cells. Well and good—but when you have too much TBG, too much of your thyroid hormone is *bound* and not enough of it is *free* to enter your cells. That's why birth control pills and hormone replacement therapy can make thyroid dysfunction worse.

In fact, any fluctuations in estrogen or the other sex hormones can undermine your thyroid's function, just as any disruption in thyroid function can go on to disrupt sex hormones. This is why restoring healthy thyroid function can often enable a woman to get pregnant or help her carry a child to term. It's also why pregnancy, postpartum, perimenopause, and menopause can throw thyroid function out of whack.

I thought this was part of what had happened to Martina. Her second child had pushed her system to where she needed a small dose of supplemental thyroid hormone. Now perimenopause was pushing her further, to the point where that small dose was no longer enough.

Last but by no means least, I thought that the stress of Martina's campaign was making too many demands on her thyroid. Many people think of stress as a psychological issue, but I'm here to tell you that when you feel stressed, anxious, or overwhelmed, your body responds to it physically, through both your thyroid hormones and your stress hormones. Your thyroid, sex hormones, and stress hormones are all interrelated, so that any shift in any part of this system can disrupt everything else.

When I talked to Martina about the problem of stress, she bristled, insisting that she was not going to give up her campaign. On the contrary, I told her. I live a busy, demanding life and so do most of my patients. The goal is not to eliminate stress but to *relieve* it; to alternate stressful times with relaxing ones. That way, your body has a chance to recover, your stress hormones rebalance, and both your thyroid and your immune system benefit immensely. That's why "relieve stress" is such an important part of The Myers Way Thyroid Connection Plan.

Physical and Emotional Stressors That Can Disrupt Your Thyroid

Emotional

Abuse

Aging parents

Birth of a child

Children undergoing problems

Death of a loved one

Divorce or a painful breakup; the loss of a friend

Family conflicts

Financial difficulties

Illness

Layoff or loss of work

Marriage

Moving

New job, promotion, new project, other work challenges, including welcome ones

New relationship, falling in love (yes, that can be stressful!)

Trauma

Work pressures

Physical

Illness

Insomnia, sleep problems; not enough sleep for any reason

Missing meals

Overexercise (exercise that is too intense or goes on too long)

Physically demanding work that requires lifting, standing for long periods, or other exertion

Pregnancy and postpartum

Trauma

Fourteen days later, Martina e-mailed my office and said she had already lost three pounds and was feeling calmer. She was sleeping better and had much more energy. "And all without medication!" she marveled.

Just about then, I got Martina's labs results. They might have looked fine to her doctor, but they looked very far from fine to me. First, I had more data than her doctor had. Most conventional doctors test for only a couple of types of thyroid hormone. I go for a far more detailed picture.

I also interpret the lab values differently. Conventional doctors look for normal reference ranges, which are very wide. I have higher standards for your health: I look for *optimal* ranges, which are much narrower. I don't just want you able to function—I want you functioning at the highest possible level.

If I'd been in charge of Martina's thyroid care after the birth of her second child, we might have been able to manage her thyroid just by making changes in her diet and lifestyle. But after eighteen years of dysfunction, her thyroid could no longer produce the right amount of hormone by itself. So now, in addition to having Martina follow The Myers Way, I would need to prescribe her the right dose and type of supplemental thyroid hormone. Based on the detailed lab readings, I thought that Martina did not need to increase the *amount* of supplemental thyroid hormone dose but did need to change to a more natural and effective *type*.

Martina's story is a classic example of why it's so important to get a complete thyroid panel and not rely on just one or two lab measurements. It's also a good example of how dynamic thyroid issues can be and how your physician needs to monitor your situation continually. For years, Martina had done fine on her previous dose of supplemental thyroid hormone. But then she began facing some new stresses, from perimenopause and also her campaign. As a result, her body responded differently, so her previous dose and type of supplemental thyroid hormone were no longer working.

Martina's story also makes clear how grievously conventional medicine fails people with thyroid dysfunction. Prescribing birth control pills or hormone replacement therapy (HRT) is a common response when a woman is having hormonal issues. Yet if those issues are actually caused by thyroid dysfunction, the birth control pills or HRT will frequently make things worse rather than better. That's what happens when you fail to get to the root of the problem.

I started Martina on her new supplemental thyroid hormone, and within days she e-mailed my office saying that she felt as though a light had come back on in her brain. Her mind cleared. Over the next few weeks she had more energy than she had had in years. She began to feel warm and comfortable, and she immediately became hopeful about the new treatment. Within about eight weeks, she had lost the excess weight she'd gained, and in less than three months, her hair was thicker and healthier than ever and she said she felt like she was twenty years younger.

"My previous doctor made me feel like I was just a complaining woman," Martina said on our last visit. "Like I was just being fussy or difficult or something like that. Even though I *knew* something was wrong, he wouldn't listen to *me*—he just looked at the labs. I'm a competent person—a professional and an elected official. But he treated me like some silly schoolgirl who couldn't understand science."

She took a deep breath. "I guess for all those years I really wasn't paying that much attention. I just took the pills he gave me and was glad they worked. The one good thing about this whole situation is that now I do finally understand what's going on in my body and what I can do to stay healthy."

THOMAS: "YOU'RE A MAN, SO YOU CAN'T HAVE A THYROID PROBLEM"

Thomas was head of the accounting department at a local brokerage house. A careful, methodical man, he was used to documenting and analyzing even the most minor events, and he brought the same rigor to his health care. Every time he saw the doctor, he wanted to know what was being tested, what his test results were, and what the doctor recommended. Then he wanted his doctor to keep track of how well the recommendations worked and whether they needed to be altered.

At age forty-two, Thomas went to his doctor complaining of fatigue, decline in muscle tone, and low libido. He felt that he had completely lost his motivation and that he had very little stamina, both physically and emotionally.

"I'm used to training for marathons," he told his doctor. "I run two of them a year. Now I can barely drag myself through a mile. I used to look forward to my runs. Now I dread them."

Thomas also told the doctor that he had gained seven and a half pounds in the last three months, "even though I've started keeping a food log to make sure that I haven't been eating any more." Thomas had cut out desserts, alcohol, pasta, and potatoes, he assured the doctor. Yet his weight remained stubbornly above normal.

Finally, Thomas explained, "My sex life seems to be permanently on hold." Although he told the doctor that he and his wife had once enjoyed an active sexual relationship, "Now we're lucky if we make love once a month."

The doctor checked Thomas's testosterone levels, and, sure enough, they were low. He prescribed a small dose of testosterone supplement, which gave him a bit more energy and slightly more sexual interest. However, Thomas's weight continued to climb, and he also began reporting brain fog—times when he couldn't remember something he had just done, difficulty keeping three tasks in his head at once, even confusing two different sets of numbers at work.

"These things happen as you get older," Thomas's doctor told him. "I can increase the testosterone, but some folks get headaches or acne when the dose is too high. I can offer you an antidepressant, but that can also cause brain fog for some people. There really isn't any other remedy that I can see."

This answer did not sit well with Thomas at all. Numbers and accuracy were not only his livelihood, they were a source of pride. "If I can't do my job well, I don't deserve to have it," he told me on our first appointment. "And when my body and brain are *off*, I can't do my job well!"

Thomas had come to me on the recommendation of a friend who had read one of my blogs about optimal thyroid function. The friend understood that I offered a broader range of lab testing and that I often found solutions to problems that eluded other doctors. Thomas thought it was worth a try.

Thyroid dysfunction had been my first thought when Thomas told me his story. But when I reviewed his medical records, I saw that his previous doctor hadn't even tested his thyroid! I was horrified—but I wasn't shocked. All too often, doctors just assume that men—especially men below sixty—do not have thyroid dysfunction. As a result, they don't test for it.

Now, it *is* true that thyroid dysfunction is seven times more common among women than men. But that doesn't mean that men don't have thyroid dysfunction too. Hey, it's an equal opportunity disorder! Many conventional doctors, however, look elsewhere when they are treating men, and so men like Thomas simply go undiagnosed.

In my opinion, this is close to medical malpractice. Anyone—male or female—should automatically be given a complete thyroid blood panel if they are complaining of any of the thyroid symptoms listed on pages 20 and 21 or any of the disorders listed below. This is standard in functional medicine, but, alas, not in conventional medicine. Conventional doctors tend to be far less sensitive to the signs of thyroid dysfunction, especially when the patient is anyone other than a middle-aged woman.

Disorders That May Indicate Thyroid Dysfunction

If a patient of any age or gender presents with any of the following symptoms or disorders, I routinely run a full battery of thyroid tests:

ADHD
Adrenal dysfunction
Anorexia
Anxiety
Autism
Autoimmune disease
Brain fog or memory issues
Cardiovascular disease
Chronic constipation
Dementia
Depression
Diabetes

Erectile dysfunction

Goiter or swelling in the neck

Hives

Hormone imbalances

Irritable Bowel Syndrome (IBS)

Infertility or tendency to miscarry

Insomnia: inability to fall and/or stay asleep

Learning disability or developmental delay

Neurological issues

Obesity

"Senility" — any seemingly age-related mental or emotional issues

Small Intestine Bacterial Overgrowth (SIBO)

While we were waiting for Thomas's labs to come back, I started him on The Myers Way Thyroid Connection Plan. I told him that this could make an enormous difference to his energy levels, mood, and overall hormonal balance. When we got the lab results, then we could consider whether he needed to take supplemental thyroid hormone.

Thomas was excited about The Myers Way because he had never liked the idea of taking supplemental hormones "every day of his life," as he put it. "Can I just do everything through diet and lifestyle?" he asked me. "Will that be enough?"

I explained that often, if your thyroid dysfunction is caught early, diet and lifestyle changes *can* be enough. We can help the thyroid function better by giving it what it needs (nutrients, vitamins, minerals) and removing obstacles to its functioning (food sensitivities, leaky gut, toxins, infections, overexercising, and stress). What we can't do, though, is *regrow* the thyroid—if it has been damaged, that damage will remain, and supplemental thyroid hormone might be needed.

"So," I told Thomas, "let's start you on the plan and see what happens. The next few weeks should give us a good idea of whether you need supplemental thyroid hormone or not."

Thomas loved the idea of taking control of his health and he diligently followed The Myers Way. However, he was surprised by my recommendation that he find a less intense form of exercise than running, which I thought had punished his thyroid just a bit too much.

"I thought exercise was healthy," Thomas protested. "I was looking forward to having more energy so I could start running again."

I explained to Thomas that our bodies need a certain amount of challenge — of stress — but that there is a point of diminishing returns or even negative returns. If you are pushing your body too hard, your thyroid and adrenals rebel. You often begin producing too much cortisol, a powerful stress hormone that can disrupt both thyroid and immune function. Overexercise can undermine your thyroid, slow down your metabolism, and even cause you to gain weight. Some people's bodies are designed to be pushed very hard, but most of us do better with less demanding exercise. That's why many of my patients who run marathons or do triathlons, Ironman, or CrossFit discover that their intense exercise is burning out their thyroids and that a gentler but still effective form of exercise actually helps them feel more energized and lose more weight.

Thomas agreed to switch to walking and Pilates, which built up core strength but did not stress his body in the same way. To his surprise, he felt more energized almost immediately, and he soon began losing his excess weight. Within his first two weeks on The Myers Way, we agreed to take him off the supplemental testosterone because he clearly no longer needed it; his vitality — and his sex drive — was back to normal by the end of the month. His brain fog dissipated, and Thomas actually felt sharper and clearer than he had in a long time.

As Thomas continued on The Myers Way, his health kept improving, and his labs showed it. His thyroid function returned not only to normal but to optimal levels, and I never had to put him on supplemental thyroid hormone. Thomas rejoiced in both his improved health and his sense of control over his own body.

"What I want in a doctor is someone who helps me support my own health," he told me emphatically on our last visit. "What I like about The Myers Way is that it allows me to take my health into my own hands."

GLORIA: "WE'RE MORE CONCERNED WITH YOUR LUPUS"

Sometimes a patient presents with another serious condition, which makes a conventional doctor focus elsewhere and forget the thyroid. This is what happened to Gloria, a freelance graphic designer who for several years had struggled with lupus, an autoimmune disorder that is conventionally treated with a number of different medications, most of which have harsh side effects and a limited window of effectiveness. Many autoimmune patients find themselves switching immunosuppressive medications every six to twelve months, always hoping that the next prescription will be the one that works better and longer.

This was Gloria's story too, and over the past decade, she had been to some of the most prestigious medical centers in the country. When she finally made her way to my office, having read my book *The Auto-immune Solution,* she was skeptical but hopeful, especially when she realized how much more extensive my testing was than the tests run by her previous doctors.

We already knew that Gloria had lupus, a condition that left her feeling fatigued and listless. Those are thyroid symptoms too, so her doctors simply assumed they were caused by the lupus. Her doctors did routinely check some aspects of her thyroid function. But, as with Martina, they used only a limited panel of labs—far fewer tests than I always ask for. And, most significantly, they didn't check her thyroid *antibodies.*

Most thyroid conditions are autoimmune in nature; that is, they are caused by your immune system going haywire and attacking your thyroid. Your immune system uses antibodies to detect a foreign invader— a bacteria or virus that might cause harm to your body. When you have an autoimmune condition, your immune system makes antibodies that target a part of *you*—in this case, your thyroid.

That's why my labs always include tests for the two most common types of thyroid antibodies, thyroid peroxidase (TPO) and thyroglobulin antibody (TgAb). If I see them, I know that there is an autoimmune dysfunction brewing. Sometimes the antibodies show up years before the actual thyroid dysfunction does. That is, the antibodies are there, but the thyroid has not yet been attacked by the immune system, or not enough to cause any damage. In that case, you can often prevent damage to the thyroid by following The Myers Way and reversing the autoimmune dysfunction.

In fact, when I reviewed Gloria's blood work, I saw that some of her thyroid lab results were normal and actually even optimal—except that she did indeed have high levels of antibodies. When I shared this diagnosis with Gloria, she was astonished.

"I don't understand how this could happen," she kept saying. "I've been to so many prestigious specialists. You mean to tell me that none of them picked up this other condition?"

Although the missed diagnosis was, to me, unacceptable, I could see how it had come about. Conventional medicine believes that since an overactive immune system is responsible for autoimmune disorders, including lupus, the correct response is to suppress the immune system through an immunosuppressant. Because Gloria's doctors had been so focused on monitoring her immune system and her lupus symptoms, they had never bothered to check her thyroid antibodies.

The good news here was that I had caught the antibodies early enough to prevent damage to Gloria's thyroid. As a huge added bonus, following The Myers Way could lower the level of thyroid antibodies so that her immune system would stop attacking her thyroid. We could also reverse the symptoms of her lupus and generally improve the function of her immune system.

To Gloria's delight, our attention to her immune system, gut, and thyroid paid off big-time. The next time we checked levels of her thyroid antibodies, they were already reduced by half. After three months they were barely detectable and her lupus symptoms had greatly improved, leaving her pain-free and energized for the first time since she was a teenager. She was eventually able to stop taking her lupus medication, which to Gloria seemed like a minor miracle. And her revitalized thyroid left her with an emotional calm and mental clarity that she had never before experienced.

"For the first time I can remember, I feel truly *healthy*," Gloria told me. "We didn't just get rid of a few symptoms or even reverse a disease. We created a whole reservoir of health."

TAYLOR: "YOU JUST NEED TO RELAX"

Taylor was an enthusiastic young woman in her late twenties who worked as a paralegal at a large law firm. When she'd first started there, she'd loved her high-pressure job, but by the time she came to me, she was anxious and on edge, barely able to settle into the chair in my office.

Taylor told me that her doctor had diagnosed her with hyperthyroidism—an overactive thyroid, which caused her hands to tremble and her muscles to feel weak. She felt nervous and irritable, was set off by the slightest disagreement or problem. She had been slowly losing weight, although, she assured me, "I'm eating like a pig—I'm simply hungry *all the time.*" She was also concerned that she seemed suddenly to have frequent bowel movements. Most upsetting was that instead of being able to walk briskly for two or three miles, "which I could do my entire life," now she had to rest every block or two, "and my heart is just racing."

Taylor's conventional doctor gave her the same three choices that I had been given: harsh medications, radioactive ablation of the thyroid, or surgery to have her thyroid all or partially removed. Taylor was horrified by those choices, as I had been. When she searched online for *thyroid—natural approaches,* she found the podcast where I told the same story you read in the introduction. She decided to come to me for help because she knew I would understand what she was going through.

I told Taylor about the herbs I typically recommended to suppress an overactive thyroid naturally. I also told her about The Myers Way Thyroid Connection Plan and how it would support her thyroid function, immune system, and overall health. I let her know that trying to suppress an overactive thyroid is often more challenging than helping to optimize an underactive thyroid.

So, I told Taylor, her treatment might take several months. I sympathized with how hard the anxiety, the tremors, and the insomnia could be, but I thought that natural means could work for her if she was willing to see it through.

"You need to be patient—and very, very gentle with yourself," I told Taylor. "We'll just have to take it one step at a time."

Taylor's commitment paid off. Eight months later, she was rewarded with an end to her symptoms and a boost to her overall health. On her last visit, we talked about the difference between her experience with functional medicine and her experience with conventional medicine.

"Conventional medicine offers these sweeping solutions that sometimes work quickly but often have terrible side effects," she said thoughtfully. "And you feel like the whole thing is out of your hands—like it's the doctor who has the ultimate control. Yet doctors still can't guarantee a good outcome—you still might have side effects or your meds might stop working or whatever."

She took a deep breath. "With your approach, it took months before I felt really good again—but now I feel terrific! I feel like I know how to get myself healthy and keep myself healthy. The decisions are mine—the power is mine. In my book, that's worth a little patience."

WHY DOES CONVENTIONAL MEDICINE MISFIRE SO OFTEN?

Hey, I'm not saying that conventional medicine *never* gets thyroid right. Sometimes a thyroid patient goes to a conventional doctor, gets an effective dosage of supplemental thyroid hormone, and the symptoms go away.

But often—as Martina, Thomas, Gloria, and Taylor found out—conventional medicine misses the mark. Patients like Thomas are not properly diagnosed. Patients like Martina are not given the right dose of supplemental thyroid hormone. Patients like Gloria are not given all the tests they need. Patients like Taylor are not offered good options. And, with shocking frequency, patients are medicated for conditions other than thyroid dysfunction: given birth control pills or hormone replacement therapy to ease the problems of perimenopause and menopause; testosterone for low energy and low sex drive; beta-blockers for a racing heart; sleeping pills for insomnia; antidepressants for depression; antianxiety medications for anxiety . . . The list goes on and on.

For autoimmune patients, the problem is even worse. If you've got Hashimoto's thyroiditis—the autoimmune condition of an underperforming thyroid—you're typically prescribed supplemental thyroid hormone. But you are rarely offered any education about what's really going on in your body, let alone how you can use diet and lifestyle to reverse your symptoms and prevent another autoimmune disease from developing. (Remember, once you have one autoimmune disease, you are three times more likely to get another.) If you've got Graves'— well, you've already read my story in the introduction, so you know the three terrible options offered there: harsh medication, destroying the thyroid with radioactive iodine, or removing the thyroid entirely.

And if you've got another autoimmune condition *and* a thyroid dysfunction, as Gloria did, your options are even worse. The immunosuppressive medications conventionally prescribed for many autoimmune conditions can work to relieve some symptoms, but they are often accompanied by debilitating side effects. Moreover, these medications actually suppress your immune system, which can leave you more likely to develop another autoimmune disease or worse, possibly even cancer. These medications might not work for you at all, or they might work for only a few years or even just a few months. Then you've got to increase the dose or switch to a new immunosuppressive medication. It can be a demoralizing process—sometimes a devastating one.

Meanwhile, what virtually no conventional doctor offers—for any type of thyroid or autoimmune condition—is a diet and lifestyle that can get to the root of the problem. As I showed in *The Autoimmune Solution,* you can make extraordinary improvements in an autoimmune disorder by following the diet and lifestyle changes laid out in The Myers Way. As Thomas and many other patients have discovered, you can make similar improvements in a thyroid disorder (although in some cases you might need some supplemental thyroid hormone as well).

So what's going on? In my opinion, it all goes back to the differences between conventional medicine and functional medicine. Let's take a closer look.

CONVENTIONAL MEDICINE VERSUS FUNCTIONAL MEDICINE: WHAT'S THE DIFFERENCE?

Conventional medicine is what the vast majority of U.S. doctors practice and what is taught in medical school. It's most likely what your doctor practices as well. Conventional medicine tends to focus on coming up with a diagnosis for a specific disease. Then that disease — or maybe only its symptoms — are treated with a specific medication. If that medication has side effects, conventional doctors often prescribe more medications to treat the side effects. If a patient has two different disorders — say, lupus and a thyroid issue — conventional medicine would likely send that patient to two different specialists, perhaps a rheumatologist and an endocrinologist.

Functional medicine takes a vastly different approach. Instead of dividing the body into separate systems and specialties, functional medicine approaches the body as a whole, integrated system. Instead of trying to treat symptoms only, functional medicine focuses on addressing the root cause of illness, on prevention, and on achieving total health — that is, achieving the optimal *function* of every aspect of your body.

Now, let's be clear: both conventional medicine and functional medicine are science-based. While some functional practitioners are chiropractors, naturopaths, and osteopaths, many of us are MDs, and we went to the same medical schools as the conventional doctors. For example, I went to medical school, then completed a three-year residency in emergency medicine. I was even an attending physician in a major trauma center and pediatric emergency department for several years. And then after all of that, I spent two years doing additional training through the Institute for Functional Medicine.

In fact, functional medicine often relies on cutting-edge medical research that has yet to make its way into the practice of conventional medicine. Most research takes an average of a shocking eighteen years to become part of what an ordinary doctor routinely does. But functional medicine physicians tend to be pioneers, finding new ways to incorporate medical discoveries into their practice.

The diagnosis is the endgame for the conventional MD: find the diagnosis and the right pill to treat the disease or the symptoms. In functional medicine, the diagnosis is just the starting point. We then focus on finding the *why:* Why did you get this particular disease? What's the root cause? How can we fix the root cause and reverse the disease, and how can we prevent future illness?

Another key difference is the type of treatment we focus on. Conventional doctors rely largely on medications tailored to specific disorders and symptoms. Functional medicine doctors use natural means as much as possible to improve total body function as well as to target specific organs and systems. We rely largely on diet, supplements, herbs, and lifestyle, including healing the gut, taming the toxins, healing infections, and relieving stress. We also use prescription medications and surgery when those are the best choices.

For thyroid conditions, functional medicine uses state-of-the-art lab tests to come up with the most accurate diagnosis. We use the same thyroid labs that are available to conventional doctors, but we run a more complete panel and interpret them differently. Most conventional doctors are satisfied if your labs fall within a standard reference range deemed to be normal. Functional medicine physicians aren't looking for normal — they're looking for excellent, optimal, the best possible health and function of every part of your body.

This still leaves me wondering about why conventional medicine does such a shockingly poor job of treating thyroid conditions. Why aren't they running the same labs we are? Why aren't they availing themselves of a wider range of treatment options? These are all based in hard, cold science, and they would make a huge difference, even without the extraordinary benefits of diet and lifestyle.

Should we blame the medical schools, which teach almost nothing about the effects of diet and lifestyle changes? Or the insurance companies, which don't like paying for a lot of tests and allow doctors only fifteen minutes for every visit? Is the problem that conventional physicians tend to be extremely busy and overworked, making it hard for them to keep up with the latest research? Why haven't they at least changed their reference ranges, which the American Association of

Endocrinologists recommended all the way back in 2003? I don't know, but most of them haven't done it.

Thyroid dysfunction is certainly hard to diagnose for any of us. The symptoms can mimic those of other illnesses, and often they are intertwined with other disorders. Depression, anxiety, brain fog, fatigue, weight gain, and insomnia can have multiple causes, as can muscle weakness, tremors, and heart palpitations. Compounding the problems, many medications have side effects that resemble thyroid dysfunction. And if you're being treated by a conventional doctor—especially as you get older—you are likely to be on one or more medications. (The average American between the ages of sixty-five and sixty-nine takes nearly fourteen prescriptions each year; from age eighty to eighty-four, the figure goes up to eighteen.)

A huge advantage of functional medicine is that it is *personalized*—an individual approach to each patient. Consequently, we spend a great deal of time listening to every single person who comes in for help, making sure that we've heard the whole story and identified all the many factors that could be playing a role. My first-time appointment with a new patient lasts eighty minutes so that we really have time to cover every possible element that might affect his or her health. Conventional medicine is keyed toward a few readily identifiable diagnoses, so many overworked doctors tend to want to jump right to the problem they recognize, pushing patient concerns and opinions aside. This can be a particular problem for female patients, especially older women, who might trigger for some doctors the stereotypes of "hysterical," "always complaining," and "worried about trivial things."

Perhaps most important is the way that many conventional physicians have bought into the myth that our bodies are *meant* to break down and that radiant, vibrant health is a truly unreachable goal, especially as we get older. If you're a doctor and that's your vision of health, then you're going to settle for less.

Functional medicine is way more optimistic. We know that age isn't the main issue—function is. If you give your body the food and activities that support it and protect your body from the toxins and unhealthy foods that undermine it, you're going to remain vital and energetic your entire life. We *know* you can achieve optimal health and function at any age, and we're not going to stop until you get there.

Certainly for autoimmune diseases — which include a large portion of thyroid disorders — the differences are striking. As I explained in *The Autoimmune Solution,* most conventional doctors accept a very low standard of improvement when it comes to autoimmunity. They've bought into the notion of the broken immune system that can't ever be fixed, and so all they try to do is medicate your symptoms, with all the problems that entails: medications that don't work well, medications that stop working, annoying or disturbing or devastating side effects that themselves have to be medicated.

By contrast, The Myers Way can reverse autoimmune conditions and symptoms through natural means, even if it can't reverse any damage already done to your thyroid. Still, even if you have to take supplemental thyroid hormone, The Myers Way enables you to achieve a pain-free, symptom-free life of energy, vitality, and well-being. It's happened for thousands of my patients and tens of thousands of my readers. It can happen for you too.

Part Two

UNDERSTANDING YOUR THYROID

CHAPTER 3

What Is the Thyroid?

If I gave out prizes to different body parts, I'd give the thyroid the Most Important Yet Most Underappreciated Award. This small, butterfly-shaped gland is the true powerhouse of your entire body because the hormones it produces create power for each and every one of your cells. Without exactly the right amount and type of thyroid hormone, your cells can't reproduce properly. Your organs cannot function at optimal levels. And your metabolism goes completely out of whack, either slowing down to a crawl (*hypo*thyroidism) or speeding up to a frantic rate (*hyper*thyroidism).

In fact, your thyroid produces not one but four types of thyroid hormones, two of which convert into still other types of hormones. We can be grateful that this system is so complex, because getting exactly the right type and amount of thyroid hormone to each cell is a hugely important task. Just a little imbalance, and you feel lousy.

Your need for thyroid hormone is also complex and dynamic. On days when you are superactive, extra stressed, or fighting off a cold, your thyroid works harder. When you don't get enough sleep, your thyroid struggles. When you eat foods that stress your gut, your immune system, or your adrenals, your thyroid suffers. And when your hormonal balance changes—as happens for women during pregnancy, postpartum, in perimenopause, and during menopause, and for men during andropause—your thyroid also takes a hit.

The good news is that once you understand how to support your thyroid, you can make sure this vital organ gets everything it needs to do its complex and demanding job. So let's take a closer look at how your body creates, regulates, and delivers your thyroid hormones—an intricate process that begins deep within your brain.

THE HYPOTHALAMUS: YOUR MASTER GLAND

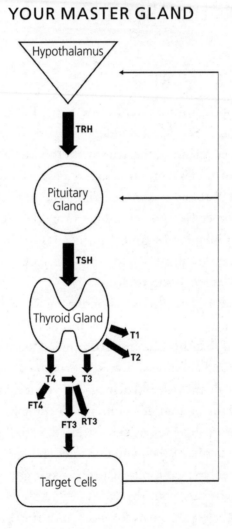

Your hypothalamus, which resides in your brain, has a lot of vital regulatory tasks to perform. It determines when you feel hungry—and how hungry you feel. It regulates your thirst. It manages your sleep, controls your body temperature, and directs the production of a number of hormones, including all forms of thyroid hormone.

I picture the hypothalamus as a busy manager sitting at a huge control panel, sort of like your body's air traffic controller. Data is constantly coming in that your hypothalamus must interpret. Then, based on its understanding of the data, it sends out the command for various biochemical responses, much as an air traffic controller might alter the flight path of an incoming plane.

In order to manage your thyroid properly, your hypothalamus is constantly monitoring the levels of thyroid hormone in your blood. If blood levels seem low, your hypothalamus releases a biochemical messenger, thyrotropin-releasing hormone, or TRH. The ultimate goal of thyrotropin-releasing hormone is—as the name suggests—to make sure that some thyroid hormone gets released into your bloodstream. But the hypothalamus can't communicate with your thyroid directly. It has to go through channels via another vital organ known as the *pituitary*.

YOUR PITUITARY: SECOND IN COMMAND

The pituitary is a pea-size gland located at the base of your brain. It takes a lot of orders from the hypothalamus and indeed sits just below it. Your pituitary is charged with regulating several key processes, including growth, reproduction, lactation, and stress.

So when your hypothalamus sends out its TRH to the pituitary, your pituitary releases a hormone of its own, thyroid-stimulating hormone, or TSH. This hormone goes directly to your thyroid, *stimulating* it to release some thyroid hormones into your bloodstream.

So far, you've got two takeaways:

• *Whenever you think about your thyroid, you have to think about a whole network of organs, glands, and biochemicals.* Proper thyroid function doesn't depend on just one organ but on three—your thyroid, your hypothalamus, and your pituitary. As we shall see later in this chapter, sex hormones and stress hormones also come into play, and as we shall see in chapter 4, the immune system and the gut are involved as well. So don't think *thyroid*—think *network*. That will help you visualize all the many ways your thyroid needs support—and all the ways you have the power to provide that support.

• *Your TSH levels are an important source of information about your thyroid.* Even though your TSH is produced by your pituitary, it's a crucial indicator of how your thyroid is doing. If TSH levels are too high, that suggests that your thyroid needs extra stimulation, which in turn suggests that maybe something is wrong with your thyroid. That's why many practitioners test TSH levels, even though TSH isn't produced by the thyroid itself.

Your Thyroid Glossary: Key Terms at a Glance

TSH (thyroid-stimulating hormone): the hormone released by your pituitary to stimulate your thyroid to produce thyroid hormone

T4: the storage form of thyroid hormone

Free T4: the storage form of thyroid left *free* rather than bound

T3: the active form of thyroid hormone

Free T3: the active form of thyroid left *free* rather than bound

TBG (thyroxine-binding globulin): the protein that binds to thyroid hormone so that the hormone can move through your bloodstream

Reverse T3: a type of thyroid hormone that prevents free T3 from attaching to your cells, thereby blunting or preventing its effects

Thyroid resistance: a disorder wherein your cells have difficulty receiving free T3, so even when blood levels of free T3 are optimal, not all of the hormone is able to enter your cells

Thyroid antibodies (thyroid peroxidase [TPOAb] and thyroglobulin antibody [TgAb]): biochemicals produced by your immune system to attack your thyroid

YOUR THYROID: FUELING AND
ENERGIZING YOUR BODY

Now, when your thyroid feels that little jolt of TSH, what happens? From your bloodstream it pulls in *iodine* (a mineral) and *tyrosine* (an amino acid) and uses them to produce *thyroid hormones,* which it then releases into your bloodstream.

To be more specific, your thyroid converts the tyrosine into *thyroglobulin* and then attaches to it either one, two, three, or four iodine atoms. We call these four types of thyroid hormones T1, T2, T3, and T4, accordingly.

To be honest, we don't really know much about T1 and T2. They make up only a tiny percentage of your thyroid gland's output. But I must admit, they have me really curious. The body doesn't do anything without a very good reason, so perhaps someday we'll discover a whole new frontier of thyroid health when we learn more about these mysterious hormones. Meanwhile, unless you're a research scientist, you can pretty much forget about them and focus on T3 and T4.

T4—thyroglobulin plus four iodine atoms—is the primary output of your thyroid gland. This is the *storage* form of the hormone, circulating throughout your bloodstream and stored in your tissues. However, T4 doesn't actually enter your cells, so it doesn't really affect your energy, your metabolism, or your symptoms. For that, you need T3, the *active* form of the hormone: thyroglobulin plus three iodine atoms.

You've got two sources of T3. Some is released by your thyroid itself, but some is converted from T4. This is a really elegant and effective system. The constant presence of T4 in your bloodstream and tissues means that any time your body needs a little more T3, it can pull some T4 out of storage and convert it into T3. Think of T4 as cash in the bank and T3 as cash in your hand. When your thyroid signaling system is working optimally, you've got cash in your hand instantly, any time you need it—but you've never got *more* cash than you need. Like any wise money manager, you keep all your extra cash safely in the bank.

Too little T3 in your cells, and you get *hypo*thyroidism, putting you at risk of the symptoms on pages 20–21. Too much, and you get *hyperthyroidism*, marked by the symptoms on page 21. (And of course, sometimes you get unusual symptoms for each condition, such as the people who *lose* weight when they are hypothyroid. That's another example of how complex and intricate your thyroid signaling system can be.)

BOUND OR FREE: HOW MUCH THYROID HORMONE IS ACTUALLY AVAILABLE?

Now, we could talk about the intricacies of the endocrine system all day long, but what you really want to know is how much T3 is available to power your cells and how much T4 is available to be converted into T3. This seems like it should be a simple question, but it too can get quite complex.

What if we ran labs on a blood sample to find out how much total T4 and T3 was there? Well, that wouldn't really tell us how much thyroid hormone is available to power your cells because so much thyroid hormone is not free but *bound:* bonded to proteins that help transport it through your blood.

The key protein to which thyroid hormone attaches is called *thyroxine-binding globulin* (TBG). T4 and T3 bind to TBG (as well as other proteins), making them unavailable to your cells and tissue until your body is ready to use them. In fact, 99 percent of the thyroid hormone in your bloodstream is bound, which is another really elegant way for your body to make sure that it *never* runs out of hormone. This might go back to when we first evolved as humans, when people couldn't always rely on getting the nutrients their bodies needed to make thyroid hormone.

A healthy body has the right level of TBG—that is, the level that enables your thyroid hormone to operate most efficiently to power your cells. However, certain factors can alter your body's production of TBG. And again, it's a question of balance. With too little TBG, *not enough* hormone will be bound; hyperthyroidism could be the result. With too much TBG, *too much* hormone will be bound, and you could develop *hypo*thyroidism.

A number of factors can affect your body's level of TBG, most commonly the following:

- *Estrogen levels.* This is sadly a common problem because way too many of us—both male and female—are overexposed to estrogen. Women taking birth control pills or getting hormone replacement therapy are at risk of excess estrogen, as are all of us who are exposed to *xenoestrogens:* industrial chemicals that mimic the behavior of estrogens. These chemicals abound in the air, food, and water, as well as in many personal-care products (shampoo, deodorant, moisturizers and lotions, cosmetics).
- *Corticosteroid levels.* If you are being treated with *corticosteroids*—powerful anti-inflammatory medications such as cortisone, hydrocortisone, and prednisone—your TBG levels are also affected. Since this type of medication is frequently prescribed to autoimmune patients, they are at increased risk of TBG disruption.

Because bound hormone does not affect your body while free hormone does, I always measure *free* T4 and *free* T3. Some conventional physicians do as well, but many measure only the total numbers, which don't give you nearly enough information. And many don't measure these hormones at all. This is one reason why it's so important for you to understand what labs your doctors are ordering to make sure that they are ordering all the labs you need.

THE CONVERSION PROCESS

Okay, so you've got all that storage T4 in your tissues. How does your body bring it *out* of storage and convert it to T3?

The first thing to understand about the conversion process is that it is triggered *locally* by whatever part of the body needs more thyroid hormone. However, the actual conversion is made primarily in the gut, liver, skeletal muscle, brain, and thyroid. This is one of the awesome aspects of the thyroid signaling system, and it allows for fine-tuned responses to a wide variety of conditions. If your stomach is challenged by the need to digest a particular food, your stomach cells need more thyroid hormone. If your brain is challenged by a particularly stressful demand—your annoying coworker says something insulting, and you're mustering your self-control to keep from snapping back with your own rude retort— your brain cells need more thyroid hormone. If your legs are challenged by an unusually intense workout in spin class, the cells in your leg muscles need more thyroid hormone. Because thyroid hormone powers every single one of your cells, your body's need for thyroid hormone is urgent, specific, and ever-changing.

This is also why the thyroid signaling system is so intricate. Different parts of your body are continually facing different challenges throughout the day and night. And each of those challenges requires a different amount of thyroid hormone. Digesting a salad requires less energy than digesting a piece of steak. Walking to the corner requires less energy than going for a run. Coping with your coworker requires less energy than a major fight with your spouse. So your body has developed this remarkable system to address a wide variety of physical, mental, and emotional demands.

But just as a computer can break more easily than an abacus, so can your thyroid signaling system break down in a wide variety of places. Its very complexity, flexibility, and specificity mean there are many ways for something to go wrong.

Now how, exactly, does your body convert T4 into T3?

Essential to the process is an enzyme called *deiodinase*. This enzyme needs selenium, zinc, and iron to function properly, which is one reason that diet is so crucial to proper thyroid function. It strips one of the *outside* iodine atoms off the T4, turning it into free T3. And that free T3 is now poised and ready to enter your cells and power them up.

THE ENTRY PROCESS

Wait, not so fast! T3 might be all set to enter your cells, but that, too, is a complex process.

In order to pass through the membrane of each cell, T3 needs help from *cortisol*. Cortisol is an incredibly powerful and important biochemical involved in a number of vital functions, and we'll have more to say about it when we look at the relationship between thyroid function, adrenals, and stress. For now, let's just note that if your cortisol levels are low, your T3 will have a harder time moving from your tissues, where it doesn't really help you, into your cells, where it does. Your takeaway:

• *Cortisol is vital to healthy thyroid function.* Without enough cortisol in your system, you won't get enough T3 into your cells, and you'll end up with the debilitating hypothyroid symptoms listed on pages 20–21.

Another factor in this entry process is the health of your cell walls. Strong, healthy cellular walls or *membranes* vastly improve cellular function. They allow your cells to *take in* the hormones and nutrients they need while enabling them to *keep out* toxins and other substances that might interfere with function.

A number of nutrients are helpful in supporting cellular health, but chief among them is healthy fat. That's because your cell walls are made of fat, so you want to make sure you are giving them high-quality building materials! Eating unhealthy fats, especially trans- or hydrogenated fats, destroys the health of your cell walls as well as disrupting gut health. You'll learn more about this in part 4.

THE ENERGY WITHIN YOUR CELLS

You've successfully converted T4 into T3, and you've used cortisol to move T3 into your cells. Now what?

Here's where the rubber meets the road, so to speak, because it is where your thyroid actually governs your metabolism. Within each cell are structures known as *mitochondria*. These are the true power plants of your cells, taking in glucose (a form of sugar) and oxygen and then converting these basics into energy. T3 helps regulate this process.

Take a moment and imagine the trillions of mitochondria pulling the sugar and oxygen out of your blood and transforming them into energy, cell by cell by cell. Think of all those tiny power plants working together to keep you energized. Then visualize your thyroid sending just the right amount of thyroid hormone into every single cell, keeping the mitochondria humming at just the right level. That's you, vital and energized.

These micro-level reactions work together to control all your crucial metabolic processes: heart rate, weight regulation, energy levels, brain function, and many more. So when your thyroid isn't working properly, it disrupts cellular function in any or all of these systems. The result is a wide array of symptoms that might seem unrelated (which is why thyroid dysfunction often goes undiagnosed) but that can all be traced back to your thyroid.

REVERSE T3: PUTTING ON THE BRAKES

The thyroid signaling system has one more way to regulate the delicate balance of thyroid and energy production in your cells. There is another hormone, called reverse T3, which, like T3, is made from T4. You'll recall that T4 becomes T3 when one of its *outside* iodine atoms is stripped away. T4 becomes reverse T3 when one of its *inside* hormone atoms is stripped away.

Like T4, reverse T3 is *inactive;* that is, it does not regulate or stimulate energy production within your cells. What it does do is attach to the receptors within your cells where free T3 would normally lodge. If reverse T3 is taking up a receptor, that leaves less room for free T3. That's your body's clever way of modulating the amount of free T3 in your cells. If free T3 is the fuel revving up those mitochondrial engines, reverse T3 is the brake pedal, slowing the whole thing down.

You can see why it's important to measure your reverse T3 as well as the ratio between free T3 and reverse T3. Both measurements are a crucial indicator of what is actually going on inside your cells, letting you know whether they are getting the right amount of fuel or too much brake. Unfortunately, most conventional doctors fail to test reverse T3.

What Stimulates Your Body's Production of Reverse T3?

- Heavy metals—particularly arsenic, cadmium, lead, and mercury—which make their way into your body through a variety of environmental factors (For more on heavy metals and other toxins, see chapter 8.)
- Overexercise, because your body can't distinguish between CrossFit, Ironman, and marathons and the kinds of grueling exertion that threatened our primitive ancestors' survival
- Starvation diets or other extremely low-calorie weight-loss plans. In another throwback to primitive times, your body thinks it's starving and mobilizes all its resources to retain fat and avoid expending energy.
- Stress, including physical, mental, and emotional (For more about stress, see chapter 10.)

SUPPORTING YOUR THYROID SIGNALING SYSTEM

As you can see, I marvel at the beauty and complexity of the thyroid signaling system. And when I'm treating a patient, I know I have to look at every aspect of that system to see where things might be going wrong:

- Your pituitary can release the wrong amount of TSH—too much or too little.
- You can have too much TBG in your bloodstream, so too much T4 and T3 are bound and not enough is free.
- Your thyroid can release the wrong amount of T3—too much or too little.
- Your thyroid can release the wrong amount of T4—too much or too little.
- Your body can have difficulties converting T4 to T3, creating a shortage of free, active T3.
- Your cells can have difficulties receiving T3, so even if they are

getting enough hormone, they aren't using it properly. This is known as *thyroid resistance,* and it can lead to all sorts of problems.

• Your body might be converting too much T4 into reverse T3, so the excess reverse T3 is blocking the effectiveness of your free T3.

Now, here's the good news. Although you still might need supplemental thyroid hormone, to compensate for a damaged thyroid, or herbs, to slow down an overactive thyroid, you can make huge strides in supporting your entire thyroid signaling system and promoting optimal thyroid, cellular, and mitochondrial function through The Myers Way Thyroid Connection Plan. You'll be giving your thyroid everything it needs to function at its peak and removing all the obstacles on the way to optimal health.

How The Myers Way Thyroid Connection Plan Supports Your Thyroid Signaling System

- Provides the nutrients your body needs to produce, convert, and regulate thyroid hormone—*iodine, selenium, B vitamins, zinc, iron, vitamin A, vitamin D*—and sufficient protein for your body to make the amino acid *tyrosine*
- Supports cellular function with healthy fats
- Promotes overall hormonal balance (so your thyroid doesn't have to contend with excess estrogens that might stimulate too much binding hormone)
- Reduces exposure to toxins and promotes your body's ability to detox (again, so your thyroid doesn't have to contend with excess estrogens)
- Reduces inflammation (so you'll have no need for corticosteroids and similar medications that stimulate too much binding hormone)
- Promotes healing your gut, a key factor in reducing inflammation
- Supports your immune system (for autoimmune thyroid conditions)
- Heals infections, another key factor in reducing inflammation and supporting immune response
- Ensures you get the sleep your thyroid needs
- Ensures you get the right amount and type of exercise
- Promotes stress relief

WHEN YOUR THYROID FUNCTION GOES AWRY

As we have seen, your thyroid can go out of balance in two ways:

- Hypothyroidism (an underactive thyroid). See the list of symptoms on pages 20–21.
- Hyperthyroidism (an overactive thyroid). See the list of symptoms on page 21.

Hypo- and hyperthyroidism are how thyroid dysfunction manifests, but there are several possible underlying causes for each. Most patients' thyroid disease is caused by an autoimmune disorder. We'll look more closely at autoimmunity in chapter 4. But you might have thyroid issues for other reasons, including:

- Insufficient nutrients
  - tyrosine or iodine, needed to create thyroid hormone
  - selenium, zinc, vitamin A, or iron, needed to convert T4 to T3
  - vitamin B or D, needed to regulate metabolism and hormones
- Adrenal system imbalances (which we'll look at in a moment)
- Pituitary disease. We'll take a closer look at this possibility in part 3.
- Eating inflammatory foods or foods that disrupt your immune system (which we will look into in the next chapter)
- A condition known as leaky gut (also in the next chapter)
- Insufficient sleep (which we'll look at in part 4)
- Overexercise (also in part 4)
- An overload of toxins (again, part 4)
- Persistent, chronic low-grade infections (part 4)

THE STRESS CONNECTION

Another hugely important factor in thyroid function is your *adrenal glands,* which produce stress hormones. These hormones are a crucial part of your metabolism, which they affect both directly and via their impact on your thyroid.

What Do Your Stress Hormones Regulate?

Blood pressure

Blood sugar

Digestion

Electrolyte balance

Immune response

Mood and cognition

Stress response: your reaction to both acute, short-term stress (the fight-or-flight response) and chronic, long-term stress

---

Just like the thyroid, your adrenal glands are regulated by the hypothalamus and the pituitary gland along a pathway known as the HPA axis. (*H* is for *hypothalamus, P* is for *pituitary,* and *A* is for *adrenals.*) When you experience stress, whether emotional, mental, or physical, your hypothalamus releases a chemical that sends a signal to your pituitary gland. Your pituitary sends its own signal to your adrenal glands, which respond by releasing a cascade of stress hormones.

Your body makes a number of different stress hormones, including adrenaline and noradrenaline (aka epinephrine and norepinephrine), dopamine, and cortisol. These are the hormones that define your physical, mental, and emotional experience of stress.

But what is stress? This condition is such a major factor in your thyroid and immune health that I want to take some time to define it properly, because there are a *lot* of misconceptions about stress.

As we saw in the previous chapter, stress can be positive or negative, and it can be emotional, mental, or physical. Any challenge that your body must rise to meet is a stressor: a deadline at work (emotional), multitasking (mental), a heavy load of groceries to bring into the house (physical). Some stressors can be fun and exciting: receiving the promotion you've wanted for so long, skiing through fresh powder on a beautiful mountain, planning a honeymoon with the love of your life. Some stressors can be painful or unpleasant: finding an assisted-living facility for an aging parent, helping your child cope with being bullied, dealing with a demanding boss. (For a list of typical stressors, see page 45.)

What all stressors have in common is that they involve the mobilization of your *sympathetic nervous system,* which is half of your *autonomic nervous system.* Your autonomic nervous system regulates bodily functions that happen automatically, without your having to consciously control them; for example, blood pressure, breathing, digestion, heartbeat, reproduction, and sexual response. When these autonomic functions need to be revved up to meet a challenge, your sympathetic nervous system controls them. When they need to be calmed down to restore, relax, and heal, your parasympathetic nervous system controls them.

So what happens when your body needs to key up and respond to a challenge? Your sympathetic nervous system springs into action. It directs blood away from your digestive system—who needs to eat when there's work to be done or an emergency to deal with?—and toward your muscles so they can run, push, lift, or perform however you need them to (as we'll see later, your sympathetic nervous system originally evolved to deal primarily with *physical* challenges). It deprioritizes your immune system—yes, protecting your body from infection and injury is important, but not nearly as important as coping with this immediate threat. Sex and reproduction—not so important at the moment. Thyroid function—ditto, because as important as your thyroid is to your long-term health and vitality, in that instant, your body is ignoring the long-term to focus on the short: how to protect you *right now,* through fight or flight. Yes, this is the famous fight-or-flight reaction, aka the *stress response.*

In the face of an immediate fight-or-flight emergency, the stress response pushes up your blood pressure, so you can have more power to fight or run away. Your sympathetic nervous system gets you breathing harder and faster so you can get ready to run. It makes your palms sweat so your body can regulate its temperature even when it's fighting or fleeing. As you can see, the stress response generally leaves you feeling keyed up, alert, and ready to go.

So far, so good—but what happens next? In a healthy body, the *stress response* is followed by a *relaxation response*. This counteracts the stress response and allows your system to calm down. Your blood shifts back to your digestive system so you can effectively digest your food. Your sexual function returns. Your thyroid and immune system get the support they need. Your blood pressure drops to normal and your muscles relax. If the stress response is nicknamed "fight or flight," the relaxation response is called "rest and digest." Just as the stress response is governed by the sympathetic nervous system, the relaxation response is governed by the *parasympathetic nervous system*—the other half of the autonomic nervous system.

Take a moment and visualize these two halves making a contented whole. See how during the working day, your sympathetic nervous system takes over, revving you up and helping you stay alert, focused, and on point. Feel the surge of energy you get in response to the stressful challenges of the day and note how you mobilize your resources to deal with them.

Now picture the end of the day, when your parasympathetic nervous system takes over. See yourself winding down to enjoy a delicious meal, the company of loved ones, a favorite activity, a relaxing bath. Feel the pleasure of your demands ending for the day, as your body prepares for sleep (and perhaps also for sex!).

This is an image of health—an ongoing alternation between stress and relaxation, between fight-or-flight and rest-and-digest, between your sympathetic nervous system and your parasympathetic nervous system. Stress is fine—as long as it is balanced by relaxation. That's our goal on The Myers Way Thyroid Connection Plan, because that balance offers your thyroid and your immune system the support they need to function at their best.

I want to make one thing superclear: When I talk about stress relief,

I am not saying, "Strive for a life with no stress" or "Give up the activities that stress you out." First of all, many of your stressors may be beyond your control: money worries, demands at the office, concerns about sick or aging parents, the needs of your children or your partner. Second, you don't *have* to live a stress-free life—you only need to balance your stresses with relaxation.

As I said in the previous chapter, I lead a busy, demanding life that I would never call stress-free. But that's okay, because I've learned to balance that stress with relaxation: acupuncture, mindful breathing, heart-rate variability (HRV), neurofeedback, float tanks, a wonderful relaxation technique called HeartMath, saunas, hot baths, time with my loved ones, time in nature. In chapter 8, I'll share with you my best stress-relieving secrets. Meanwhile, let's find out what happens when you *don't* de-stress.

STRESS AND YOUR THYROID

Now, what if the stress never really goes away? What if instead of a marauding leopard, the stress takes the form of a months-long trek across the desert to migrate to a new home? What if instead of a short-term deadline, you have endless duties and obligations, at work, at home, with relatives, friends, coworkers, and your constantly demanding boss? Now we have what is called chronic stress, and it is about the worst thing possible for your hormonal health.

For one thing, your adrenals go into overdrive for extended periods, continuously flooding your body with cortisol until they can no longer keep up with the constant demand for more and more stress hormones. Now you're in a state of adrenal dysfunction, where your poor, overworked adrenals are no longer able to produce enough stress hormones or where they are producing the wrong types of hormones at the wrong times.

In a healthy body, you get a burst of cortisol in the morning, which wakes you up. Then cortisol levels taper off gradually throughout the day and evening until finally your cortisol levels are so low that you drift off to sleep. But when you're suffering from adrenal dysfunction, you might wake up exhausted and not really rested, drag yourself through a long miserable day—and then suddenly, when it should be bedtime, you're wide awake, wired and anxious and completely unable to sleep.

Feeling constantly wired and on edge is another form of adrenal dysfunction, and feeling absolutely depleted and unable to muster even a little bit of energy to rise to the occasion is yet another. In all these cases, your adrenals are out of balance, and your body is suffering.

And so is your thyroid. Why? It all goes back to your hypothalamus and pituitary.

Remember how those two glands are in a feedback loop with your thyroid gland? When your blood levels of thyroid hormone drop, the hypothalamus tells the pituitary to signal the thyroid to make more hormone.

Well, cortisol is in a *negative* feedback loop with the hypothalamus and pituitary. When your blood levels of cortisol reach a certain point, your hypothalamus and pituitary slow down so as not to trigger any more stress hormones. But the high cortisol also signals your hypothalamus to slow down thyroid production.

This makes sense when you think about the primitive conditions under which our bodies evolved. Stress in prehistoric times usually meant two things: Not enough food and too much energy expenditure. Stress meant "I'm about to starve to death," or "I might die of hypothermia—my body fat is melting away," or "We've got to trek across the desert for weeks and maybe months, and that's going to take a lot of energy." What do we want in those conditions? A slow metabolism that will cling to every extra ounce of fat and keep us from burning off those dangerously scarce calories. And your thyroid is the governor of your metabolism.

So when you feel stressed, the cortisol in your bloodstream tells your master glands that danger is still close at hand and you'd better start storing up those calories and conserving every possible bit of energy. Ultimately, the message reaches the thyroid and tells it to stop producing so much thyroid hormone, which will cause your metabolism to slow down and become sluggish. You'll hold on to all the fat you've got and maybe even gain some weight. You'll probably also feel foggy, unmotivated, and fatigued, but at least the whole process kept you from expending energy that you might not be able to replace.

Of course, in modern times in developed countries, most of us are not in danger of freezing to death or overexerting ourselves in a hunt to find food. But when your stress never goes away—when it is never replaced by the relaxation response in the steady, regular alternation that your body likes best—then your primitive body can only think, *Hypothermia! Exhaustion! Starvation!* And in trying to prevent your imminent death, it slows your thyroid down.

While all that stress is going on, your digestion, reproductive function, and immune function are being slowly but surely drained of resources, because your body is trying so hard to remain in fight-or-flight mode. So your thyroid dysfunction is likely to be compounded by problems with digestion, sex hormones, and your immune system. For good or bad, it's all connected.

But wait, there's more! There are so many ways that stress hormones can disrupt thyroid function, and here's another: Stress hormones affect the enzymes that convert T4 to T3. So under stress, more of our thyroid hormone remains in storage and less becomes available to power our cells.

Your body has yet another trick up its sleeve. When stress is high, you convert more of your T3 into reverse T3—the brake that slows your metabolism even further.

We're not done yet. The stress response also triggers a slew of inflammatory immune cells called *cytokines*. Cytokines have many functions, one of which is to make thyroid receptors less sensitive to thyroid hormones. Less sensitive receptors mean that you need more thyroid hormone than usual to have the same impact. Yet another way that stress slows your body down—*and* another way your lab results can be tricky to interpret. Because if you have thyroid resistance, you can have the right levels of thyroid hormone in your bloodstream, but your actual cells are being deprived. Your labs will look normal, but your thyroid symptoms persist.

This can occur even if you are already taking supplemental thyroid hormone. Your doctor checks your labs, prescribes accordingly, and your blood work shows that everything is normal. But you are still suffering—because the hormone in your bloodstream is not making it into your cells.

One more thyroid issue before we're done. Stress can cause excess estrogen to accumulate. As we have seen, this extra estrogen increases levels of thyroxine-binding globulin, the protein that carries your thyroid hormones through your bloodstream. When thyroid hormones are attached to TBG they remain inactive, so T4 can't be stored in your tissues or converted to free T3. Once again, stress slows down your metabolism, impairing thyroid function in multiple ways.

You can see why relieving stress and supporting your adrenals is such a crucial aspect of thyroid health. In chapter 8, you'll learn how to test your adrenal function and how to find the ways of relieving stress that are right for your personality and lifestyle. Don't worry—no matter how busy you are, there are always ways to pause and release stress. I'll share with you the techniques that have worked for both my patients and myself.

Now, because most thyroid dysfunction is autoimmune in nature, I'd like to move on to the immune system so you can understand how it, too, is crucial to your thyroid health.

CHAPTER 4

The Autoimmune Connection

My patient Vanessa had been to four doctors by the time she came to me, and each one left her more frustrated than the last. Now in her midforties, Vanessa had been struggling with hypothyroidism since she turned thirty, when her conventional MD first put her on fifty micrograms of a type of supplemental thyroid hormone called Synthroid, a version of the hormone manufactured in a laboratory and probably the most commonly prescribed conventional response to hypothyroidism.

Here's how it went for fifteen years. Vanessa showed up at her doctor's office, tired, overweight, depressed, and overwhelmed by brain fog. Her doctor tested her TSH, prescribed Synthroid, and sent Vanessa on her way. The supplemental thyroid hormone helped some, but never enough—Vanessa hung on to an extra fifteen pounds, felt "kind of" tired, mildly depressed, "sort of" foggy. Two or three years later, the symptoms shifted from unpleasant to unbearable, and Vanessa dragged herself back to her doctor. The doctor tested her TSH again, increased her dose of Synthroid, and Vanessa stumbled through another couple of years.

On and on it went, year after year. Vanessa went from doctor to doctor, desperate to find someone who would make her feel great instead of "just better enough so that I can keep functioning," but no one ever really seemed to make much difference.

Vanessa had heard of Hashimoto's thyroiditis, a form of hypothyroidism that is caused by the immune system's attacking the thyroid. She wondered whether that was why her thyroid symptoms kept getting worse and worse, and she asked each of her doctors whether she had auto-immune thyroid dysfunction. Each assured her that the autoimmune factor didn't really matter. For one thing, in conventional medicine, the treatment is the same no matter what causes the hypothyroidism: supple-mental thyroid hormone in the form of Synthroid. Then, too, Vanessa was told that autoimmune conditions could not be reversed. "Once you have them, you have them," she heard from one doctor after another. "There's really nothing you can do about it."

One day, Vanessa saw my book *The Autoimmune Solution* in her local bookstore. She was struck by the promise in the word *solution,* and since she lived in Austin, she made an appointment with me, wary but hope-ful that maybe I could get her from *lousy* to *terrific.*

My first step was to run a complete panel of tests on Vanessa. Sure enough, her instincts were right: she indeed had thyroid blood dysfunction.

"THERE'S NOTHING YOU CAN DO ABOUT IT": THE MOST DANGEROUS AUTOIMMUNE MYTH I KNOW

Of all the destructive myths conventional medicine has about autoim-mune conditions, this one is probably the most dangerous. As I told Vanessa, *of course* there's something we can do about autoimmune disorders—there's a *lot* we can do about them! Whether your autoim-mune disorder is lupus, multiple sclerosis, rheumatoid arthritis, Graves' disease, Hashimoto's, or something else, The Myers Way can help you reverse your symptoms, support your immune system, and live a vital, pain-free life.

Now, let's be clear. Nothing we know about so far can *cure* an auto-immune condition—not even The Myers Way. Once you are autoim-mune, your immune system will always have the potential to attack your own body, destroying vital cells, damaging organs, and otherwise wreaking havoc.

What we *can* do is help *reverse* autoimmunity, which we accomplish by lowering the inflammation in your body and supporting your immune system. We can achieve these goals by eliminating inflammatory foods, healing your gut, reducing your toxic burden, healing infections, and relieving your stress. Your immune system might always have the *potential* to rage out of control, but with the right diet and lifestyle—the one embodied by The Myers Way—you can keep that potential in check.

By contrast, conventional medicine takes a two-part approach to autoimmune disorders—and both parts are problematic. First, conventional MDs often try to suppress immune function, reasoning that if the immune system is overactive, suppressing it makes some kind of logical sense.

The problem is that immunosuppressants are harsh medications with powerful and often disturbing side effects. Plus, if you are suppressing your immune system so that it won't attack your own body, you're also disabling it from attacking genuine invaders—the viruses and unhealthy bacteria that can actually pose a threat to your health.

Part two of the typical conventional approach involves medicating symptoms—both the symptoms of the disorder and the symptoms of the medications used to treat it. Painkillers, antinausea meds, laxatives, steroids, sleep aids, and a host of other pharmaceutical wonders are all part of the polypharmacy used to mitigate the dire effects of prescription medications.

When it comes to thyroid, the conventional medical protocol follows this basic pattern with some small differences. For Hashimoto's thyroiditis, conventional doctors leave the immune system alone. They basically just prescribe supplemental thyroid hormone to compensate for what the damaged thyroid cannot produce—and that's it. No diet or lifestyle changes to support thyroid function or immune function. No effort to stop the immune system's attacks on the thyroid. Instead, the immune system is left to continue its assault. And as Vanessa found, that means that you have to keep increasing your dose of supplemental thyroid hormone to compensate for an increasingly damaged thyroid.

For Graves' disease, as you read in the introduction, the conventional protocol is to leave the immune system alone but to try to suppress thyroid function, with either harsh medications, radioactive ablation, or surgery.

Once the thyroid has been suppressed, damaged, or destroyed, conventional doctors prescribe supplemental thyroid hormone to compensate for what the thyroid can no longer produce. They might also offer medications to counter the dreadful side effects: beta-blockers to slow a racing heart, sleep aids to overcome insomnia, Xanax for the anxiety, and so on.

These dreary and sometimes devastating alternatives speak to the profound pessimism of conventional medicine with regard to autoimmune disorders. Functional medicine is far more optimistic, and I am excited to share that optimism. When Vanessa asked me, tentatively, whether I truly believed she could reverse her symptoms and improve her thyroid function — whether she could halt the damage and the downward spiral, so that she was not feeling terrible while continuing to increase her dose of supplemental hormone — I was happy to tell her that I *did* see a lot of room for hope.

Following The Myers Way offers you a solution to autoimmune disorders: reverse the downward trend, eliminate your symptoms, and live a vital, energized, pain-free life without medication (although many patients will often continue to need some amount of supplemental thyroid hormone).

MEET YOUR IMMUNE SYSTEM

To understand why functional medicine is so effective for autoimmune conditions, you have to understand how your immune system works. Your immune system's job is, quite simply, to protect you from the bacteria, viruses, and parasites that try to enter your body through your skin, lungs, and GI tract. Toward this end, it has developed two parts: innate and adaptive.

Your **innate immune system** is your first responder. If you eat something toxic or if a wound becomes infected with unhealthy bacteria, your innate immune system rushes to the rescue with its chief weapon: acute inflammation. *Inflammation* is the hot, fiery reaction that your body mobilizes in order to destroy invading bacteria, viruses, and parasites. *Acute* inflammation is specific and limited: it rushes to the scene of the attack, douses the invader with killer chemicals, and then disappears.

Your innate immune system is swift and powerful, but it has no memory. It responds to every single attack as though it were the very first. By contrast, your **adaptive immune system** remembers the most destructive invaders and constructs an alert system so it can attack them the next time they show up.

Suppose you encounter a disease, such as measles. The first time the measles virus enters your system, your body doesn't realize it's a threat. You start to develop the illness, and your adaptive immune system says, "Oh, I see—we don't like this." Your innate immune system rushes to fight off the initial attack while your adaptive immune system prepares a long-term strategy for defense. The next time the measles virus tries to enter your body, the weapons of the innate immune system are poised and ready.

You probably recognize this process from vaccines. You're injected with a small amount of a disease-causing virus or bacteria, your innate immune system fights off the minor threat (so you might get some flu-like symptoms or a sore arm), and meanwhile, your adaptive immune system is preparing antibodies designed to recognize and target intruders. If you're ever threatened with another attack of the disease, your antibodies will mobilize your immune system to protect you. You have *immunity* against the disease, one of the miracles of modern science.

Some antibodies trigger a reaction against not just their own disease but other diseases that seem similar. Back in the eighteenth century, physician Edward Jenner discovered that by inoculating patients with a small amount of cowpox, he could provide them with immunity against smallpox as well. At the first hint of either cowpox or smallpox, the antibodies triggered a firestorm of inflammation that knocked out the virus before it had a chance to do any harm.

Note that both your innate and your adaptive immune systems rely on inflammation as their chief weapon. So far, we've been talking about only the good kind of inflammation—the acute kind that shows up when there's an invader and leaves when the invader leaves. But even acute inflammation creates problems for your body: *redness, pain, heat,* and *swelling,* which you will recognize from how your body responds when you have an injury, an infection, or an illness of any kind. So what happens when inflammation becomes chronic and those problematic effects never really go away?

CHRONIC INFLAMMATION: THE ROOT OF AUTOIMMUNITY

In my previous book, *The Autoimmune Solution,* I describe chronic inflammation as a condition when your immune system is on never-ending alert. If you've got too much chronic inflammation for too long, it can trigger any genetic potential you might have to develop auto-immunity. In response, your immune system goes rogue, attacking imaginary enemies as well as real ones, with disastrous consequences for your body.

In *The Autoimmune Solution,* I ask you to picture the members of a security squad sitting in Command Central. A host of invaders—infections, toxins, stressors, harmful bacteria, and many others—continue to assault the building, so the squad never has a moment to take a break, even for a meal or a good night's sleep. At first, they're selective about whom they fire at, because the inflammatory response is a powerful one and it can destroy good guys as well as bad. But when the threats just keep coming, the poor, beleaguered security squad begins to lose control. Their shooting—at first carefully calibrated and targeted—now becomes random and desperate. They just start spraying the surrounding area with everything they've got, not noticing that some of their targets aren't actually dangerous or that they themselves are causing a huge amount of destruction by their uncontrolled fire.

Now picture your immune system in place of that security squad, assaulted again and again and again. If the attacks *on* your immune system keep coming, the attacks *from* your immune system keep coming. This is the point at which you might develop an autoimmune condition, a disorder in which your poor, beleaguered immune system begins attacking *you.*

What's the solution? Bring down chronic inflammation. You trigger inflammation in a number of ways—by eating certain foods, by having a leaky gut, high toxic burden, or constant low-grade infections, by overexercising, and by not having enough stress relief. You can bring down inflammation by healing your gut, since 80 percent of your immune system is located there (makes sense, given that the vast majority of threats to your system come in through what you eat or drink).

The Myers Way Thyroid Connection Plan (as well as The Myers Way Autoimmune Solution laid out in my previous book) will help you bring down inflammation to the point where your immune system has the chance to take a deep breath, calm down, and stop overreacting. However—and this is what I mean when I say that you can't *cure* autoimmunity—if your inflammation levels rise again, your immune system is likely to go right back on the attack. Put simply:

- Chronic inflammation can trigger an autoimmune response
- Chronic inflammation helps *maintain* an autoimmune response
- Only by lowering your inflammation levels *and keeping them low* can you hope to reverse an autoimmune condition

Conditions Associated with Chronic Inflammation

Autoimmune disorders of all types
Bone and joint disorders (back pain, muscle pain, arthritis)
Cancers of all types
Cardiovascular diseases (heart disease, atherosclerosis)
Digestive disorders (acid reflux [GERD], irritable bowel syndrome, ulcers, gallstones, fatty liver, diverticulitis, food sensitivities, food allergies)
Emotional and cognitive disorders (anxiety, brain fog, depression)
Hormonal disorders (fibrocystic breasts, endometriosis, fibroids)
Metabolic disorders (obesity, diabetes)
Neurological disorders (ADD/ADHD, Alzheimer's, autism, dementia)
Psychiatric disorders (bipolar disorder, schizophrenia)
Respiratory disorders (sinusitis, seasonal allergies, asthma)
Skin conditions (acne, eczema, rosacea)

DIAGNOSING AUTOIMMUNITY

Now that you know *why* it's important to diagnose autoimmunity, let's talk about *how* to diagnose it.

Vanessa was more fortunate than most; at least she had been accurately diagnosed with an autoimmune condition. Far too many thyroid patients never find out if their condition is autoimmune or not, largely because conventional medicine doesn't treat the two types of thyroid dysfunction any differently.

As you already know, I don't hold with that at all, and I'm excited to help you reverse your condition and eliminate your symptoms. My first step is an accurate diagnosis, which begins by including a test for *thyroid antibodies* in my complete thyroid panel of blood work.

Thyroid antibodies are just what they sound like—creations of your adaptive immune system designed to target your thyroid. Why did your immune system decide your thyroid was a threat? That remains an unsolved mystery, although we do know it has something to do with the constant inflammatory assault that causes your immune system to feel so harassed and overwhelmed that it just starts firing at the wrong targets.

The two most common thyroid antibodies are thyroid peroxidase antibody (TPO) and thyroglobulin antibody (TgAb), and there are lab tests available to measure both. Remember, once you have one autoimmune disease, you are three times more likely to develop another one. So if you are diagnosed with thyroid dysfunction, *please* make sure your doctor checks your thyroid antibodies in addition to your thyroid hormone levels. (More about working with your doctor in part 3.)

YOUR GUT: THE KEY TO YOUR IMMUNE SYSTEM

Vanessa knew she had an autoimmune condition, but she didn't realize that she had a condition known as *leaky gut*. I would say that just about everyone with an autoimmune condition has leaky gut, and many more people besides, so let's take a closer look at gut health and how it affects your immune system.

As you might guess by its name, leaky gut occurs when your gut (specifically your small intestine) becomes too permeable, allowing particles to leak from your digestive tract and travel freely through your bloodstream. (The more formal name for leaky gut is "intestinal permeability.")

Now, here's where your gut and your immune system intersect. The lining of your gut wall—known as the *epithelium*—is only one cell thick. And right on the other side of that oh-so-thin wall is roughly 80 percent of your immune system.

When your gut wall is healthy, everything is great. Your immune system never has to deal with anything potentially dangerous or inflammatory seeping through the wall; all that can fit through the tightly joined cells are tiny portions of nutrients that have been fully digested and broken down to their smallest, most essential components.

But when your gut wall is leaky—specifically, when the *tight junctions* that hold its cells together remain open—small amounts of partially digested food can pass through, and this alarms your immune system to no end. It hasn't been trained to recognize partially digested dairy or gluten or any other food item, and after a while, it begins to consider them foreign invaders, much like the measles virus. And then watch out, because—you guessed it—your adaptive immune system develops antibodies to target the invaders. Now every time you drink milk or eat a bite of bread—every time you encounter even a tiny portion of dairy or gluten in any form—your antibodies go on alert, and those guys in Command Central go nuts again, spraying your entire system with all the firepower available. That's not in itself an autoimmune response—it's actually a *food sensitivity*. But enough inflammatory response, and now you are at risk for autoimmunity. That's one of the reasons why diet is such an important part of The Myers Way. So here's your takeaway:

- *To have a healthy immune system, you've got to have a healthy gut.*

Factors That Contribute to Leaky Gut

Alcohol

Challenging foods and food sensitivities

Dairy

Eggs

Gluten

GMO foods

Grains and pseudograins

Legumes

Nightshades

Sugar

Chemotherapy

Gut infections and imbalances

Parasites

Small intestine bacterial overgrowth (SIBO)

Yeast overgrowth

Medications

Acid-blocking medications

Antibiotics

Birth control pills

NSAIDs (aspirin, ibuprofen, and prescription NSAIDs [nonsteroidal
   anti-inflammatory drugs])

Prednisone

Mycotoxins (toxic mold)

Radiation

Stress

Physical stress (illness, lack of sleep, overexercise)

Emotional stress (family, personal, and work pressures)

Surgeries

THE GLUTEN CONNECTION

Besides suffering from leaky gut, Vanessa consumed a lot of gluten — a type of protein found in such grains as wheat, barley, rye, and spelt. Gluten is obviously found in breads, baked goods, and pasta, but it also appears in a shocking number of processed foods, including ones you might never associate with grains: soups, gravies, hot dogs, soy sauce, and even supplements and medications, which use gluten as a binding and preservative. Gluten also shows up in lots of personal-care products, so even when you are standing in the shower or rubbing moisturizer on your skin, you may be dosing your body with gluten.

This is a problem, because gluten is one of the main causes of leaky gut for people with thyroid dysfunction and autoimmune diseases. The most extreme reaction to gluten occurs in celiac patients — gluten literally destroys a portion of their gut, impairing their digestion and putting them at risk for a number of health problems. A less extreme and more common response comes from non-celiac *gluten sensitivity* — that is, your adaptive immune system makes antibodies to the gluten and generates an inflammatory response any time you consume some (or rub some on your skin!).

The pioneering work of Dr. Alessio Fasano has identified another problem that is even worse. When anyone with gluten sensitivity eats gluten-containing food, the gluten proteins make their way through the stomach and arrive at the small intestine, where the body responds by producing zonulin. No, that's not a villain from *Star Wars;* it's a chemical that triggers the tight junctions of the intestinal walls to open up, creating permeability. Other causes of leaky gut include gut infections such as Candida overgrowth, medications like antibiotics or birth control pills, and stress.

So now your permeable small intestine has allowed partially digested food to leak into your bloodstream, along with toxins and microbes that would otherwise have remained behind a secure gut wall. No wonder your immune system goes on high alert! The threats just keep on coming, putting your body in a state of chronic inflammation and you on the path to develop an autoimmune disease. Unfortunately, the gluten that caused your gut to become leaky also makes it more likely that you will develop thyroid disease in one of the most dangerous cases of mistaken identity that I know.

MOLECULAR MIMICRY: A CASE OF MISTAKEN IDENTITY

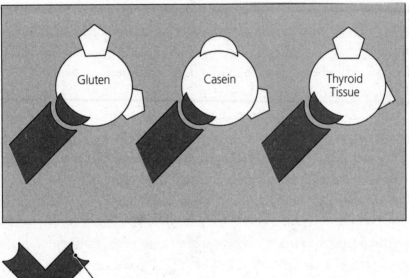

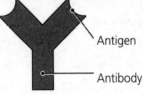

Antigen

Antibody

Every time your body is exposed to a dangerous outside invader, your immune system memorizes its structure, specifically its protein sequence, so that it can develop the perfect defense to that pathogen and recognize it in the future.

But as we have seen, the immune system's recognition system isn't perfect. After all, it confused smallpox with cowpox, right? If one molecule's structure and protein sequences are similar enough to another's, the immune system can be fooled into attacking the look-alike molecules—even if they're part of your body's tissue. Molecular mimicry is one of the most common triggers for an autoimmune response—the confusion of your body's tissue with some foreign invader.

Unfortunately for the thyroid, it has a common doppelgänger that puts it at risk for rogue autoimmune attacks. You guessed it: gluten. This protein is structurally similar to your thyroid tissue, so when your immune system wants to attack it, guess what it does to your thyroid? It's not pretty. In addition, 50 percent of people with gluten sensitivity also experience molecular mimicry with casein, a protein found in dairy products. (This is also known as *cross-reactivity*—when you react to your original trigger and to another trigger that resembles the first one.) One of the key researchers in the field, Dr. Aristo Vojdani, believes the figure is closer to 100 percent.

Even worse, the more permeable your intestinal wall, the more likely that partially digested gluten and dairy will leak into your bloodstream. From your immune system's point of view, this is like that man in horror films who comes running through the room crying out, "They're everywhere! They're everywhere!" Your poor, overworked immune system begins to see enemies on all sides, and so it attacks the dairy, the gluten, and your thyroid tissue with equal force.

Interestingly, those attacks on your thyroid can have two vastly different results. If you've got Hashimoto's, immune system assaults disrupt your thyroid's ability to work properly, slowing your entire metabolism to a crawl. This was Vanessa's experience, and it explains why her symptoms kept getting worse and worse over the years. As her thyroid tissue was bombarded by her immune system, her thyroid became more and more damaged and less and less functional. Accordingly, it produced less and less thyroid hormone, so Vanessa had to keep upping her dose of the supplemental hormone.

If you have Graves' disease, as I did, your immune system messes with your thyroid in a different way. In that disorder, your thyroid antibodies behave as though they were molecules of thyroid-stimulating hormone, causing your thyroid to overproduce its hormones and sending your metabolism into overdrive.

By the way, even if your thyroid disease is *not* autoimmune, you can fall prey to molecular mimicry. That's why I recommend that all of my patients with thyroid dysfunction remove gluten and dairy from their diets, even if they are not autoimmune.

Molecular Mimicry: Bacteria and Viruses

Although gluten and casein (dairy protein) are the most common threats, researchers have also noted molecular mimicry triggered by the bacteria *Yersinia enterocolitica,* which makes its way to the gut via contaminated food or water. As a result, the *Yersinia* causes Graves' disease by its cross-reactivity with the thyroid-stimulating hormone receptor. Other examples of potential triggers for molecular mimicry include Epstein-Barr and other herpes viruses. See chapter 9.

STRESS AND YOUR IMMUNE SYSTEM

There is one more significant factor that suppresses your immune function: stress. To some extent, your body responds this way to stress so it can focus fully on overcoming the stressor. Stress causes inflammation too, so your immune system slows down to prevent a state of chronic inflammation. A suppressed immune system can also trigger latent viral infections, some of which can in turn trigger autoimmune thyroid disease.

Furthermore, if you experience multiple episodes of chronic stress, causing your immune system to rev up and slow down repeatedly, you are at greater risk of your immune system overreacting and triggering an autoimmune response.

As part of suppressing your immune system, cortisol weakens your immune system's primary barriers—the blood–brain barrier, lungs, and gut barrier. And as we just saw, a weakened gut barrier leads to leaky gut, which sets you on the path to autoimmune disease, releasing gluten and dairy (among other things) into your bloodstream, setting you up for molecular mimicry. Yep, it's a vicious, vicious cycle—but as Vanessa learned, you *can* turn it around.

FINALLY FEELING TERRIFIC

Once Vanessa understood the huge difference she could make by changing her diet and lifestyle and by getting the right type and dose of supplemental thyroid hormone, she was excited to move forward. She eagerly began The Myers Way Thyroid Connection Plan. She removed inflammatory foods from her diet, taking special care to avoid gluten and dairy so as not to provoke reactions caused by molecular mimicry. She took supplements to support her thyroid function and her immune function. She followed the rest of the protocol as well: healing her gut, reducing her toxic burden, treating underlying infections, doing the right type of exercise, getting deep, restful sleep, and relieving her stress. (You'll learn all about these factors in part 4.)

Over the next three months, I could read the benefits in her labs. When she first came to me, Vanessa's TSH was 2.3 μIU/mL, her free T4 was 1.1 ng/dL, her free T3 was 2.4 pg/mL, her reverse T3 was 19 ng/dL, and her TPO level was 640 IU/mL. She didn't have any thyroglobulin antibodies, but her high level of TPO antibodies made it clear that she did in fact have Hashimoto's. Although by conventional standards, her TSH was normal, it was a little outside of the optimal range that I like to see, between 1.0 and 2.0 μIU/mL for most people. Although her free T4 was optimal, her free T3 was less than ideal—I look for an optimal reading of 3.2 pg/mL.

As you have seen, there are two striking differences between my approach to labs and that of conventional doctors. One, conventional doctors often neglect to test for thyroid antibodies, whereas I consider that test of supreme importance. Two, they look for normal ranges, whereas I look for *optimal* ones: the ranges that ensure you are functioning at the best possible level of health you can achieve. As Vanessa had learned, normal ranges can still leave you feeling lousy.

I thought Vanessa needed more free T3, so I changed her from Synthroid—which is composed entirely of T4—to a type of supplemental hormone that also includes T3. The type I used for Vanessa was Nature-Throid, which is made from desiccated porcine hormone. I started with a dose of 1.5 grains or 90 mg.

The results of the diet and lifestyle program combined with the changes in supplemental hormone were quite dramatic. Within a few days, Vanessa was already feeling the impact of the free T3. Her mood lightened and she felt energized and hopeful. A few weeks later, she was feeling better and brighter all around. She was steadily losing weight and feeling that her energy levels were finally what she had known as a young woman. I was excited for Vanessa—and her labs affirmed that there was much to be excited about:

- Her TSH was at an optimal level of 1 μIU/mL.
- Her free T4 had risen slightly to 1.3 ng/dL.
- Her free T3 was at a very healthy 3.2 pg/mL.
- Her reverse T3 had dropped to 16 ng/dL.
- And her TPO antibodies had fallen to 320 IU/mL—half of what they had been.

As we continued to work together, she maintained optimal thyroid levels while her antibodies kept falling, indicating that she was indeed reversing her autoimmune condition.

To me, Vanessa's story embodies the promise of The Myers Way Thyroid Connection Plan: not settling for okay or even fine, but finding a way to get to terrific. I always say that optimal health is your birthright. I was thrilled that Vanessa had managed to claim this birthright so she could feel terrific for many years to come.

Part Three

WORKING WITH YOUR DOCTOR

CHAPTER 5

Why Your Doctor Gets It Wrong

By the time she came to me, Susannah had been to three different doctors over the past three years—yet none of them could accurately diagnose or appropriately treat her thyroid dysfunction. "They kept telling me I was fine because my labs were normal," Susannah told me on her first visit. "But I'm exhausted and depressed and gaining weight, and I can't even think straight. I *can't* be okay if I'm feeling like this!"

When I reviewed Susannah's medical records, I could see the problem. Each doctor she'd seen had looked at only part of her condition. The blood tests they ran showed Susannah's thyroid hormone levels to be within normal range—but those tests were incomplete. She *did* have thyroid dysfunction, but her doctors could not see it in the labs they ordered.

Susannah's first doctor had tested only her TSH. As you recall, TSH—thyroid-stimulating hormone—is a biochemical produced by the pituitary gland to trigger the release of thyroid hormone as needed. Many conventional MDs test only the TSH and look no further. If TSH readings are high, this suggests that the thyroid needs extra stimulation, indicating potential dysfunction. But if the readings are within the normal range, most conventional doctors assume that the thyroid doesn't need extra stimulation and is therefore performing normally. Susannah's doctor looked at the seemingly normal reading and told her she was fine. But Susannah was far from fine.

Susannah's second doctor tested both her TSH and her free T4. As you recall, T4 is the storage hormone, produced by your thyroid in response to the stimulation of TSH. Some doctors test free T4 in addition to TSH and leave it at that. Since Susannah's readings for these two figures were also within the normal range, her doctor didn't detect her thyroid dysfunction. But because Susannah was struggling with debilitating symptoms, he agreed to put her on a very low dose of Synthroid (25 mcg). Susannah followed up again in three months, and her TSH and free T4 had improved—but her symptoms were no better. Because her labs were normal, however, the doctor was unwilling to increase her dose of Synthroid. So, even more frustrated, she looked for yet another doctor.

Her third doctor, a holistic practitioner, was more thorough. She tested Susannah's TSH and free T4, which by now were actually optimal since Susannah had been taking Synthroid. But because she was still having symptoms, the holistic doctor also tested her free T3. As you recall, free T3 is the *active* and *unbound* form of the thyroid hormone—the portion of the thyroid hormone that actually makes its way into your cells. A free T3 reading often gives the most immediate portrait of what's going on with your thyroid, but here again, Susannah's readings were within the normal range.

The doctor was confused, because she had expected to see a low free T3 reading. When she didn't, she wondered if maybe the other doctors had been right. Perhaps Susannah didn't have thyroid dysfunction at all but rather was depressed, in perimenopause, or just getting older. "I looked for a thyroid issue, but I didn't find anything," the doctor told Susannah. "All of your thyroid labs are completely normal, even your free T3."

At this point, Susannah was in despair. A friend who had had a similar experience with doctors referred her to me. After talking extensively with Susannah, I was convinced she did have thyroid dysfunction, because her symptoms were classic (see pages 20–21). Of course, as a scientist, I don't go only on the symptoms a patient reports. I also needed to see Susannah's labs.

When I did, I found out two things.

First, although Susannah's TSH and free T4 were *optimal,* her free T3 numbers were only *normal.* That is, they were okay but not great. Every blood test has a *reference range*—an upper and lower limit of what is considered normal. And as you've learned, the standard reference range for thyroid labs is way too wide. Technically, yes, Susannah's free T3 was within the normal range. But I felt her reading was too close to the lower end of the scale, making it far from optimal.

In addition, none of Susannah's other doctors had ever tested her reverse T3. As you recall, free T3 is your body's gas pedal, revving up your metabolism and powering you with energy, while reverse T3 is your body's brake, slowing down your metabolism and helping your body conserve energy rather than expend it. In a healthy body, free T3 and reverse T3 are perfectly balanced so that your engine runs neither too hot (excess weight loss, diarrhea, racing heart, anxiety) nor too cold (weight gain, constipation, sluggishness, depression). But occasionally, especially in times of excessive stress, the balance is off.

In fact, Susannah had been hit by a triple wave of stress — her elderly father had just been diagnosed with Parkinson's disease, her child was struggling with dyslexia, and rumors of layoffs were circulating in her department at work. As you recall from part 2, unrelieved stress cues your body to *slow down, hold on to fat,* and *conserve energy.* Your body responds in many ways, including by increasing its production of reverse T3. And indeed, Susannah's reverse T3 levels were elevated, overpowering her free T3 and slowing down her metabolism. I believed this was at least part of the reason behind her exhaustion, weight gain, and brain fog.

Besides looking at her reverse T3, I also tested Susannah for the most common thyroid antibodies — thyroid peroxidase antibody (TPO) and thyroglobulin antibody (TgAb). If your thyroid antibodies are high, that's an indication that your immune system is routinely attacking your thyroid. It became clear to me that Susannah had Hashimoto's thyroiditis.

I adjusted Susannah's supplemental thyroid hormone. In addition to Synthroid, which consists only of T4, I put Susannah on a specially compounded formula of time-release T3 so that we could quickly increase her levels of free T3. That would counterbalance her excessive reverse T3, restoring her energy levels, clearing her brain fog, and allowing her to lose weight.

Adjusting her dose of supplemental hormone was important. But Susannah also needed to follow The Myers Way Thyroid Connection

Plan, so that the fundamental problems that had been disrupting her thyroid and immune system would be resolved:

• Diet and supplements supplied Susannah's thyroid with the nutrients she needed to make enough thyroid hormone and convert T4 to T3. We also got her on a grain-free and dairy-free diet. I explained to Susannah that her immune system had begun reacting badly to gluten and dairy, poised to attack even tiny amounts of either food. And because her immune system had confused her thyroid gland with those foods—the molecular mimicry you learned about in chapter 4—she needed to remove those two foods 100 percent from her diet to stop the attacks.

• Helping Susannah heal her gut—which had become leaky through stress and other factors—went a long way toward convincing her immune system to calm down and stop attacking her thyroid.

• Lowering Susannah's toxic burden was also important. Many industrial chemicals have this weird effect on your body—they act just like estrogen, which is why they are called *xenoestrogens,* literally, "foreign estrogens." Too much exposure to the toxins routinely found in water, air, food, and such common household items as plastics, personal-care products, and cleaning products has the same effect as giving your body a massive overdose of estrogen. (You'll learn more about that in chapter 8.) Excess estrogen—whether in the form of your body's own estrogen or in the form of xenoestrogens—is bad for a whole lot of reasons, including that it promotes thyroxine-binding globulin (TBG), which leads to too much *bound* rather than *free* thyroid hormone. Reducing toxic exposure and improving Susannah's ability to *detoxify* her body—to rid it of those industrial chemicals—meant that she would bind less thyroid hormone and restore healthy levels of free T3 and free T4.

• Making sure that Susannah was infection-free was also important, so that infections did not trigger inflammation and undermine her immune response. Most important, stress relief helped Susannah restore a healthy balance between reverse T3 and free T3. As you saw in part 2, excess stress means excess cortisol, which disrupts thyroid function in all sorts of ways, contributing to brain fog, exhaustion, and weight gain. Techniques such as HeartMath, acupuncture, massage, meditation, and nature walks eased some of her stress burden, lowered her cortisol, and restored optimal thyroid function. (You'll learn more about stress relief in chapter 9.)

And indeed, Susannah showed rapid improvement on The Myers Way. Within a few weeks, she felt significantly better, and by her third month on the program, she was full of energy, clearheaded, and optimistic. Her labs showed so much improvement that she no longer needed as much of the compounded time-release T3. Her body was making more free T3 and less reverse T3, creating a healthier balance.

Unfortunately, since this had been going on for several years before I met Susannah, her thyroid had already been damaged to the point that she would always need to take some supplemental thyroid hormone. The good news, though, was that she was now symptom-free and would remain so as long as she stayed on The Myers Way. And her thyroid was now functioning so much better, we could get the same results with a smaller dose of hormone.

So what's your takeaway?

• *Even when your doctor tells you that your thyroid labs are okay or normal or just fine, you might* **still** *have thyroid dysfunction.*

That's why it's so important to know which thyroid labs your doctor is ordering for you, what they mean, and which other lab tests you might need. In this chapter, I'll walk you through conventional treatment and help you understand its shortcomings. In the next chapter, I'll help you figure out how to get an accurate diagnosis and effective treatment.

THE TESTING TANGLE

As you can see from Susannah's story, most doctors miss a *lot* of thyroid dysfunction, largely because of the way they test for it and because of how they interpret those tests. I'm even surprised by how many alternative and holistic practitioners miss some important labs that are needed to get a complete picture. Here are the most common reasons doctors are not picking up your thyroid dysfunction from your lab results:

1. They don't order blood tests for thyroid dysfunction at all

What? How could that happen? Well, as we saw in chapter 2, men are generally believed to be at low risk for thyroid dysfunction, so they are often not tested. And although it's true that women are seven times more likely to develop thyroid disorders than men, men *do* get thyroid dysfunction. But if they're not tested, who's going to know?

Likewise, both women and men under forty are believed to be at low risk for thyroid dysfunction. So people in that category might also be underdiagnosed.

Finally, thyroid dysfunction is frequently confused with other conditions. So if your doctor has diagnosed you with another condition, particularly if you're under forty or you're a man, the biggest problem with your thyroid blood test is that no one ever did it in the first place.

Conditions Frequently Confused with Thyroid Dysfunction

Aging

Anemia

Anxiety

Brain fog

Chronic fatigue syndrome

Constipation caused by gastrointestinal disorder

Dementia, including early-onset Alzheimer's

Depression

Diarrhea caused by gastrointestinal disorder

Heart condition

Infertility or miscarriages

Insomnia caused by sex hormone imbalance or psychological issue

Obesity caused by diet, genetics, or another factor

Sex hormone issues: andropause, postpartum, perimenopause, menopause, menstrual irregularities

Stress

2. They test only your TSH

As Susannah discovered, many conventional MDs think that a TSH test is really all you need. What can I tell you? It isn't. While the information we get from TSH can be important, it reflects only what's going on between the pituitary and the thyroid. It doesn't tell you anything about what's happening on a cellular level or whether your thyroid hormone is actually entering your cells.

Moreover, if you are taking supplemental thyroid hormone that contains T3 (Armour, Nature-Throid, Westhroid, and other forms of desiccated thyroid hormone), the T3 can artificially suppress your TSH. So if you're taking any form of T3, your TSH readings will be even less reliable as a guide to your overall thyroid health.

3. They test your total T4…but not your *free* T4

You already know the problem with this: Only the free T4 is metabolically active and able to convert as needed to free T3. Bound T4 does not affect your metabolism, so a total T4 reading—a single number that includes both free and bound T4—gives a really inaccurate picture of what's actually happening within your body.

So why do so many doctors measure total T4 and not also free T4? I don't know—but they do.

4. They test your free T4…but not your free T3

Okay, so the obvious problem here is that T3 is the form of thyroid hormone that is metabolically active—that actually produces results in your body. If we don't know how much T3 you have, we really don't have a good idea of your thyroid status.

This might seem obvious, but some aspects of this issue are *not* so obvious. For instance, some people respond to an underproducing thyroid by relying on their adrenals to pick up the slack. If that's you, your body is relying on stress hormones for the energy and focus that you should be getting from your thyroid hormone. You could end up with an odd collection of symptoms that don't *seem* to indicate an underperforming thyroid—but do. For example, although most people with an underperforming thyroid gain weight and feel sluggish, I've had hypothyroid patients who lost rapid and unhealthy amounts of weight, felt anxious and wired, and struggled with insomnia. That sounds more like an *over*performing thyroid, doesn't it? (See the symptoms on page 21.) But when I looked at their labs, their free T3 levels were dangerously low. Adrenaline, cortisol, dopamine, and other stress hormones were fueling their bodies, compensating for low free T3. No way could I have diagnosed their condition just by looking at TSH or free T4. The only way I could have known what was really going on was to accurately measure their free T3.

Low free T3 levels might also mean you aren't converting enough free T4 into free T3. Often this is a nutritional issue — to make the conversion, you need iodine, tyrosine, vitamin A, B vitamins, zinc, and selenium, which most people don't have enough of. To diagnose that problem, though, you need to know what the free T3 levels are.

5. They test your total T3…but not your *free* T3

Again, you know the problem with this: Only the free T3 is metabolically active. Bound T3 does not affect your metabolism, so a total T3 reading—a single number that includes both free and bound T3—gives us an inaccurate picture.

Why do so many doctors measure total T3 and not free T3? Again, I just don't know. But they should—and now *you* know which tests you need, even if they don't.

6. They test your T3 uptake…but not your *free* T3

T3 uptake is an indirect measure of thyroxine-binding proteins that is supposed to give us an indication of how much of your T3 is *free* and how much is *bound*. I've seen this lab in some of my patients' medical records, and frankly, I don't find it very useful. What we really need to know is a direct measure of free T3 itself.

7. They test your free T3…but not your reverse T3

You saw what a problem this was for Susannah. Often, reverse T3 is the missing piece of the puzzle — the explanation for why someone's symptoms are severe when their labs look fairly normal. Even some functional medicine physicians and alternative/holistic practitioners don't check reverse T3; again, I don't know why. I do know that a number of stressors can cue your body to increase its production of reverse T3, which can then create thyroid dysfunction for you. Measuring your level of reverse T3 levels gives us a full picture of the problem.

8. They don't test your antibodies

You learned what's wrong with that in chapter 4: without knowing a patient's antibody status, we have no way of knowing whether his or her thyroid dysfunction is caused by autoimmunity.

For me, diagnosing an autoimmune disorder is crucial, because I know how to support the immune system and reverse the condition so that your immune system stops attacking your thyroid. Conventional MDs don't go along with me on this; they believe there is no way to support your immune system or to reduce its attacks on your thyroid— all they know how to do is medicate symptoms. From that point of view, the root cause doesn't matter.

I've even found that thyroid antibodies can *precede* diagnosis of an autoimmune condition by up to five years. If you find that you have high levels of antibodies on your lab test—even before you show any signs of thyroid dysfunction—you can use The Myers Way to support your thyroid and your immune system, helping to reverse the autoimmunity and prevent any thyroid dysfunction down the road. There's a big prize for being successful: by preventing autoimmune damage to your thyroid early on, you'll have no need for medication or supplemental hormones.

So even if your conventional MD doesn't care about knowing your autoimmune status, *you do.* Because once you know, you can follow diet and lifestyle recommendations that will help you reverse your symptoms, support your immune system, and keep you in optimal health.

9. They don't test for the nutrients needed for optimal thyroid function

As you saw in part 2 and will see more completely in part 4, your thyroid needs certain nutrients to manufacture thyroid hormone. Your body also needs specific nutrients to convert T4 to T3, receive T3 into its cells, and otherwise promote optimal thyroid function. Last but not least, your immune system depends on certain nutrients for proper immune function. If my patients are low in any of these key nutrients, I prescribe supplements. But if your conventional MD isn't testing for blood levels of these key nutrients, how can he or she prescribe them for you?

Key Nutrients Your Body Needs for Optimal Thyroid and Immune Function

B vitamins

Essential fatty acids

Iodine

Iron

Selenium

Tyrosine

Vitamin A

Vitamin D

Zinc

You'll learn more about why these nutrients are crucial in chapter 7.

---

10. They don't test your sex hormones or stress hormones

You saw in part 2 that stress can promote the accumulation of excess estrogen, which in turn increases TBG, binding more thyroid hormone and reducing your levels of free T4 and free T3. You also saw the multiple ways in which cortisol, a key stress hormone, can disrupt thyroid function.

That's why I test sex hormone and stress hormone levels for my thyroid patients, especially if there is any mystery at all about why they're having symptoms. Most conventional MDs don't consider these hormones' effects on thyroid function important. Even endocrinologists, whose specialty includes hormones of all types, tend to view each type of hormone separately rather than seeing all of them as part of one interrelated system. Failing to test for the different types of hormones can once again prevent proper diagnosis and treatment.

DIAGNOSING HYPERTHYROIDISM

Doctors are less likely to miss hyperthyroidism. That's because they typically use TSH as a screening marker, and when you are hyperthyroid, your TSH is almost invariably low. So, in contrast to hypothyroidism, TSH readings alone often will give you an accurate diagnosis.

But not always. Be aware that in the early and middle stages of hyperthyroidism, you might actually have normal concentrations of free T4 and free T3—even though you are having overt symptoms. Remarkably, even though my own symptoms were so bad I could barely function, my Graves' was considered subclinical based on my lab results. Once again, your labs won't necessarily tell the whole story.

Often MDs will not test your antibodies. They must test your TPO and TgAb to know if you are autoimmune. If you are having hyperthyroid symptoms and your labs are normal and antibodies are negative, then they will need to test Graves' specific antibodies are negative, then they will need to test Graves' specific antibodies—TSH receptor antibodies (TRAb) and thyroid-stimulating immunoglobulins (TSAb)—to confirm the diagnosis.

Now, there is one more problem here: What if no one checks for hyperthyroidism in the first place? If your doctor thinks that your condition is caused by something else, he or she might fail to test you. Your hyperthyroidism might be misdiagnosed as one of the conditions in the list on page 21.

Make sure you get your thyroid tested with a complete thyroid blood panel if you have many of the symptoms on page 21. You'll learn more about which lab tests to request in chapter 6 and there's a handy Checklist on pages 124–125.

Diagnostic challenges: Why even laboratory tests aren't enough

Now, even when we've run every available lab test, coming up with a clear picture of what's going on with your thyroid can still be quite challenging. As you've seen throughout this book, the thyroid and its network—the thyroid signaling system—is an incredibly complex and intricate arrangement, with every element *affecting* and *affected by* multiple other elements.

To make it all even more complex, each element within the system is on its own schedule, so to speak. TSH, for example, operates by a negative feedback loop—it doesn't really get going until it detects low levels of thyroid hormone in your bloodstream. So it might take a few days before TSH springs into action. As a result, on any given day, TSH levels might or might not convey an accurate portrait of what's going on.

Free T4 and free T3, by contrast, are constantly fluctuating in response to the stresses and demands of your day. If you're stressed and anxious as you arrive at the doctor's office, that could affect your thyroid blood levels. If while you are sitting in the waiting room you get an angry e-mail from your boss or a worrying text from your kid, that could affect your stress hormones and thyroid hormones as well. If your breakfast that morning was unusually hard to digest, if you picked up a cold or the flu, if your entire week has been a stress bomb, if you're looking ahead to a crucial meeting or an unpleasant family confrontation, your thyroid is going to feel it—and show it.

I tell my patients that their thyroid activity is like a movie—and when I test their blood, I'm getting only a single frame from that movie. Maybe that frame accurately conveys the essence of the whole film, but maybe it doesn't. Maybe you're living at a super-high level of thyroid hormone, but for some reason, when we draw your blood, your levels are uncharacteristically low. Maybe you're living with significantly low thyroid, but just before we take your blood, something causes your thyroid to spike. Testing is crucial, and I'd never diagnose a patient without it, but let's be clear: it has its limits.

Moreover, even if a lab test reading is accurate—or, let's say, *representative*—it's not always obvious what that reading means. The TSH reading tells us what's going on with the pituitary; the free T4 test tells us how much storage hormone is available; the free T3 results show us how much active hormone is present in your blood. But what we really want to know is what's happening on a cellular level: How much free T3 is entering each cell, unimpeded by reverse T3 or thyroid resistance?

Unfortunately, there isn't a test for that—only a series of labs that, put together, allow me to deduce what I think is going on with the whole system. It's as though I walked into a burglarized office and was able to observe a set of clues—a broken door, a few footprints, some fingerprints, and the bank accounts of some key suspects. I can *probably* put a good picture together of what happened from that evidence, especially if I have a long talk with the key witness to the crime—the patient. But the whole process is often more of an art than a science.

You've seen throughout this book how many non-thyroid factors are involved in your thyroid and immune function: diet, gut health, exercise, stress levels, toxic burden, and (as you'll learn in chapter 9) such low-grade infections as yersinia, Epstein-Barr, and herpes simplex. To give you the right diagnosis and treatment, your MD needs to look at all those factors—some of which can be tested only imperfectly, some of which can't be tested at all. Again, it's more an art than a science. My concern is that conventional doctors aren't being thorough about the science or complete about the art. If I've got only a few pieces of suggestive evidence, they have even less—only a single footprint and half a fingerprint to find that office burglar. And, as you probably know from your own experience, they are rarely interested in interviewing the witness before proceeding on to their standard diagnosis.

What's your takeaway?

- *Know which lab tests to ask for.* I'll go through all of this in the next chapter. For some lab tests, you will need a doctor's order. Others you may be able to order yourself, and I'll explain that too. If you'd like to find a functional MD, check out the website of the Institute for Functional Medicine (www.functionalmedicine.org).
- *Support your own optimal health through The Myers Way Thyroid Connection Plan.* I wish I could treat every one of you individually. But since I can't, I can offer you the next best thing: a way to take your health into your own hands. You may need a doctor to prescribe supplemental thyroid hormone, but you yourself can make sure you get

the diet, supplements, gut healing, detox, infection healing, exercise, sleep, and stress relief you need to make a difference to your thyroid, your immune system, and your overall health.

Derailed by reference ranges

When Gerald came to see me, he was confused and frustrated. An architect in his midfifties, Gerald had been diagnosed about fifteen years earlier with hypothyroidism. His doctor had prescribed Synthroid, and over the years, Gerald's dose had slowly but steadily been going up. Gerald had always felt good enough—until this year. Then, suddenly, he was thoroughly exhausted, quickly put on twelve pounds, and felt overwhelmed with depression.

Gerald's doctor reviewed his labs and insisted that Gerald was getting the right dose of supplemental thyroid hormone. He suggested that Gerald might simply be depressed and offered to prescribe antidepressants.

Gerald couldn't see why such debilitating depression and exhaustion would overtake him out of the blue. In fact, his firm had just landed a couple of assignments that offered Gerald some exciting challenges, and he *had* been feeling hopeful and inspired.

Gerald happened to see me on *The Dr. Oz Show,* talking about the profound effect that diet—especially gluten—can have on our physical and emotional selves. Instead of starting on the antidepressants, he decided to give me a call.

When I ran labs on Gerald, I discovered an all-too-common situation. Gerald's numbers might have been within the *normal* reference ranges—but they weren't *optimal.* For several reasons that I'll discuss below, the standard reference ranges used by most conventional MDs are highly problematic. It's very common to have your lab results fall within the normal reference range even though you still have thyroid symptoms and feel lousy in real life.

Now, as we've seen, the thyroid signaling system is complex and intricate, and it doesn't work in a linear way. A tiny change in your hormone levels—a slight move away from optimal—doesn't necessarily have a tiny effect on your symptoms and well-being. Even a very small departure from optimal can have huge negative effects, leaving you exhausted, depressed, and miserable—just like Gerald. And even a slight change in your type and/or dose of supplemental thyroid hormone can make an enormous change as well.

So when I compared Gerald's lab results not to normal ranges but to *optimal* ones, I could see that he needed more support. For example, his TSH was 3.5 µIU/mL, well within the normal reference range—but *optimal* ranges are much narrower, especially for someone who is already taking supplemental thyroid hormone: between 1.0 and 2.0 µIU/mL. His free T4 was 0.89 ng/dL, whereas I wanted an optimal range of greater than 1.1 ng/dL. And his free T3, normal at 2.7 pg/mL, was very far from the optimal range of greater than 3.2 pg/mL. You can see how much room there is to be suboptimal, even when your doctor insists that your labs are normal.

I decided to try him on Armour, a prescription-only natural hormone that contains both T4 and T3. Previously, Gerald had been on Synthroid, which contains T4 only, and I thought the additional T3 would lift him out of depression and fatigue.

Well, it actually lifted him *too far,* into anxiety and overdrive. The additional T3 caused Gerald's heart to race as though he'd just had three cups of strong coffee. So I decided instead to try him on Tirosint, a different form of synthetic T4 but one without the binders and fillers that make Synthroid problematic for some people. That new form of supplemental thyroid hormone hit the perfect balance, helping Gerald regain his energy and spirits without pushing his metabolism too hard or too fast.

As you can see, there's no one right answer when it comes to diagnosing and treating thyroid dysfunction. I had to analyze Gerald's labs based on what ranges were right *for him,* not on some generalized conventional ranges, which in any case are far too broad. I also had to keep tweaking Gerald's supplemental thyroid hormone to get just the right balance and amount of T3 and T4.

This personalized approach is sadly foreign to most conventional MDs, who seem to believe that one-size-fits-all is an effective way to diagnose and treat thyroid dysfunction. Of course, sometimes the standard approach works, and then everyone is happy. But when it doesn't, you need to insist that your doctor keep trying alternatives until you finally get the optimal health and well-being that you deserve. (More on how to do that in chapter 6.)

Gerald and I had a long talk about what triggered his sudden drop into depression and exhaustion. When I reviewed his diet, I could see that he consumed a lot of gluten in the form of breads, pizza, bagels, and pasta. Although Gerald told me he wasn't a sweets person, I explained to him that sugar is far from the only problem in the modern Western diet. For many people, gluten is a highly inflammatory protein that weakens gut integrity and undermines the immune system.

Furthermore, Gerald had had a sinus infection that would just not go away. In the last six months he had been on three different month-long courses of antibiotics. These antibiotics, along with his high-carb diet, had destroyed most of the friendly bacteria in his gut, making room for an overgrowth of intestinal yeast. Don't confuse intestinal yeast with the yeast you use in baking! Intestinal yeast is a fungus that disrupts gut activity. And the gut is where your body makes 95 percent of its *serotonin,* a feel-good biochemical that helps protect against depression. So some of Gerald's depression almost certainly resulted from the way his high-carb diet and his heavy use of antibiotics had altered his gut bacteria. His underfunctioning thyroid made his depression even worse. That's the classic vicious cycle in which every factor makes every other factor worse . . . and worse . . . and worse.

Fortunately, we could reverse this downward spiral by taking several key steps:

- Remove the gluten and other inflammatory foods from Gerald's diet
- Put him on a lower-carb diet to starve the yeast
- Treat the yeast with herbs and supplements
- Heal his gut with supplements
- Get him on the right type and dose of supplemental thyroid hormone
- Support his thyroid with good sleep and stress relief.

Within a month, Gerald felt like his old self. And within three months, Gerald told me, he felt *better* than his old self; he was thinking more clearly, reacting more calmly, enjoying a more balanced and reliable energy. When gut, immune system, and thyroid all work together, the results can be amazing.

What's Wrong with Reference Ranges?

When I tell people how off base conventional medicine has gotten when it comes to the thyroid, they find it hard to believe me.

"Really?" they reply. "I must be missing something. It can't be *that* bad."

Oh yes. It can. And here is one of the most startling problems.

When doctors and laboratories developed what would later become the standard reference ranges for thyroid readings, they used readings taken from people with thyroid dysfunction.

That's right. As labs and doctors were putting those ranges together, they didn't go out and recruit healthy people. Instead, they used patients who had come to them with thyroid dysfunction. Which means that right from the start, the numbers were out of whack, because the readings from people with thyroid dysfunction were the ones that were tagged as normal. As a result, the reference ranges were way too wide. It would be as if someone went into a group of people who were all ten to fifty pounds overweight—and tagged those as the normal reference ranges for weight. Normal—maybe. Healthy? No. But that's exactly how standard thyroid reference ranges were developed.

I find this so hard to believe I most likely *wouldn't* believe it if I didn't know for sure it was true. Among many others who have criticized this practice is the National Academy of Clinical Biochemistry, which as far back as 2002 concluded that standard reference ranges were probably "skewed by the inclusion of persons with occult thyroid dysfunction." In other words, including too many disordered thyroids was throwing off the thyroid ranges, just as including too many overweight people would throw off healthy weight ranges. Had the thyroid reference ranges been based only on the readings of people with healthy thyroid function, they would have been much narrower—and a much better goal for us physicians to try to get our patients to attain.

So as you can imagine, many patients who visit their doctors might be told that they are within those normal ranges—the ranges *taken from people with thyroid dysfunction*. But because the normal ranges included so much dysfunction, a lot of people who are told they are fine still don't feel completely well. And instead of questioning the ranges—instead of saying, "Wow, so many of my patients fall within those ranges and they still feel lousy; something must be wrong with the ranges"—most conventional doctors say, "If our patients feel lousy, it can't be thyroid, because, look, they're within the ranges! It has to be something else—depression, sex hormones, anxiety, stress, aging, dementia, heart problems, blood pressure issues; there are certainly lots of choices. But the problem can't be thyroid, because, look—the ranges are normal!"

So if you have had the feeling that either you or your doctor must be missing something, if you keep saying how awful you feel and your doctor keeps telling you that it can't be thyroid because your labs don't lie, well, now you know one all-too-frequent explanation for what's been going wrong.

In 2003, the American Association of Clinical Endocrinologists (AACE) decided that maybe the reference ranges weren't as accurate as they might be. So they issued a press release urging doctors to narrow the ranges and to consider patients who fell outside the narrower ranges as genuinely suffering from thyroid dysfunction. In case you're interested, the old TSH ranges were 0.5 µIU/mL to 5.0 µIU/mL, which is pretty darn wide. And the new ones recommended in that press release were narrowed to 0.3 µIU/mL to 3.0 µIU/mL. I consider this still too wide, but at least it was an improvement. The association said "AACE believes the new range will result in proper diagnosis for millions of Americans who suffer from a mild thyroid dysfunction but have gone untreated until now."

Those millions of Americans might then have been properly diagnosed and treated, except for one thing. Most conventional doctors simply ignored the AACE press release and went right on using their old reference ranges, as did most labs. That's right. Even though the chief organization of specialists in all types of hormone treatment told them to narrow their reference ranges—the ranges that, from the beginning, had been developed in a problematic way—most conventional doctors failed to follow the recommendation. I don't believe they were even aware of it. After all, it was only a press release. And it's not like there's some national organization that e-mails doctors, telling them about recent research or new national standards that would require them to change their daily practice. Once they've left medical school, doctors are pretty much on their own when it comes to research. As I've said previously, it takes an average of eighteen years for research to make its way into standard medical practice, a shocking but accurate figure.

However, here's something I truly don't understand. Despite the 2003 press release, in 2012 the AACE published an article recommending yet another number as the upper range of TSH readings: not the 3.0 µIU/mL of the press release, but rather 4.12 µIU/mL. In other words, they presented a recommendation even worse than their first one — though both were still much better than what most physicians were currently doing. Nevertheless, most doctors were unaware of *both* the press release *and* the article — and continued to use reference ranges that were much too high! So as a result of either ignorance or confusion, you're being told your labs are well within the reference ranges, even though you feel lousy. (By the way, the 2012 AACE recommendation for TSH in pregnant women is even lower — <2.5 µIU/mL — and as we just saw, most doctors don't follow them anyway.)

Here is what I want for my patients — the optimal lab values that I'd like to see you hit:

- TSH 1.0 to 2.0 µIU/mL or lower (dessicated thyroid or compounded T3 can artificially suppress TSH). Pregnant women <2.5 µIU/mL
- FT4 >1.1 ng/dL
- FT3 > 3.2 pg/mL
- RT3 < than a 10:1 ratio of RT3 to FT3
- Thyroid peroxidase antibodies < 9 IU/mL or negative
- Thyroglobulin antibodies <4 IU/mL or negative

I also listen — a *lot* — to my patients. If their symptoms don't match what their labs are saying, and if I can find no other disorder to account for those symptoms, then I typically will treat them for thyroid dysfunction, because I know that the labs don't always tell the full story.

Few conventional MDs will go that far to find the right diagnosis and treatment. In the next chapter, I'll advise you on how to work with your own doctor.

RAISE YOUR EXPECTATIONS

I think my greatest quarrel with conventional medicine has to do with how pessimistic its vision is. Most conventional MDs aren't looking to get you feeling great. They aren't trying for optimal reference ranges or the best possible balance of thyroid hormones for your particular body. For most of them, getting you to feel good enough is good enough.

It's not completely their fault. Our whole society has bought into the myth that getting older means you gain weight, slow down, feel foggy, lose energy, and suffer from aches and pains and all sorts of little complaints that sometimes turn into big complaints. You may have bought into it too. I hope, by this point, I've inspired you to aim higher.

No matter how old you are, no matter what your medical history, no matter how lousy you feel right now, *you can feel better.* No matter what your doctor tells you, no matter what your friends and neighbors and family tell you, *you can feel better.* If you are willing to support your body and commit to the food, sleep, exercise, detox, and stress relief that every human body needs, I urge you to go with a far more optimistic view than your doctors might have. As we move into the next chapter, that's the vision I want to leave you with: Glowing, radiant health *is* possible. And it can be yours.

CHAPTER 6

How to Ask Your Doctor for More

If you've read my story in the introduction, you know that I've been where many of you are now. I've been in the hands of a doctor who disregarded my experience and insisted that I couldn't possibly be as sick as I thought I was. I was told I had only three choices, all of which were distressing, none of which were how I wanted to treat my body, and none of which promised me optimal health. I heard—more times than I care to remember—that there was nothing I could do to support my own health, that my only option was to follow the doctor's orders, be obedient and submissive and uncomplaining.

Now, I had one big advantage that most of you probably don't have: I was in medical school. In fact, I had chosen to go to medical school precisely to do the kind of work that I now do: to empower people to find the root cause of their illness and then to reverse that illness through holistic and natural means—diet, supplements, exercise, lifestyle. That vision kept me searching for something better, even when my conventional doctors told me I couldn't have it. I also have a strong personality, and I had been raised by my mother never to accept the status quo. So when the doctors pushed me, insisting that I was suffering only from stress or that I should immediately follow the invasive treatments they recommended, I pushed back.

I spent years fighting with conventional MDs, and I remember that period as one of the most awful in my life. But I have to be glad I went through it, because now I know what *you're* going through—and now I am equipped to help you.

In the previous chapter, I took you through the basics of what your conventional doctor is likely to offer, with all the pros and cons. In this chapter, I'm going to teach you how to ask for what you want and, hopefully, how to get what you deserve from a system that often doesn't work very well. The good news is that you *can* speak up, and you can make a difference in your own health by doing so. So let me give you my best advice — exactly what I'd tell you if you were my friend or family member and couldn't come to me yourself.

TAKE CHARGE OF YOUR OWN HEALTH

Look at it this way. The doctor is supposed to be the expert on health and medicine. But you will always know your body best. *You* are always the expert on *you*. You don't necessarily know more than the doctor about science, medications, supplemental hormones, or anything requiring a medical degree (although, having read this book, you might be surprised at how much you *do* know!). But you do know the most about *you:* how you feel, what you're willing to do, what you want. The doctor is there to help, support, and advise. But you can take charge of your own health.

As I see it, that's a three-step process:

Step 1: Get committed.
Step 2: Set your objectives.
Step 3: Develop a strategy.

Let's take a closer look.

Step 1: Get Committed

Hey, I hope you have a smooth, easy time dealing with your doctor and your insurance company. Some people do. But many don't, so if you're going to take charge of your own health, you might have to get ready to conquer the doctor! The best way I know to take on a tough challenge is to get real clear about why you're doing it. So I want you to figure out exactly *why* you want to get healthy. What's in it for you?

Are you sick of feeling tired, run down, and overweight? Are you having trouble waking up and getting to work each day? Are you so tired and out of shape that you can't play with your children or make it through a full day in the park with your grandkids? Is your heart racing out of your chest and your stomach clenched with anxiety, and do you want a more natural alternative than the harsh medications with their scary side effects that your doctor has told you about? Have you already had your thyroid ablated and now you're miserable every day, and you'd give just about anything to feel normal again?

Maybe you haven't felt like yourself for a long time, and you *know* something is wrong. You keep telling your doctor but he or she just won't believe you. Maybe your family and friends can't quite understand why you seem to feel exhausted all the time. Perhaps they have trouble believing that you really are sick, especially since the doctor says you're fine. You might be desperate for some real answers so that they finally believe you.

Maybe you want a better sex life. Or you want to get pregnant. Or you want to be able to carry your child to term without another miscarriage. Maybe you just want to feel well enough to socialize with your friends, or go for a jog, or go out to a movie without falling asleep in your chair. Maybe you'd love to take that dream vacation—if only you weren't so fatigued or anxious or sick.

Maybe you know that having one autoimmune condition makes you three times more likely to get another. You know the second one might be even more debilitating—lupus, multiple sclerosis, scleroderma, rheumatoid arthritis—and you're anxious to prevent it.

Perhaps you're tired of being depressed or anxious all the time. Maybe you just can't stand the brain fog another day—you want to think clearly, the way you used to. Maybe you can't bear to see any more of your hair fall out, or you're just so tired of feeling cold all the time. Maybe you just want to live a long, happy life, full of energy, vitality, and joy.

Whatever goals you'd like to reach, I want you to use them to solidify your commitment. I want you to become *unwavering* in your pursuit of optimal health so that when you run into obstacles, you won't take no for an answer. Hey, it might be smooth sailing—I hope it is. But often, with conventional medicine and the insurance companies that are part of the system, you've got to push hard for what you want. *Get committed* so you will be ready to push as hard as you need to. A properly functioning thyroid and immune system are your birthright, and that's what I want for you. Now, what do you want for yourself?

Step 2: Set Your Objectives

Now that you're committed, what are your objectives? Here are a few recommendations for how to proceed. I encourage you to add any objectives that are personal to you and your situation.

Objective #1: Get the Right Tests

Here are the lab tests that you would ideally get to determine the state of your thyroid. Although, as I've explained, we might get different results under different conditions, there's no way to correct for that—you just need to be aware that if your symptoms and experience say one thing (such as that you don't feel well) and the tests say another (such as that you are fine), you should believe your experience and not the tests.

I measure each of the following items for my patients. Do what you can to see that your doctor does the same for you.

BLOOD WORK FOR THYROID HORMONES
- TSH
- Free T4
- Free T3
- Reverse T3
- Thyroid peroxidase antibody (TPO)
- Thyroglobulin antibody (TgAb)

For optimal reference ranges, see page 119.

BLOOD WORK FOR THE NUTRIENTS NEEDED FOR OPTIMAL THYROID FUNCTION
- Iron/ferritin (serum): normal 12–150 ng/mL; optimal 75–100 ng/mL
- Vitamin D (serum): normal 30–100 ng/mL; optimal 50–70 ng/mL
- Vitamin A (serum): normal 0.30–1.20 mg/L; optimal 0.8–1 mg/L

- Homocysteine (serum): normal 4–15 mmol/L; optimal 7–8 mmol/L
- Selenium (RBC): 120–300 mcg/L; optimal 200–250 mcg/L
- Zinc (RBC): normal 790–1,500 mcg/dL; optimal 1,000–1,200 mcg/dL
- Magnesium (RBC): normal 1.5–3.1 mmol/L; optimal 2.5–3.0 mmol/L

Which Part of Your Blood Are You Testing?

When your doctor takes a blood sample, that sample contains both red and white blood cells as well as other components of your blood. Usually, a lab will spin your blood in a centrifuge to separate out the red blood cells (RBCs) and work only with the *serum* that remains. However, the red blood cells are where you want many of the nutrients to actually penetrate. I'm less interested in the level of nutrients in your serum and far more interested in the level in your red blood cells themselves. Conventional labs don't offer RBC tests for all nutrients—sometimes they just test the serum—but they do offer RBC tests for zinc, selenium, and magnesium, so make sure you get those.

You might have noticed that I didn't put iodine on that list. You do need iodine, but unfortunately, there's no good way to test for iodine deficiency. One test has you putting iodine or mercurochrome (a form of iodine) on your skin. In theory, the more quickly it gets absorbed, the more urgently your body is taking it up, suggesting that your body needs more iodine. However, so many different factors can affect the way you respond that I don't consider that test especially reliable.

Another test—known as an iodine challenge test—has you consume a high dose of iodine and then collect your urine over the next six hours. Presumably, the more iodine in your urine, the less your body needed the iodine. This test also has its limits, because everyone has a different clearance rate for urinary excretion. Plus, if you don't have a thyroid because of surgery or ablation, you don't have any thyroid tissue to take up the iodine, which makes it even more difficult to interpret the results.

Yet another test measures the iodine in your blood—the so-called serum test. This is even less reliable than the urine test because iodine is cleared so efficiently from the blood that the test isn't sensitive enough to give us the measurement we need.

What's the solution? I'm sorry to say that there simply is no good way to know exactly how much iodine you need. I give you my recommendation in The Myers Way Thyroid Connection Plan. If that doesn't seem to be right for you, work with a functional medicine practitioner to help you adjust the dose. (For more about iodine levels, see "The Iodine Controversy" on pages 177–178.)

Monitoring Your Own Thyroid Function

Between labs, you can monitor your own thyroid function by taking your basal body temperature (BBT), which you do with a basal thermometer. Your thyroid is like the motor that keeps your body running, and your BBT is a measure of how hot your motor is running. By taking your BBT, you can get a sense of whether your thyroid is burning too hot (hyperthyroidism), too cold (hypothyroidism), or just right: between 97.2 and 98.6 degrees Fahrenheit.

What I like about the BBT is that it helps you monitor your progress day by day. After all, your temperature doesn't lie. Sometimes my patients complain that they don't notice any difference during the first few weeks of treatment. But when they check their temperature, they see that their numbers are moving closer to optimal. It's good to know something's working, even if you can't immediately feel it.

How to Take Your BBT

Buy a basal thermometer, available at your local drugstore or online. Put it by your bed where you can easily reach it upon awakening.

As soon as you get up, before sitting up or exerting yourself in any way, reach for the thermometer. Follow the directions that come with it. Record your temperature.

Repeat sometime between 2:00 p.m. and 4:00 p.m. Be sure to do this at the same time each day. This afternoon measurement is not strictly a *basal* body temperature, but since your temperature is often lower in the morning than in the afternoon, I like to know if my patients' temperature ever gets into the optimal range.

Women: Be aware that your BBT will rise before ovulation and remain more elevated in the second half of your cycle, which will affect your numbers. You'll need to take your BBT for a month or two so you can see what your own baseline is for these fluctuations.

A temperature frequently below 97.7 can indicate that you have hypothyroidism. Share this information with your doctor. If your temperature is frequently about 98.6, you might have hyperthyroidism or an underlying infection. For more about infections, see part 4.

Checking for Goiters and Nodules

A goiter is a swelling in your neck from an enlarged thyroid, and it can be caused by hypothyroidism, hyperthyroidism, or other conditions. Nodules can develop due to a number of factors. The condition should be treated by a doctor, so you might want to do a self-exam on your thyroid gland from time to time. Here's what you do:

- Face a mirror.
- Take a sip of water.
- Tilt your head back while still looking in the mirror.
- When you swallow the water, look for any lumps or areas that are not the same on both sides of the thyroid.

You might have swelling—a goiter—on one side or on both. A thyroid nodule is usually round and you can feel it moving with your thyroid gland when you swallow, or it might roll beneath your fingertips. If you find either a goiter or a nodule, please schedule an appointment with your doctor.

How do you get your doctor to run these tests? If she is open to it—and if your insurance company is too—you're best off just getting them all run at once.

I understand that running a complete thyroid panel may be new for your doctor, and she might be resistant to doing it. Hopefully, you can convince her to at least run tests for TSH and free T4. If that doesn't uncover thyroid dysfunction or if the prescription you get is not giving you the results you want, then I highly recommend that you go back and urge your doctor to run a complete thyroid panel.

If you do get a second run of tests, be sure it is a *complete* thyroid panel. You don't ever want her to run, say, *just* free T3 or *just* reverse T3—you need the whole picture to really understand what every number means. If you decide at some point that you want to get your own lab work done (see page 358), then you, too, need to get the *complete* thyroid panel, not just one or two tests.

The nutritional tests are important too, but I get that you're going to be working step by step with a doctor who won't necessarily run every test you ask for right away but who might run them after you develop more of a rapport. Ideally, you'd run all the nutritional tests at once, but they *can* be run piecemeal if necessary—selenium on one visit, ferritin on another. It's only the thyroid tests that need to be run as a group, because every element interacts with every other.

If your doctor is unwilling to run any of the tests I recommend, I have partnered with a lab company where you can order your own labs online at a significantly reduced cost and get them drawn at a local laboratory. You can then work with me or one of my wellness coaches to review your labs. Check the Resources section for the lab website.

Objective #2: Get the Right Treatment

Once you've got your labs, your objective becomes to get the right treatment. Let's break it down based on hypo- and hyperthyroidism.

IF YOU ARE HYPOTHYROID...

If you are hypothyroid and have not yet begun taking supplemental thyroid hormone, you may be able to prevent taking it by starting The Myers Way Thyroid Connection Plan. Regardless of your lab results, I would recommend that you follow this plan for twenty-eight days. If you notice significant improvement, you might not need supplemental hormone—as long as you continue to maintain this diet and lifestyle.

If you are already taking supplemental thyroid hormone, I would recommend that you follow the plan for twenty-eight days before going back to your doctor. If diet and lifestyle changes solve your problem, terrific! You might even need to ask your doctor to *lower* your dose of supplemental hormone if you start feeling hyper or jittery.

Either way, if twenty-eight days of The Myers Way aren't enough to make you feel completely terrific, continue following the plan—you want to keep giving your thyroid and immune system maximum support. But now you should also ask your doctor for the full panel of thyroid blood work. Based on the results, your doctor might prescribe a different type and/or dose of supplemental hormone. Here are your choices:

Option 1: Levothyroxine (brand names are Levothroid, Levoxyl, Synthroid, Tirosint, Unithroid)

Levothyroxine is a synthetically produced form of thyroid hormone that contains only T4. You need to allow at least ten days before the T4 is converted into T3, which is when you will feel the effects of the hormone. This slow action might be just what you need, especially if your body can manage the conversion. If you have difficulty converting T4 to T3, however, or if you need a bigger, quicker boost, levothyroxine might not be enough—you'll know, because even after a month or two, your labs will show low free T3. (And you still won't feel energized and terrific!) In that case, option 2 or 3 might work better for you.

You should also be aware that all forms of levothyroxine are not created equal. Studies have shown that the generic form does not perform as consistently as any of the brand-name products, so make sure your doctor prescribes a brand-name version. Usually, I'm all for saving my patients money, but supplemental thyroid hormone is a prescription where I insist that my patients make sure they get one of the brand names. You should too.

Another potential concern is that many forms of levothyroxine—the generic and most of the brands—are made with lactose, a milk protein used as a binder. As we have seen, dairy can trigger inflammation, and if your condition is autoimmune, it might also cue your immune system to start attacking your own thyroid.

Don't panic; for the vast majority of people, the amount of lactose in a daily dose of levothyroxine is small enough to do no harm. But if you have a strong dairy sensitivity, you might do better with Levothroid, Levoxyl, or Tirosint, all of which seem to be lactose-free. (I say *seem* because it's hard to get a complete answer about what exactly is in those pills!)

Likewise, Synthroid and Unithroid use corn as fillers. Again, probably no big deal, but if you have a super-sensitivity to corn, you might react.

Except for Tirosint, the brands and the generics of all of these have dyes; each is a different color, depending on the dose. Though I do not advocate eating packaged foods with coloring and synthetic dyes, most people are fine with the small amounts of dye in each daily pill. However, some might react with digestive issues, skin problems, or brain fog.

I'll say it again: The vast majority of people are fine with each of these pills. If you happen to be part of the tiny minority that can't tolerate a particular additive, work with your doctor to switch to another form.

By the way, Tirosint, which is new on the market, contains only thyroid hormone, gelatin, glycerin, and water. Because it has no dyes or potential trigger foods, the manufacturer claims that the actual hormone is more bioavailable (available for your system to absorb), especially for people with such gastrointestinal conditions as gastroesophageal reflux disease (GERD, aka acid reflux), lactose intolerance, celiac disease, gluten sensitivity, irritable bowel syndrome, or a prior gastric bypass procedure. Because those conditions can make it difficult to fully absorb *anything* you consume, a more bioavailable form might enable you to absorb more thyroid hormone—and that might mean you can take a lower dose.

Option 2: Desiccated Thyroid (brand names are Armour, Nature-Throid, Westhroid, WP Thyroid)

This is a natural form of thyroid hormone made from the desiccated thyroid of pigs. As a result, it contains both T3 and T4, but always in the same fixed amounts. For some people, the T3 gives a wonderful surge of energy and well-being within only a few days. If you've been dragging along for a while, feeling fatigued, unfocused, and depressed, you might appreciate the burst of vitality from this type of supplemental hormone.

A 2013 double-blind study published in the *Journal of Clinical Endocrinology and Metabolism* in which patients had no idea which form of

thyroid hormone they were getting found that about half of all partici-
pants felt better on desiccated thyroid hormone, 19 percent preferred
levothyroxine, and 23 percent had no preference.

Now, some people might assume that this study proves that natural
desiccated thyroid is better than synthetic hormone. However, that may
not be the full story. It may be that the reason the natural hormone works
so well is that it contains both T4 and T3 whereas the synthetic hormone
contains only T4. As you've read, many people have difficulty converting
T4 into T3, so getting any form of supplemental T3 may be the key to
feeling terrific. So don't be discouraged if your doctor is unwilling to prescribe desiccated thyroid hormone. There are other alternatives, such as
synthetic T3 (see option 4, below), which might work just great for you.

If you've lost all or part of your thyroid due to surgery or ablation, I
highly recommend desiccated hormone, because it also contains T1
and T2. Even though we don't know exactly what T1 and T2 do, it
seems like a good idea to replicate as far as possible the range of hormones your own thyroid would have produced.

Some people find that desiccated thyroid provides *too much* of a
boost, pushing their metabolism into overdrive and creating anxiety, a
racing heart, or insomnia. If that's you, try a lower dose. You might also
do well on option 3: levothyroxine plus some compounded T3, or even
a specially compounded formulation of both T4 and T3 (see below).

All forms of desiccated thyroid are dye-free. Nature-Throid and
WP Thyroid do contain lactose, which may trigger food sensitivities.
However, the amount of lactose in these supplemental hormones is so
small that it typically causes no problems, even to those with sensitivities. Likewise, Armour contains dextrose, made from corn, but again,
in such a tiny amount that it is unlikely to cause problems. My advice is
not to worry unless you develop symptoms, in which case you can see
about switching to another form.

Option 3: Specially Compounded Thyroid Hormone
This type of thyroid hormone must be made up in a compounding
pharmacy according to specific instructions from a physician.
Compounding pharmacies are great because they can make just about

any type of prescription medication in any dose and in many different combinations. I often prescribe sustained-release T3 in combination with Levoxyl, Synthroid, or Tirosint for those who feel jittery on desiccated thyroid hormone. And occasionally I need to create a uniquely tailored dose of thyroid hormone with the exact proportions of T3 and T4 that seem to be called for by a patient's tests.

Typically, specially compounded hormones are not covered under most insurance policies, but some companies will make allowances for it. If levothyroxine or desiccated thyroid works for you, that may be easier on many fronts. If other forms are not working for you, however, you might seek out a physician who is willing to create a custom-made prescription. Be sure that your doctor prescribes sustained-released T3 since T3 is so quick-acting. Your doctor might also be able to include T1 and T2, which, again, can help replace normal thyroid output for those of you who have lost all or part of your thyroid glands.

Option 4: Liothyronine (brand name is Cytomel)
I don't typically prescribe this synthetic form of T3 because it's so fast-acting. If you're sensitive to it, you might feel a sudden jolt, as if you just drank too much coffee. I generally prefer a specially compounded formulation of T3 that allows me to specify an exact dose tailored to my patient plus a sustained-release formula that distributes the hormone through the body more evenly throughout the day.

However, some conventional doctors will prescribe this while refusing to prescribe a desiccated or compounded form of the hormone. For some reason I have yet to understand, many conventional doctors mistrust desiccated hormone and don't see the need for specially compounded forms. I guess they are just stuck in their ways. (Many holistic and functional doctors can be equally stubborn about *only* prescribing desiccated or compounded hormone, which I also don't understand.) In addition, most insurance covers Cytomel but not the others. If that's the case, Cytomel might be a better option for you than using T4 alone, especially since not everybody has that jolting reaction. Possibly, after some months on The Myers Way Thyroid Connection Plan, your thyroid function will improve enough to enable you to go back to only Synthroid. Note that Cytomel contains starch, which might come from corn, potato, or wheat, but again, that's unlikely to cause you problems unless of course you have celiac disease.

Working with Your Doctor on Supplemental Hormone

I've always been puzzled as to why so many physicians are adamant about which type of thyroid hormone they prescribe. Conventional doctors tend to stick to levothyroxine, while many holistic, functional, and alternative practitioners swear by desiccated thyroid. Myself, I'm completely open because I have seen time and time again that everyone is different. Why become attached to a particular type of hormone and prescribe it to all your patients? Why not try to meet each patient's needs with whatever works best for him or her?

In that spirit, I would encourage you to work with your doctor to explore your options. If you can convince your physician to join you in your search, you might be able to find a type and dose of thyroid hormone supplement that fits you perfectly.

Here's how I personally proceed when prescribing supplemental thyroid hormone:

- If the person has never taken supplemental thyroid hormone and her labs are within normal but not optimal range, I generally start her on The Myers Way Thyroid Connection Plan. If her labs haven't improved sufficiently in two or three months, I consider prescribing supplemental hormone in addition to The Myers Way.
- If the person has already been taking supplemental hormone or if it turns out that The Myers Way isn't enough, I look at the labs. Depending on the free T4 and free T3 lab results, I prescribe either some form of T4 (typically Synthroid or Tirosint) or something that contains T3 (desiccated thyroid or a specially compounded form of T3).
- If I prescribe just T4 and it isn't having enough of an impact, then I move on to desiccated thyroid, usually WP Thyroid or Armour. If the person is autoimmune, however, I make sure to keep a close eye on his or her antibodies, on the off chance that the supplemental hormone is triggering attacks from the immune system. (See "Can Hashimoto's Patients Take Desiccated Thyroid?" below.)

- If the person is missing some or all of the thyroid gland, I usually start with desiccated thyroid gland like WP Thyroid or Armour, because that contains both T4 and T3 as well as some T1 and T2, allowing for a more complete replication of the hormones that his or her own thyroid gland would have produced.

- If none of my initial attempts work or if there is something about the person's blood work indicating specific needs, I then turn to a specially compounded form of thyroid hormone. For the vast majority of patients, however, the more readily available forms of thyroid hormone do just fine.

If You Have Lost All or Part of Your Thyroid Gland...

I highly recommend taking some form of desiccated thyroid hormone. That way, you can be sure of getting all four types of thyroid hormone, T1, T2, T3, and T4.

Can Hashimoto's Patients Take Desiccated Thyroid?

Recently, several articles have appeared online suggesting that Hashimoto's patients should avoid desiccated thyroid. The theory goes that since your body is already attacking your thyroid, putting more thyroid gland into your body will inspire even more attacks.

The theory might sound plausible, but out of the thousands of Hashimoto's patients I've treated, I have seen desiccated thyroid increase antibodies in only four.

Some people don't do well on desiccated thyroid for other reasons, and we switch them to either synthetic T4 or a compounded form of T4 and T3. And, of course, we always keep checking antibodies to monitor the activity of the immune system. But I find most people who take desiccated thyroid immediately feel better and continue to do so.

IF YOU ARE HYPERTHYROID...

Be aware: Left untreated for a long time, hyperthyroidism is far more dangerous than hypothyroidism, with risks including heart arrhythmia, heart attack, heart failure, hypertension, and osteoporosis. If you are hyperthyroid, you need to work with a doctor who will monitor your labs as well as the condition of your heart and bones.

That said, there is an alternative to the conventional medication used to treat hyperthyroidism. A set of herbs can, over the course of several months, help regulate an overactive thyroid, especially in conjunction with the diet and lifestyle provisions of The Myers Way Thyroid Connection Plan. So let's take a look at all the alternatives to treat hyperthyroidism, from least to most invasive.

Option 1: Herbs and Supplements
If you are diligently following The Myers Way Thyroid Connection Plan, you can treat your hyperthyroidism with the following herbs and supplements. Your improvement is likely to be gradual, you probably won't achieve full thyroid balance for several months, and you must always be under a doctor's care. But I have had a lot of success with the following protocol:

• *Bugleweed* (**Lycopus virginicus***).* A substance known as lithospermic acid, along with other organic acids, gives bugleweed its thyroid-calming power by decreasing your levels of TSH and T4 and interfering with the process by which your body synthesizes thyroid hormone. Bugleweed also helps keep antibodies from binding to your thyroid gland, which is one of the factors in Graves' disease. You can take bugleweed in the form of a tea, tincture, or pill. I recommend a liquid extract in the ratio of 1 to 2 (one part herb to two parts water). *Start with a daily dose of 2 mL. After 3 days, increase to 4 mL, and 3 days later, increase to 6 mL.*

• *Motherwort* (**Leonurus cardiaca***).* An herb from the mint family, motherwort doesn't work directly on your thyroid gland or hormones but does alleviate some hyperthyroid symptoms, including heart palpitations, anxiety, sleep problems, and, occasionally, loss of appetite. I think of motherwort as a natural beta-blocker (see below). However, it does have some side effects. Don't take it with any type of sedating medication, including antihistamines. Be aware that it might cause miscarriage, increase uterine bleeding, and potentially interact badly with many cardiac medications, so be sure to check with your doctor before taking it. I recommend a liquid extract in the ratio of 1 to

2 (one part herb to two parts water). *Start with a daily dose of 2 mL and after five days, increase to 4 mL.*

• *Lemon Balm (***Melissa officinalis***).* Another calming member of the mint family, lemon balm seems to block certain hormone receptors, preventing TSH from binding to your thyroid tissue and keeping antibodies from attaching to your thyroid. As a result, it reduces anxiety, improves sleep, eases pain, combats digestive symptoms, and restores appetite. It's a terrific herb to help you combat stress, boost your mood, and make you feel calm and alert. It's also good for migraine and hypertension. *Start with 300 mg and after seven days increase to 600 mg.*

Because these three herbs are often used together to treat hyperthyroidism, you can also find products that combine them. (See Resources.) Unless you are taking a combination herb, I recommend staggering the days you increase your doses, so you don't increase every herb on the same day.

• *Glucomannan.* I've recently started treating patients with this fiber from the konjac root, which has been supported for the treatment of hyperthyroid in research by Adil Azezli of Istanbul University. His 2007 study in the *Journal of American College of Nutrition* showed that by affecting the way your liver metabolizes thyroid hormone, glucomannan decreases levels of circulating thyroid hormone in your body. *Start with 1.5 gm twice daily and then work up to 3.0 gm twice daily.*

If you are hyperthyroid, I also want you to get the nutrients your body needs as long as your thyroid is working overtime. In fact, whether you go the natural or the conventional route, the following supplements will be part of your protocol on The Myers Way Thyroid Connection Plan. All of them will help combat oxidative stress; that is, the wear and tear on your system that results from an overactive thyroid:

• *L-Carnitine.* When your thyroid is in hyper mode, you lose L-carnitine through your urine, so you need to replace it. L-carnitine can help prevent or reverse muscle weakness and other symptoms, possibly by keeping thyroid hormone from getting into the cells of at least some of your body's tissues. It might also combat such symptoms as insomnia, nervousness, heart palpitations, and tremors. ***Start with 2,000 mg/day and work up to 4,000 mg/day as needed.***

• *CoQ10.* You have some CoQ10 in almost every one of your body's cells. A powerful antioxidant, CoQ10 helps convert food into energy while protecting the integrity of your cells. Studies have linked hyperthyroidism to low levels of CoQ10, so I recommend it to all my hyperthyroid patients. You also need CoQ10 if you're on beta-blockers or cholesterol-lowering medication, since those meds inhibit CoQ10. ***Take anywhere from 100 mg/day to 400 mg/day with a meal containing fat.***

• *Calcium Citrate and Vitamin D.* Being hyperthyroid puts you at risk of bone loss and osteoporosis, so please take both of these supplements together, as that will multiply their effectiveness: ***1,000 milligrams of calcium for adults nineteen to fifty and 1,200 milligrams for women over fifty-one and men over seventy-one, taken in conjunction with 1,000 to 5,000 IUs of vitamin D_3 for adults seventeen to seventy years old and 800 IUs for those over seventy-one.***

Option 2: Conventional Medications

If you are hyperthyroid, either propylthiouracil (PTU) or methimazole might be prescribed for you. Both stop your thyroid from producing thyroid hormone, but the side effects are challenging: dry skin, fatigue, and the loss of hair.

As you read in the introduction, I also suffered from extreme dry mouth and nostrils when I was taking PTU, as well as from the extremely rare side effect of liver damage. (See "Side Effects of Hyperthyroid Medications" on page 138.)

Your doctor might prescribe a milder conventional alternative — beta-blockers (such as propranolol) to slow down a rapidly beating heart and to stop the conversion of T4 to T3. However, I don't recommend that approach unless absolutely necessary, because it can lower your blood pressure, cause depression, and create a rebound effect when you get off it, making your symptoms suddenly become even worse. Other side effects of beta-blockers are fatigue, headache, digestive issues, sleep problems, loss of sex drive, and erectile dysfunction. If you can rely on the calming herbs I suggest above and/or follow my suggestions in chapter 9 to alleviate stress, that would likely be better for you.

If you choose to go the conventional route, either PTU or methimazole should be your first choice, whichever one your doctor recommends. Try it for six months—a year at the most. If it has not been successful in slowing your thyroid by then, your doctor is likely to offer you two alternatives: ablating (destroying) your thyroid with radioactive iodine (I-131) or surgically removing some or all of your thyroid.

Side Effects of Hyperthyroid Medications

Propylthiouracil (PTU)	*Methimazole*
SERIOUS BUT LESS COMMON SIDE EFFECTS	• nausea
• dry cough, trouble breathing	• headache
• fever, sore throat, headache, body aches, flulike symptoms	• muscle/joint/nerve pain
• severe blistering, peeling, and red skin rash	• hair loss
• pale skin, easy bruising or bleeding (nosebleeds, bleeding gums), unusual weakness	• swelling
	• drowsiness
MAY ALSO CAUSE SEVERE LIVER SYMPTOMS	• dizziness
• dark urine, clay-colored stools	• vomiting
• jaundice (yellowing of the skin or eyes)	• stomach upset
• nausea, stomach pain, loss of appetite	• mild rash/itching
• low fever, itching	
LESS SERIOUS, MORE COMMON SIDE EFFECTS:	
• upset stomach, vomiting	
• mild joint or muscle pain	
• dizziness, spinning sensation	
• decreased sense of taste	
• mild skin rash or itching	
• hair loss	

Option 3: Ablation with Radioactive Iodine (I-131)

Ablation, which I had, basically destroys your thyroid, leaving you with nothing to support and no function to restore. If a person with a functioning thyroid encounters some extra stress during the day, his thyroid can mobilize to provide extra hormone to get him through that stress. Even a partial thyroid can mobilize in that way. I, by contrast, get only the supplemental thyroid hormone that I take each morning. I can never muster any more, no matter what the stress or challenge.

Another downside to I-131 ablation is that the ovaries and testes contain high concentrations of iodine receptors, as does breast tissue. That means that some of this radioactive iodine will be taken up in these other places while the ablation process is going on. Although there are no known stated potential risks of cancer at the dose used for ablation, there are risks of lymphoma when higher doses of I-131 are used to treat thyroid cancer, so you might want to be aware of that. You might also suffer from infertility, and you will certainly need to delay pregnancy for six to twelve months after the procedure. You'll be instructed to sleep alone and to avoid intimate contact with others for three or four days after the procedure and not to prepare food that requires prolonged handling with bare hands. The reason for these precautions is that the procedure essentially makes you radioactive, and the I-131 in you could potentially harm another person's thyroid.

However, I-131 ablation is cheap and quick. Surgery requires more time and money. In general, most insurance companies don't want to pay for surgery, but they will cover the far less expensive ablation process.

Option 4: Surgery

There is always a risk with any surgery, and with thyroid surgery you run the specific risk of damage to your recurrent laryngeal nerves — the nerves that control your larynx, or throat. Surgery might also cause vocal-cord paralysis or damage your parathyroid glands, preventing your body from producing sufficient calcium.

Even so, I think that in most cases, surgery is preferable to ablation because it usually leaves you with *some* thyroid gland, which you can then support with The Myers Way Thyroid Connection Plan. You will almost certainly need to take supplemental thyroid hormone for life, but at least you can maintain some kind of thyroid function.

If you follow The Myers Way, there is an excellent chance that within months, you could have your hyperthyroidism—including Graves' disease—in remission.

Low-Dose Naltrexone: Another Alternative?

Naltrexone is an opioid antagonist; that is, it's what they give people who have overdosed on opioids, such as heroin or another type of painkiller. It basically shuts down your endorphin receptors, neutralizing the effects of the opioid and waking you up from the coma caused by the overdose.

That's *regular-dose* naltrexone, but in very *low* doses, naltrexone is sometimes used to treat autoimmune conditions as well as cancer. Both autoimmune and cancer patients seem to have very low levels of endorphins. Sometimes they are prescribed an extremely low dose of naltrexone to take at, say, 9:00 p.m. By 4:00 a.m., when they're asleep, the naltrexone blocks their endorphin receptors for a short time, after which the receptors are flooded with endorphins in response. This sudden endorphin rush produces a feeling of euphoria, and it seems to improve immune function as well.

I personally don't think this should be your first line of defense. My sense is that a lot of the physicians who are prescribing it rely on it before they turn to root causes that can be healed more naturally. I'm more apt to use it in autoimmune conditions such as multiple sclerosis, rheumatoid arthritis, or Parkinson's than for either Graves' or Hashimoto's. So let's get you on a healthy diet, heal your gut, and make sure you are getting the right dose of supplemental thyroid hormone. Then, if you're still having autoimmune-related issues, we might consider low-dose naltrexone. Even if we keep this option in our back pocket, it's good to know that it exists!

Objective #3: Keep Monitoring Your Condition

If you have any type of hyperthyroidism, you want your doctor to keep monitoring you because of the risk of heart disease or other problematic effects caused by your body being on overdrive. Basically, hyperthyroidism is like taking a stress test twenty-four hours a day, so until your thyroid is functioning normally, you need a doctor to keep an eye on your condition.

If you have non-autoimmune hypothyroidism, you want your doctor to check your thyroid levels—the complete panel!—and your nutritional levels at least every three months. That way, if you start having problems, you can respond. My first line of defense would always be to look at diet and lifestyle. If your numbers are off, have you gotten off track in food choices, exercise, sleep, stress, or toxic exposure? Do you perhaps have an infection that is stressing your system? (You'll learn more about all of these factors in part 4.) You also want your doctor to keep monitoring your antibodies to make sure you haven't developed an autoimmune condition.

If you have an autoimmune condition, whether Hashimoto's or Graves', you want to get your doctor to test your antibodies every three to six months. A conventional MD may not see the point, because in his or her view, nothing you do can make any difference to your autoimmune status. But I know otherwise, and by now, you do, too. Following The Myers Way Thyroid Connection Plan can make a significant difference in your level of antibodies. You want to keep checking in with your body to see that you are continuing to bring the antibodies down. And if they start to go up, you want to figure out why. Did you consume some gluten, dairy, or another inflammatory food? Did you skimp on sleep or overdo the exercise? Did you go through a period of stress without using any of the stress-relief tools that you'll learn about in chapter 9? If you know the level of your antibodies, you'll know what's working for you and what isn't—so do everything in your power to get your doctor to keep giving you that test.

If you have Hashimoto's and are taking desiccated thyroid, you also want to know if it drives your antibodies up. If so, you can immediately switch to another form of supplemental thyroid hormone.

If you have Graves' and are treating it with herbs, taking medication, or undergoing ablation, you want to make sure to keep checking your TSH and your free T4, free T3, reverse T3, and antibodies. All of these treatments will shut down your thyroid function, beginning by blocking the conversion of T4 to T3. Your labs might well indicate ongoing hyper-thyroidism in the classic pattern of low TSH and high free T4. (Remember, in Graves', your antibodies mimic the effects of TSH, so your own TSH can be very low even as your thyroid is being overstimulated.) Yet as the treatment takes effect, your free T3 will be low. You might feel both *hyper-* and *hypo-;* both wired and tired. Hopefully, you are also following The Myers Way, which might eventually enable you to stop taking meds and simply rely on diet and lifestyle.

Objective #4: Get the Nutrients and Supplements That Support Your Thyroid

This is the part of your health that is up to you, not your doctor. Isn't it great that *you* can fully take charge here, especially knowing the fundamental importance of nutrition? Following a healthy diet is crucial for achieving optimal health—and that is always in your control.

I'm clearly a big believer in supplements. But if you take away just one message about nutrition, let it be this: The key to good nutrition is *diet.* If you load up on supplements while relying on poor-quality foods, you are doing your body a huge disservice, and it will be nearly impossible for you to achieve optimal health.

Of course, if you have thyroid and/or immune dysfunction, you are likely deficient in some key nutrients, so we want to load you up with the right supplements. Your body needs iodine and B vitamins to make thyroid hormone, as well as tyrosine (an amino acid found in proteins), and your body can't convert T4 into T3 without selenium, and zinc. You also need vitamin A to help bring the thyroid hormone into your cells. You need vitamin D_3 and vitamin A to support your immune system and omega 3 fish oils for healthy cell membranes. Supplementing with these basic nutrients can make a huge difference.

Now, is there any part of this objective that requires a doctor's help? Not really. Some people do get prescriptions for a super-high dose of vitamin D_3—50,000 IU—but I am not a big fan of putting that much

D_3 into your system all at once, not to mention that all the prescription forms have dyes and fillers that aren't so good for you. You can buy over-the-counter vitamin D_3 in 1,000 or even 5,000 IU—I would much rather you do that.

Many conventional doctors dismiss the notion that diet, supplements, and gut healing can make a difference. Don't believe them! I have thousands of patients and followers who will testify otherwise, and I have the evidence of my own healing as well. If you are even a little bit skeptical, I'll make a deal with you. Give me twenty-eight days on The Myers Way Thyroid Connection Plan, so you can see for yourself. I'd bet anything that you'll be delighted with the results—*and* you'll enjoy the power of taking charge of a huge aspect of your health.

Step 3: Develop a Strategy

In most cases, the two biggest obstacles are your conventional MD's attitude, and your insurance company.

Dealing with Your Doctor

It's sad but true: Many doctors still have egos that lead them to insist that they know best. Even if you bring in a medical article or a reasonable explanation for your request, this type of doctor doesn't want to be told what to do. (However, I have created a "Letter to Your Doctor" that you can use as a starting point. See Appendix A.)

Even doctors who are more open-minded, however, face significant pressures from our current health-care system. Most get flagged if they order too many lab tests, and then they are at significant risk of the insurance companies dropping them from their plans.

My advice here is for you to analyze your obstacles as accurately as you can. What do you think the roadblocks are with your MD, and how serious are they? Is your doctor someone who will eventually go along with what you want, even if you don't like his attitude or the way he makes you feel? Maybe you can compromise on the bedside manner if you're at least getting the right tests and treatment. Is your doctor under pressure from the insurance companies, and if so, is there a work-around that he or someone in his office might suggest?

It's easy to get into a mind-set of defeat and frustration, especially when you feel lousy. Try your best to figure out exactly what the problem is, though, because that way you can respond effectively, regardless of how you feel about it.

Dealing with Your Insurance Company

There's actually quite a bit of good news here. The thyroid labs I recommend are not considered alternative or experimental. Even if your doctor doesn't typically order them, they are covered by most insurance companies.

If your doctor absolutely will not order the complete panel of thyroid labs that I recommend, you do have options. In many states, you don't need a doctor's order for blood work and can order the tests yourself through a conventional lab. But your insurance won't cover this, and it can be quite expensive. I have partnered with a lab company where you can order your own labs online at a significantly reduced cost and get them drawn at a local laboratory. You can then work with me or one of my wellness coaches to review your labs. (See Resources.)

On the good-news front, most forms of supplemental thyroid hormone, including both levothyroxine and desiccated thyroid hormone, are covered by virtually all insurance companies. It's possible that some of the less well-known brands of these hormones are not covered, but in most cases you will be able to get the treatment that you need.

The herbs I suggest for treating hyperthyroidism are not covered by insurance companies—but they are relatively inexpensive and you will not be taking them forever. You can get them from my website or through a number of herbal suppliers or health-food stores. So no worries there.

Most functional medicine doctors don't take insurance because we want to give our patients longer appointments and more individualized care than is typically covered by most policies. If you want to be treated by a functional medicine physician, you might choose an insurance policy with a high deductible and use the money you save in premiums to help pay for your functional MD.

Take Charge of Your Health

- Support your health with The Myers Way Thyroid Connection Plan, which will take you very far regardless of what your doctor does.
- Keep good, accurate, complete records of *everything*—every doctor's visit, every phone call to the insurance company.
- Stay positive by renewing your commitment. Remember *why* you are doing this.
- If your doctor will not order the labs I recommend, you can order them yourself. (See Resources for the online lab company I recommend.)
- Be resourceful and creative. If one thing doesn't work, try something else.
- Join my free online The Myers Way Community Forum (www.amymyersmd.com/community). Many people are going through the same types of struggles, and you can get great advice and support from them.
- Work with me, one of my partners, or one of my wellness coaches to get personalized feedback.
- Figure out which compromises you can make, and make them. When something is too important for compromise, stick to your guns.
- Never give up. Your health is too important.

EYES ON THE PRIZE

As you prepare to advocate for the health care you deserve, I really want to support you and urge you never to give up hope. There are doctors out there who will support you, work with you, order the labs, and prescribe the supplemental thyroid hormone you need. If you don't find what you're looking for right away, just keep searching. In the Resources section and on my website, I've shared some suggestions for how you can work with me, one of my partners, my wellness coaches, or a doctor in your area, and there may be undiscovered resources in your own community as well. Whatever you encounter, keep going until you find the treatment that you need—because optimal health is your birthright, and you deserve to feel terrific.

Part Four

THE MYERS WAY

CHAPTER 7

The Power of Food

Food has extraordinary power—both to heal and to harm. Imagine: the foods you put into your body can completely transform your physical health, your energy levels, and even your state of mind. Yep, you heard me, and I'm not getting all New Agey, I'm speaking as a scientist: What you eat affects how your brain processes thought and emotion, as well as how your thyroid and your gut affect your brain. On The Myers Way Thyroid Connection Plan, you'll stop eating foods that harm you while loading up on foods that heal.

Feeling skeptical? Think of how cranky and impatient you get when you miss a meal, how sad and hopeless you start to feel, how foggy your head gets. And then when you eat something, you immediately perk up, calm down, refocus, reenergize. Now multiply that good feeling by a factor of ten as you feed your body the nutrients it craves for vitality, a great mood, and optimal health.

If you need more convincing, I could tell you all about the science. I could remind you that without iodine plus proper protein intake, your thyroid gland doesn't have the building blocks it needs to make thyroid hormone—it's as if you're asking a master builder to make you a house from a sack of pebbles and some mud. Yeah, you'll probably get *some* kind of makeshift dwelling—but it won't be nearly as good as it would have been if you'd provided steel and concrete. You can't give your thyroid bad materials to work with and expect it to perform up to par— that doesn't make any kind of sense.

Or I could tell you that without enough iron, selenium, and zinc, your thyroid signaling system doesn't have the minerals it needs to convert T4 into T3. Not to mention that without zinc, your hypothalamus can't gauge how much thyroid hormone your body is making, so it can't properly regulate that whole process. And without iron, your body can't convert *iodide* (the food version of iodine) into *iodine* (the biochemical that your thyroid actually uses). I could also tell you that without healthy omega 3 fats, your cell walls lose their integrity, and without vitamin A, free T3 is going to have a world of trouble making its way into your cells. And I could talk for quite a while about why and how your immune system needs B vitamins and vitamin D to keep a healthy balance.

Even then, some of you might be skeptical about the power of food, and given the way conventional doctors talk about nutrition, I can hardly blame you. Conventional doctors often treat food as, at best, an afterthought. When asking their former doctors about nutritional approaches, many of my patients have been told, "Well, if you want to try it, it probably won't hurt." What a dismissal of one of our most powerful healing tools! This is pretty ironic, too, when you consider that Hippocrates, the actual *founder* of Western medicine, is the one who said, "Let food be your medicine and medicine be your food." They should have us physicians repeat *that* when we take the Hippocratic oath!

So how much faith do I place in good nutrition? Well, as Hippocrates knew, it's often the only medicine we need; many of my patients can restore healthy thyroid function simply through diet and lifestyle changes alone. You heard me. *With diet and lifestyle changes alone,* you can fix the problem that everyone else is taking pills for. Did you know that Synthroid is now our country's most prescribed drug, with 21.5 million prescriptions written each year, accounting for *billions* of dollars? How many of those folks could get the same or even better results from just eating better?

Now if your thyroid has already been damaged, diet alone might not be enough; you might need to give it some extra support in the form of supplemental thyroid hormone. And if you have hyperthyroidism, you will need thyroid-calming herbs until you bring your thyroid gland back into balance, plus some additional supplements to replace what your overactive metabolism burns up.

Either way, food is still your best friend—or your worst enemy. *Inflammation*—caused largely by problem foods—can tear down the walls of your house before you've even got them up. At the end of the day, eating right makes optimal health possible.

Now, the minute I start talking about food choices, some of you are going to think *diet*. And we know how much fun dieting is! For many of us, let's face it, *diet* is our least favorite word. I'll suggest you stop eating harmful foods, and you'll think, *Uh-oh, calorie counting!* or *Restrictions!* or *All those foods I'd like to have but am not allowed to!* I get it, and I'd never want you to feel deprived, if only because *deprivation* equals *stress,* and *stress* equals high cortisol levels, unbalanced stress hormones, and a whole slew of other things that are bad for you.

So let's not talk about restrictions. Let's talk about delicious food that gives our bodies what they need to function. Let's stop punishing our bodies with inflammatory foods; let's stop starving ourselves of essential nutrients needed for peak thyroid and immune function. Let's talk about how good you're going to feel when your thyroid, immune system, and entire body finally have everything they need. Let's talk about foods that power the clarity of your thoughts and the buoyancy of your mood—the fuel that enables you to sail through your day (on a good day) or slog through the challenges and overcome the obstacles (on a not-so-good day). *That's* what food can do, folks. I'm here to tell you it's true, because I've seen it in myself and in thousands of patients more times than I can count.

So welcome to the wonderful world of thyroid- and immune-friendly foods. To start, I'd like you to meet two patients: Zoe, who was hypothyroid, and Conner, who was hyperthyroid. Although these patients seemed to have opposite problems—one an underactive thyroid and one an overactive one—for both of them, food was the abracadabra that almost magically ushered them into a whole new world of health.

WHAT SHOULD A HYPOTHYROID PERSON EAT?

Zoe was an exuberant, lively woman in her early fifties who was struggling with a very challenging menopause. Contrary to her usual energetic, optimistic personality, she felt exhausted, dragged out, cranky, and short-tempered almost all the time, snapping at her husband and children, impatient with the sales team she managed, and beginning to suffer from depression, anxiety, hot flashes, night sweats, and brain fog.

Zoe had also had a bout with the flu that morphed into pneumonia. Her doctor had put her on two weeks of antibiotics, but Zoe just couldn't shake the bug, so the two weeks turned into four, and then six. Zoe found herself having more hot flashes and was now gaining weight, feeling even foggier and more miserable.

Zoe's conventional doctor ordered blood work and told Zoe that her female hormones were low and her TSH was high-normal—but still normal. Conventional medicine considers 0.5 to 4.7 μIU/mL the normal range for TSH, and Zoe's number was at the very top of that range: 4.2 μIU/mL. Zoe's doctor didn't feel that her thyroid labs warranted supplemental thyroid hormone, but he did think that hormone replacement therapy (HRT) would help her with her low female-hormone levels and her menopausal symptoms.

Zoe had read that there was some controversy over whether HRT increased the risk of heart disease and stroke, both of which ran in her family. She asked if, instead, she could rely on diet or supplements, but the doctor pooh-poohed the very notion. He did suggest, though, that exercise might help with the weight gain and maybe lift her spirits.

"It would be great to have more energy," Zoe told him with barely concealed sarcasm, "but how can I exercise if I'm too tired to move?"

Frustrated with the conventional options, Zoe Googled *menopause— natural treatments* and ended up on my website. As soon as I heard her symptoms, I thought she likely had thyroid dysfunction, and, as usual, I ran the complete panel of blood work to find out. I also thought that those six weeks on antibiotics had probably led to yeast overgrowth, because antibiotics can seriously disrupt the microbiome—the community of bacteria that we depend on for a healthy gut as well as many other bodily functions. People who take antibiotics without also taking *probiotics*—pills, powders, or capsules that contain healthy gut bacteria— often suffer from leaky gut, yeast overgrowth, and gut symptoms (nausea, gas, bloating, constipation, diarrhea) as well as weight gain, anxiety, depression, and poor immune function. My guess—based on years of observing this pattern—was that Zoe's gut and her thyroid were both functioning poorly and that each was making the other worse. They were both potentially undermining her immune system too, putting her at risk for autoimmune disorders.

Unhealthy Synergy: Each Problem Makes the Others Worse

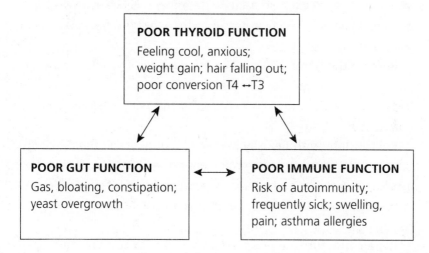

POOR THYROID FUNCTION
Feeling cool, anxious; weight gain; hair falling out; poor conversion T4 ↔T3

POOR GUT FUNCTION
Gas, bloating, constipation; yeast overgrowth

POOR IMMUNE FUNCTION
Risk of autoimmunity; frequently sick; swelling, pain; asthma allergies

I wanted to reverse this unhealthy synergy as quickly as possible. So while we were waiting for the labs to come back, I suggested that Zoe begin The Myers Way Thyroid Connection Plan.

Your Myers Way Thyroid Connection Food Plan at a Glance

Here are the basics of what you'll be doing with food and supplements on The Myers Way Thyroid Connection Plan.

Through diet and supplements, **consume the nutrients your body needs for optimal thyroid function:** iodine, protein (to provide you with tyrosine, another essential amino acid), selenium, zinc, iron, vitamin D, vitamin A, omega-3 fatty acids, and a variety of B vitamins.

Avoid the foods that disrupt thyroid function: inflammatory foods and raw *goitrogens.*

Use the 4R program to heal your gut: *remove, restore, reinoculate,* and *repair.*

Remove the bad: Get rid of anything that negatively affects your gastrointestinal environment, especially inflammatory and toxic foods, which you avoid on your Thyroid Connection Plan. You'll also take the quizzes on pages 258–263 to see whether you have such common gut infections as small intestine bacterial overgrowth (SIBO) and yeast overgrowth. If you do, you'll take healing herbs and supplements as part of your plan.

Restore the good: You can't digest efficiently if you don't have the biochemicals that you need: digestive enzymes, hydrochloric acid, and bile acids. If necessary, you'll take supplements with these components on your plan.

Reinoculate with healthy bacteria: Your gut can't function without a healthy microbiome (the community of helpful bacteria that is an essential aspect of digestion and many other functions). A probiotic— pill, powder, or capsule loaded with friendly bacteria—is part of your plan as well.

Repair the gut: You need certain nutrients to help your gut repair itself, including *L-glutamine,* an amino acid that will help mend your gut lining. That's part of your plan too, along with Gut-Healing Bone Broth, omega-3s, vitamin A, vitamin D, zinc, and herbs such as slippery elm and aloe vera.

I told Zoe that she had to avoid inflammatory foods and raw *goitrogens,* foods that suppress thyroid function. To make sure Zoe got all the nutrients she needed, I recommended a complete multivitamin that included zinc, iron, iodine, vitamin A, vitamin D, selenium, and B vitamins.

I also had Zoe take gut-healing supplements to repair leaky gut, and I started her on probiotics to replenish healthy gut bacteria. We added in some extra vitamin D for immune support. Another gut problem emerged when Zoe took the questionnaire on pages 258–259 and we discovered she had intestinal yeast overgrowth, or Candida—probably because of all the antibiotics she had taken, which had disrupted her intestinal bacteria. So we started her on my protocol for yeast control.

Last but not least, I shared with Zoe The Myers Way guidelines for reducing the toxic burden and relieving stress. These are also crucial for thyroid and immune function, as you'll learn in the next two chapters.

Zoe was relieved that she could take her health into her own hands without having to rely on treatments with potentially dangerous side effects. And sure enough, within a couple of weeks on The Myers Way Thyroid Connection Plan, she began feeling much more like her old self. She lost eight pounds, felt her mental clarity beginning to return, and found that she had more energy. She also realized that she had been suffering from mild indigestion and nausea that had grown so constant, she barely noticed it. But after two weeks of taking supplements for yeast control and gut healing, her stomach felt much better. Her hair, too, was beginning to seem thicker and healthier.

When I got Zoe's labs back, I could see that she had indeed been struggling with suboptimal thyroid. Her TSH was 3.5 µIU/mL, her free T4 was 0.95 ng/dL, her free T3 was 2.8 pg/mL, and her reverse T3 was 20.0 pg/mL. Fortunately, her thyroid antibodies were negative, indicating that she did not have an autoimmune condition.

Although her numbers showed suboptimal thyroid function, Zoe had had such a rapid response to The Myers Way that I believed she could achieve optimal health from diet and lifestyle changes alone. Her numbers and her quick improvement led me to believe that she hadn't yet suffered any permanent damage. With the right support, her thyroid gland could probably produce all the hormone she needed.

Zoe had followed The Myers Way Thyroid Connection Plan diligently for twenty-eight days (just as you will do!). Then she gradually began to add some foods back: non-gluten grains, legumes, nightshades, eggs, even an occasional cup of coffee. If she reacted badly to those foods, she'd have to avoid them for a few more months. She might be able to tolerate some down the line; some she might have to avoid for life.

Two foods would stay permanently out of Zoe's diet: gluten and dairy, which are so inflammatory that I think we all should just avoid them. Gluten is also a significant contributor to leaky gut. And both gluten and dairy promote thyroid dysfunction through the molecular mimicry we spoke about in chapter 4 (see pages 94–96).

Zoe was thrilled to know that food could help to reverse her condition. Over the next few months, she continued to improve, and within three months, she was back to her former energetic self: cheerful, patient, and enjoying life. Giving her thyroid the nutrients it needed, avoiding the foods that inflamed it, and healing her gut had all made a huge difference.

Goitrogens: The Thyroid Suppressors

Goitrogens are foods that suppress thyroid function. Some goitrogens—notably broccoli and kale—have no goitrogenic effects when cooked but do suppress thyroid function when eaten raw. Some goitrogenic foods also lose their effects when fermented. On pages 94–96, you'll find a list of common goitrogens.

Now, you might see other lists on various websites, and you might hear a lot of alarmist talk about how these goitrogens are behind the thyroid epidemic. Sorry—I just don't buy it. I certainly haven't seen any evidence of this in my clinical practice. Even if you are hypothyroid, I believe that the benefit of eating these foods *far* outweighs the risk; in fact, we include some in our twenty-eight-day plan to show you how they can be incorporated into your diet.

You'll be monitoring your thyroid function with your doctor, and by taking your BBT, and you'll be paying close attention to your symptoms. If you feel that these foods are affecting you, you can figure out what your own body can tolerate. However, in the vast majority of cases, I would *so* much rather you load up on healthy foods than cut out vegetables and fruits that can do great things for your body. Following your twenty-eight-day Myers Way Thyroid Connection Plan will give you a great start in using these foods in a healthy and sensible way.

WHAT SHOULD A HYPERTHYROID PERSON EAT?

Connor was a skinny, intense guy in his thirties who was just starting his own veterinary practice. A true animal lover, Connor had dreamed of being a vet for as long as he could remember. Now, it seemed, his dream was finally coming true.

Then Connor ran into one obstacle after another. His new office space unexpectedly became uninhabitable when a water main broke in another part of the building. The woman he'd planned to go into practice with fell in love with a man who lived on the West Coast and abruptly told Connor that she was moving out there to be with him. Connor's best friend, a man he'd known since childhood, suddenly developed a rare form of cancer, and Connor arranged with several other friends to help see him through the treatment, signing up to visit and run errands one day a week. From being on the verge of achieving his dream, Connor felt as though he'd stumbled into a nightmare.

To make matters worse, he started having unexplained symptoms — at first just disturbing and then downright scary. His hands shook. His muscles trembled. Always thin, he quickly lost fifteen additional pounds, even though he was constantly hungry and eating more than he ever had. He couldn't fall asleep without waking a few hours later seized by panic attacks that made his heart pound and his mind race.

Connor's conventional doctor quickly diagnosed him with Graves' disease, an autoimmune condition that produces an overactive thyroid. As you recall, the conventional protocol for Graves' is usually to start the patient on medication, which can have severe side effects. If the meds aren't effective, the patient is given a choice between I-131 ablation and surgery, each of which has its own side effects and risks.

None of the conventional options sounded good to Connor. While looking online for information about Graves', he came across my book, *The Autoimmune Solution*. When Connor learned that I, too, had had Graves' and that I had treated it successfully in other patients, he decided to schedule an appointment with me. This was no small commitment, because my practice is in Austin but Connor lived in New York — quite a ways away! But he was desperate to avoid the harsh conventional treatments and wanted to try natural means to restore his health.

When I ran Connor's labs, I confirmed his doctor's diagnosis. His TSH was < 0.1 μIU/mL, his free T4 was 2.5 ng/dL, his free T3 was 5.0 pg/mL, and his TPO antibodies were > 5,000 IU/mL. In other words, his antibodies were through the roof, so high that our lab couldn't measure them. Connor did indeed have an autoimmune condition, and it was causing his thyroid to go haywire. I speculated that the avalanche of stress—his office space, his partner, his friend—had overburdened his adrenal glands, which in turn had disrupted his immune function. I also knew that ever since Hurricane Sandy, many New York buildings had toxic-mold issues, which can further disrupt immune function.

As with Zoe, I didn't want to wait for Connor's labs before starting to reverse the negative synergy that was undermining his health. So we hit the ground running with The Myers Way Thyroid Connection Plan, addressing food, toxins, and stress.

Now, here's the part that might seem counterintuitive: I gave Connor a very similar diet and gut-healing plan as the one I gave Zoe, even though she was hypothyroid and didn't have an autoimmune condition. True, Zoe needed to avoid goitrogens, and she needed to follow a special protocol for her yeast condition. And Connor was hyperthyroid, so he needed to take some extra supplements to replace all the nutrients that his body was burning through while on overdrive. Basically, though, their dietary needs were almost identical.

Why? Because food is fundamental, and at some level, most of us need the same thing. Food isn't medicine in the sense that you take aspirin for a headache. Instead, it gives your body the basic nutrients it needs to function. Yes, our bodies are all different. But every thyroid gland needs tyrosine and iodine to make thyroid hormone. Every body needs zinc and selenium to convert T4 to T3, and omega-3s to maintain a healthy cell wall. Every immune system needs vitamin D, vitamin A, B vitamins, and so on.

Likewise, although each of us might respond differently to different foods, some foods just tend to be inflammatory—and inflammation is bad for every single one of us. We'll look at inflammation later in this chapter, and in part 5, you'll learn how to test the foods I have asked you to avoid so you know exactly which foods your own body can tolerate. But both the scientific literature and my clinical experience have convinced me that gluten and dairy are highly inflammatory for just about everyone, especially if you have thyroid dysfunction. It all goes back to molecular mimicry, which we talked about in chapter 4; when your immune system mounts a panicky counterattack against gluten and perhaps also dairy, it tends to attack your thyroid as well. Pull the gluten and dairy from your diet, and your immune system calms down.

So even though Connor's thyroid was overactive and Zoe's was underactive, even though Connor was autoimmune and Zoe wasn't, both of them needed to add in the same thyroid-friendly foods and basic nutrients. They also needed to avoid the same inflammatory foods as well as goitrogens. The Myers Way got them back on track—and it will help you do the same.

Feed Your Thyroid: The Basics

You'll get all of these nutrients on your first twenty-eight days of The Myers Way Thyroid Connection Plan. You can find more menus to help you feed your thyroid on my website, www.amymyersmd.com.

Nutrient	Why You Need It	Where You Can Find It
Iodine	One building block used to make thyroid hormone	seaweed saltwater fish high-quality multivitamin or supplement
Tyrosine	Another building block used to make thyroid hormone	red meat and chicken fish and seafood seaweed supplement
Selenium	Needed to convert T4 into T3 Helps prevent and reverse autoimmune thyroid	red meats, including liver chicken and turkey fish and shellfish

Nutrient	Why You Need It	Where You Can Find It
Selenium (cont.)		Brazil nuts (avoid these for your first twenty-eight days on The Myers Way, then add in gradually if you are not autoimmune and can tolerate them) spinach high-quality multivitamin or supplement
Zinc	Needed to convert T4 to T3 Triggers your hypothalamus's thyroid hormone receptors, so your hypothalamus can accurately gauge your levels of thyroid hormone and regulate its production	red meat and liver pork chicken spinach seafood high-quality multivitamin or supplement (because zinc can deplete your body's copper levels, pair your zinc supplement with a copper supplement)
Iron	Needed to convert iodide to iodine Needed to convert T4 to T3	beef and beef liver pork poultry seafood dark leafy vegetables high-quality multivitamin or supplement
Omega-3 fats	Needed to maintain cell integrity so free T3 can effectively enter your cells	fatty fish nuts and seeds (avoid these for your first twenty-eight days on The Myers Way, then add in gradually if you are not autoimmune and can tolerate them) fish-oil or flax-oil supplements
Vitamin D3	Needed for healthy immune function Needed to bring T3 in the cells	sunlight fatty fish pork portobello mushrooms fish oil high-quality multivitamin or supplement

Nutrient	Why You Need It	Where You Can Find It
B vitamins	Needed for healthy immune function	leafy green vegetables (*make sure to cook the goitrogens*) broccoli (*cooked only, please!*) beets red meat and liver supplement
Vitamin A	Needed for healthy immune function Needed to bring T3 into your cells	orange fruits and vegetables, including carrots, sweet potatoes, winter squash, mangoes, apricots liver kale (*cooked, not raw*) high-quality multivitamin or supplement

The Selenium Story

As you saw in part 2, selenium is a must; without it, your body can't convert T4 to T3. Moreover, in the right amounts, selenium can help prevent autoimmune thyroid conditions. And if you already have an autoimmune condition, selenium can help reverse it.

Why is selenium so important? It starts with *iodide*—the form of iodine that you ingest, such as the type of iodine that is frequently added to table salt to make iodized salt. When your body converts iodide to iodine, the process produces hydrogen peroxide, an oxidant, which damages thyroid cells and can trigger an autoimmune response. You need selenium to neutralize the hydrogen peroxide.

As a super added bonus, research has shown that patients who have autoimmune thyroid disease can reduce their level of thyroid peroxidase antibodies (TPO) by increasing their intake of selenium to at least 200 mcg a day. That's why on The Myers Way, I've loaded you up with selenium-rich foods and I also have you taking a multivitamin with 200 mcg of selenium.

Now, you may have heard that Brazil nuts are full of selenium and that eating too many is bad for you because you get *too much* selenium. That's true—it's hard to know exactly how much selenium is in any individual nut, so with that particular food, it is possible to go overboard. However, we don't include Brazil nuts on The Myers Way Thyroid Connection Plan, so don't worry. Please *do* enjoy the selenium-rich foods that we have included and make sure to take a multivitamin that includes this vital mineral (see page 251).

WHY DO WE NEED SUPPLEMENTS?

Oh, how I wish we didn't! In a less polluted world, with organic farms and humanely raised animals, we probably wouldn't. If our soil wasn't so depleted by farming that strips minerals and other nutrients, if our bodies weren't so burdened by toxins and industrial chemicals, if the food we ate was as rich in vitamins and minerals as nature intended, then, in fact, we would *not* need supplements.

But in this world, alas, we do. Most of the food you eat has suffered from the toxins of the environment and the overall degradation of the soil due to past farming practices, industrial runoff, toxic rain, and a host of other challenges. Even organic food is affected by these factors. Moreover, your body, burdened by all these challenges (as we'll see in chapter 8), needs extra help in coping with these physical stressors, as well as with all the emotional stressors we face. Plus we've got a lot of other factors creating nutrient depletion, including the amount of time your food spends in transit, on the grocery shelf, and in your refrigerator. Sadly, these factors decrease the nutrient value of your food even if you eat 100 percent organic.

Many people have asked me why we can't just follow the USDA's RDAs, the recommended dietary allowances. Great question, and here's the answer: The RDA is the *absolute minimum* of something that you need to take in order to avoid becoming ill, not the *optimal* amount you need to attain optimal wellness. By now, that distinction should sound very familiar!

In addition, some of you might have one or more genetic mutations that affect the way your body uses various vitamins and minerals (you'll read more about this in chapter 8). If so, you will need to supplement even more than someone who doesn't have them. These mutations are commonly associated with autoimmune conditions, although people without autoimmunity have them too. That's another reason supplements can be crucial in preventing and/or treating various conditions. Supplements are by no means a one-size-fits-all affair!

There's a whole lot of talk on the Internet about how supplements are a waste of time and money. Don't believe it. Sure, you can go overboard and take bigger doses or more supplements than you need. Sure, there are plenty of supplements out there made by companies that don't maintain the highest standards. But my recommendations in your plan and in the Resources section will help you sort through the confusion and make the right choices. Believe me, you don't want to send your body out into the world without the right support—and supplements are a critical part of that support.

HEAL YOUR GUT

As you saw, both Zoe and Connor needed to heal their leaky gut—and so does just about every patient I see. If you're having trouble with either your thyroid or your immune system, you are almost certainly having trouble with your gut. How can I be sure? Because, as Hippocrates probably suspected, the gut is basic to our survival. If you have any kind of systemic problem—any illness or disorder that lasts more than a day or two or that recurs frequently—it either started in the gut or migrated to the gut.

Gut health is absolutely key to your overall health, so we want to heal your gut as quickly as possible. If we don't, it's going to be hard to get anything else right. When you're not in peak health, your gut is like the sailboat you depend on to get you to safety. You want to focus on rowing, setting up a sail, finding the wind, steering a homeward course. But if there's a huge leaking hole in the boat and you have to keep stopping to bail it out, and it keeps dragging water and threatening to bring you down at the first sign of a little rain—well, nothing else you do is going to matter much. Till you have a healthy, impermeable gut, you can't do much to heal your thyroid, your immune system, or just about anything else. That's why gut healing is an integral part of your twenty-eight-day plan.

GET RID OF GLUTEN, GRAINS, AND LEGUMES

Once your gut is in good shape, we want to *keep* it in good shape. One key way to protect your gut is to keep gluten, grains, and legumes out of your diet. Removing gluten will prevent further intestinal damage, inflammation, and molecular mimicry with your thyroid. Grains and legumes likewise contain lectins and other proteins that irritate the gut lining, creating inflammation and leading to leaky gut. They also pose other health risks, so they won't be in your diet when you begin your twenty-eight-day plan. If you've got an autoimmune disorder, you'll keep gluten, grains, and legumes permanently out of your diet. If you don't, you might be able to slowly reintroduce grains and legumes after twenty-eight days. You'll learn more about that on pages 314–317.

I know gluten, grains, and legumes seem like standard healthy foods, but believe me, few things are worse for your gut and your immune system. Let's take a closer look.

What's wrong with gluten?

Gluten is a group of proteins found in grains such as wheat, semolina, spelt, rye, kamut, and barley. It's also used as an additive in practically every processed food from salad dressing to ketchup.

Gluten is what makes bread so sticky and fluffy. It's also a factor in more than fifty-five diseases, largely because of the disastrous effect it has on your gut and your immune system, as we saw in chapter 4. To remind you, gluten stresses your digestive tract, prompts your immune system to attack your own tissues, and contributes to gut imbalances like yeast overgrowth and SIBO. Most damaging of all is the way gluten promotes leaky gut by triggering the production of *zonulin,* the protein that can signal the tight junctions between the cells in your intestines to open and remain open.

Gluten is especially harmful to people with autoimmune conditions, but honestly, it's pretty terrible for just about everybody. I'd like you all to get rid of it 100 percent. Your gut, thyroid, and immune system will thank you for it!

What's wrong with grains and legumes?

Grains, pseudograins (like quinoa and corn), and legumes also promote leaky gut. They damage intestinal cells, feed the unfriendly bacteria that throw your microbiome out of balance, and cause the tight junctions of your intestinal walls to open and remain open.

The edible portion of these plants is the seed, which contains the embryo. In order to protect this embryo, a plant produces its own natural insecticides to repel pests. The chemicals help the seeds pass undigested through an animal's system so that when they are expelled with the animal's feces, they remain intact and can produce more plants. The chemicals that enable the seed's survival under those circumstances can be very damaging to those of you with autoimmune disease.

Grains and legumes also contain *lectins,* plant proteins that bind to carbohydrates. Two types of lectins are especially challenging: *agglutinins* and *prolamins.*

Agglutinins are another type of natural insecticide that can aggravate autoimmune disease. This is why genetically modified organisms (GMO) are especially harmful and inflammatory; they've been specially engineered to produce even *more* of their natural insecticides! If you do eat grains and legumes, make sure they are heirloom or non-GMO.

Prolamins are also hard to digest. In fact, gluten is a type of prolamin, and even gluten-free grains contain a prolamin similar in structure to gluten. Accordingly, prolamins—and the grains that contain them—can cause an immune response in anyone who is sensitive to gluten.

Grains also contain *phytates* and *phytic acid,* which inhibit digestion and bind to zinc, iron, and calcium, preventing their absorption. As you know, these minerals are crucial for both thyroid and immune system function, so you don't want to be eating any foods that keep you from absorbing them. GMO grains contain an even greater concentration of phytic acid.

Finally, pseudograins and legumes contain *saponins,* also known as glycoalkaloids, another natural insecticide produced by these plants. If you've got a leaky gut, glycoalkaloids can pass through your gut lining into your bloodstream, where they destroy red blood cells.

If you have an autoimmune condition, non-gluten grains and legumes should basically stay out of your diet, although you might be able to make an occasional exception—say, once or twice a month—as long as you don't notice any ill effects. If you don't have an autoimmune condition, you should be able to reintroduce these foods gradually, and if you don't notice any problems, keep them in your diet. However, go easy; no more than one serving a day of either grains or legumes, and less if you have trouble tolerating them. How will you know? If you start to gain weight, show signs of indigestion, or develop other troubling symptoms, your body is probably telling you to cut back on them or cut them out.

DITCH THE DAIRY

What's wrong with dairy? Oh, so many things! First and foremost, it too might trigger molecular mimicry. It's also highly inflammatory. That right there should be enough. I will add that if you eat any type of convention-ally farmed dairy, you are subjecting your body to antibiotics (terrible for the gut), bovine growth hormone (talk about an endocrine and thyroid disrupter!), and loads of unfriendly bacteria (because of the way the animals are raised, they get sick a *lot,* despite all those antibiotics). Please, skip the milk and pass on the cheese and yogurt. Your body deserves better. And you can get just as much calcium from the leafy green vegetables you will be eating on The Myers Way Thyroid Connection Plan.

SOME OTHER FOODS TO AVOID

Nightshades (eggplants, peppers, tomatoes, white potatoes) are high in lectins. They can easily damage your gut lining and impair gut func-tion. All of you should avoid them for twenty-eight days on The Myers Way Thyroid Connection Plan and cautiously reintroduce them after-ward only if you can tolerate them.

Eggs contain a protective enzyme, *lysozyme,* as their natural defense against predators. Lysozyme can be inflammatory to people with auto-immune conditions. All of you will avoid them for twenty-eight days, after which you might be able to reintroduce them.

Sugar is highly inflammatory and has absolutely no nutritional value. You will be happier and healthier if you let it go, with maybe a few exceptions. The doctor in me would love to say permanently, and if you can do that, all the better. But I can't tell you to do what I don't do myself! I do like to celebrate my birthday; I had a wedding cake when I got married; and I do indulge in a little treat on special occasions. I also enjoy very dark chocolate—at least 85 percent cacao. Let's start with taking sugar out of your diet for twenty-eight days. You can see how you feel afterward when you add in sugar in very limited amounts.

Caffeine in the right amounts is okay for some people, although even if you can tolerate it, too much of it can still disrupt your sleep and challenge your adrenals. If you are using caffeinated drinks to compensate for that morning grogginess or that midafternoon slump, you are almost certainly sleep-deprived and struggling with adrenal dysfunction. Please, cut out the caffeine during the twenty-eight-day plan, get the sleep you need, and support your adrenals. After they are back in shape, you can consider whether to add small amounts of caffeine back into your regimen (at most, sixteen ounces of coffee or thirty-two ounces of caffeinated tea).

Alcohol is okay as a very occasional beverage. A distilled liquor is preferable to beer (loaded with gluten) or wine (fermented, which can be a problem if you have intestinal yeast). I do want you to cut out alcohol for twenty-eight days. It can be inflammatory and it's full of sugar. It can worsen gut infections such as SIBO and yeast overgrowth. Last but not least, it stresses your liver, which needs all of its available resources to free your body of toxins (see chapter 8). But hey, my wedding drink was a Moscow mule, made from vodka, ginger beer, and lime. An occasional drink or two every month or so can be okay once your thyroid and immune system are working as they should.

Packaged foods are almost always full of additives, dyes, and preservatives—how else can they remain in those cardboard boxes and not go bad? Gluten, sugar, dairy, corn, soy, and other inflammatory foods are often added as well, not to mention tons of extra salt. Even gluten-free products are chock-full of ingredients that will stress your body, challenge your immune system, and, ultimately, burden your thyroid. Do your body a favor and pass—for good.

For Vegans and Vegetarians

As a physician, I have to be honest with you: Your diet is really not good for your body, especially if you have any type of thyroid or immune dysfunction. First, you will find it very hard to get the amino acids that your thyroid gland needs to make hormone as well as the B_{12} that is also vital to your thyroid.

To make matters worse, grains, legumes, and dairy products are highly inflammatory, and once you take those items from your diet, what are you going to eat? Your immune system and your thyroid depend on protein—you need amino acids to assist them as well as to build muscle, replenish your brain chemicals, and support all your body's functions.

Some vegetarians do eat a little fish and seafood. If you do, you'll find plenty of dishes in The Myers Way Thyroid Connection Plan that you can enjoy, and you can substitute them for any of the meat dishes. If you are a strict vegetarian or vegan, you can still follow the plan by removing the most inflammatory foods from your diet. You can also enjoy the delicious recipes in this book and exclude the animal protein, though this is not optimal. I hope, in time, you will choose the path of health and eat the foods that are more suited to your body.

THE POWER OF FOOD — AND THE JOY

So now you know which foods will help you achieve thyroid and immune system health.

What you don't yet know—but will by this time next month—is how *great* you're going to feel when you eat this way. Your thyroid will be healthy, your immune system robust, and your whole body will feel vibrant and energized. Your metabolism will be revving up to optimal speed, your hair and skin will be on their way to glowing health, and your mind will be clear, sharp, calm, and buoyant with optimism. That is the power — and the joy — of food. I can't wait for you to experience it for yourself!

The Power of Food: The Basics

Make sure your thyroid gland gets the nutrients it needs to

- produce thyroid hormone
- convert free T4 to free T3
- allow free T3 to enter your cells
- heal your gut, because a leaky and unhealthy gut
  - fails to absorb and digest the nutrients needed by your thyroid — and your body
  - allows partially digested food to pass through gut walls, triggering an overactive immune system
  - fails to produce enough serotonin and other vital brain chemicals, putting you at risk of anxiety, brain fog, depression, and other sleep problems
  - stresses your body, creating disruption in stress hormones and sex hormones, which in turn disrupt thyroid and immune function

Support your immune system so that

- it stops attacking your thyroid (if you are autoimmune)
- you prevent a first or additional autoimmune condition

Establish positive synergy, where your gut, immune system, and thyroid are all supporting rather than disrupting one another.

CHAPTER 8

Tame the Toxins

My patient Jenny was a hard-driving, no-nonsense corporate lawyer who showed up at my office with a debilitating case of Hashimoto's thyroiditis. Jenny already had a diagnosis from her conventional MD, but she was frustrated that her treatment didn't seem to be fully successful.

"I noticed *some* difference after taking the Synthroid," she told me. "But not enough. I'm still five pounds over my normal weight, and I would say at about fifty percent of my normal energy. My mind isn't as sharp as I would like it to be either—maybe only seventy to eighty percent. I think I can do better—and from everything I've read on your website, I think you're the one to get me there."

I appreciated Jenny's commitment to total health as well as her businesslike attempts to give me as clear a picture as possible. As with any patient, I ran a complete thyroid blood panel on her to see exactly where we were. While waiting for her labs to come back, I told Jenny that to achieve full health, she would need to make some significant changes in her diet and lifestyle.

Jenny was mostly vegetarian; she ate fish a few times a week. Just as I had been, she was shocked to find out that the supposedly healthy grains and legumes she relied on were actually undermining her health. I encouraged her to add animal protein to her diet, since her thyroid needed amino acids, iron, and B vitamins, which are hard to get in sufficient quantities if you don't eat meat.

But when I began explaining to Jenny that we had to tame the toxins, she balked. "I live in a very clean area, and I work in an office," she told me briskly. "I don't see how toxins can possibly be a problem."

This is a super-common response, and I understand why many people think this way. If you live in a nice environment with no landfills or factories in the immediate area, why would industrial chemicals and toxins ever be a factor in your health?

Unfortunately, they are, and I looked for an efficient, no-nonsense way to convey this fact to Jenny. "Do you eat sushi, tuna sandwiches, or grilled swordfish?" I ask her. "Do you have any mercury amalgams — silver-colored fillings — in your mouth? Do you cook with nonstick pans? Do you store your food in plastic containers? Do you drink bottled water? Do you work in an office where they use toner in the photocopier and where they clean with conventional products? Do you use conventional beauty products — shampoo, shower gel, moisturizer, deodorant, toothpaste, cosmetics? Do you shower in unfiltered water?"

Jenny looked at me in astonishment. "All of the above."

"Then I'm sorry to inform you that toxins are almost certainly a factor in your thyroid and immune health," I told her. "Luckily, there are lots of ways to protect yourself. And just a few significant changes can go a long way toward supporting your thyroid and immune function."

HOW DO WE TAME THE TOXINS?

In the previous chapter, I showed you that food is medicine, one of the most powerful healing tools we have. It seems obvious to me that everything we absorb into our bodies has a crucial impact on how well our bodies function and how healthy we can be.

Unfortunately, there's a downside to that principle — and it's toxins, the industrial chemicals that saturate our air, our water, and our soil. Every day, along with food, water, and air, we take into our bodies hundreds of toxic elements that disrupt our thyroid, our immune system, our digestion, and our overall health. If we don't take steps to combat this threat, our body's toxic burden can sabotage all the good effects of our other healthy choices.

I'll be straight with you: In our current world, there's a limit to what we can do to prevent and recover from toxins. There are so many of them, and they are *everywhere*. No matter where you live—city or country, suburb or village, next to a factory or beside the ocean—you are vulnerable to the millions of pounds of toxic chemicals that we keep dumping into our environment. If you accept a receipt from a store clerk, you've just made contact with toxic BPA (bisphenol A) plastic. If you clean your house with conventional products, you've exposed yourself to toxic chemicals. If you use shampoo, moisturizer, deodorant, or toothpaste, you've likely exposed yourself as well. And, on a truly sad note, indoors might be even more toxic than outdoors, given the chemicals that go into our wood floors, cabinets, mattresses, furniture, carpeting, and cookware.

That's the bad news. Now, here's the good news: Even though you can't *completely* rid your personal environment of toxins, you can make a significant difference. You can also improve your body's ability to *detoxify*—to rid itself of the toxins you accumulate each day. I don't want you to give up hope; I don't even want you to stress. As you'll see in the next chapter, stress is also not great for your thyroid and immune system! What I do want you to do is listen up, learn the basics, and make a few simple but powerful changes, creating a toxin defense plan that can make a world of difference in your health.

Sound good? Let's get started.

We'll begin by zeroing in on the toxins that pose the greatest risk to your thyroid.

Your Toxin Defense Plan at a Glance

Here are the basics of what you'll be doing to tame the toxins on The Myers Way Thyroid Connection Plan.

Step 1: Prevention—Reduce the Number of Toxins You're Exposed To

- Clean your air with a HEPA filter.
- Purify your water with filters on all your sinks, showers, and tubs or a whole house system.
- Eat clean food by buying organic and pasture-raised.

- Protect your body by choosing only "clean" body products.
- Care for your mouth by avoiding and/or having removed mercury-based dental amalgams.

Step 2: Detoxify — Support Your Body's Ability to Rid Itself of Toxins

- Know your SNP status so that you can take the supplements you need to support your detox pathways. (SNPs are single-nucleotide polymorphisms — genetic mutations that affect your ability to absorb certain vitamins that you need to detoxify.)
- Love your liver by eating the foods and supplements that enable it to filter toxins out of your blood.
- Heal your gut by following the gut-healing protocol that is part of The Myers Way Thyroid Connection Plan (see chapter 7).
- Cleanse your body through natural detox; pee, poop, and sweat away your daily accumulation of toxins.

Malicious mercury

When you consider how toxic mercury is to human health, it sure makes you wonder why it shows up in so many places:

- Your dental fillings, which means that mercury could leak continually into your bloodstream
- Vaccines — and why should the treatments meant to make us safe actually put us at risk?
- Fish, especially the larger saltwater varieties
- Pesticides, inadvertently targeting not just insects but also us humans
- Cosmetics, such as skin-lightening creams or creams to lighten age spots
- Your air, because coal-burning plants emit more than seventy thousand pounds of mercury into the air each year
- Your water, because all that mercury emitted into our air then settles in our water

Bottom line: Even if you take precautions to avoid mercury, you're still being exposed. That's why your toxin defense plan has two steps: prevention and detox, so you can keep as much mercury as possible *out* of your body and then help your body get rid of whatever you couldn't prevent.

Besides being generally toxic, mercury is particularly dangerous for your thyroid because, as luck would have it, mercury and iodine are strikingly similar. This unfortunate resemblance means that your thyroid—exceptionally good at absorbing any available iodine in your body—is also quick to absorb and store mercury.

This presents your thyroid with a twofold problem. First, any space your thyroid gland gives to storing mercury isn't available for storing iodine, compromising its ability to produce T3 and T4. No wonder hypothyroidism is on the rise!

Second, mercury and many other heavy metals increase your risk of developing an autoimmune disease. No one knows exactly how or why, but research is clear that the link exists. A 2011 study found that women with a high exposure to mercury were more than twice as likely to have thyroid antibodies.

Maybe the mercury damages the cells of your thyroid gland— along with other cells in your body—to the point that your immune system no longer recognizes those cells as self. Another possibility is that your immune system starts blaring, "Danger! Danger!" when it encounters high levels of mercury—a response that triggers inflammation. If the mercury is always present, the inflammatory response becomes chronic, which in turn sends your immune system into auto-immune hyperdrive.

In any case, mercury is a significant factor in Hashimoto's, and when I shared this information with Jenny, she was shocked—and furious. "Is exposure to mercury why I developed this condition?" she asked me. I couldn't give her a definite answer—but I could urge her to begin a toxin defense plan like the one you will read about later in this chapter.

Pernicious perchlorate

Here's another iodine look-alike that your thyroid eagerly absorbs. In fact, perchlorate is so good at competing with iodine for available space in your thyroid that in the 1950s and 1960s, it was actually used to treat Graves' disease, in the hope that blocking iodine absorption would slow down a hyperactive thyroid. Sadly, the cure was worse than the disease, since perchlorate also causes death by aplastic anemia, a condition in which your bone marrow stops producing enough red blood cells, white blood cells, and platelets.

Perchlorate is used to make rocket fuel, fireworks, and sometimes fertilizers. You wouldn't think you'd have much contact with it unless you worked for NASA or lived on a farm, but, alas, industrial runoff means that this toxic chemical is commonly found in our water supply as well as in fruits or vegetables that have been irrigated with perchlorate-contaminated water.

A 2006 study by the Centers for Disease Control found that even very low levels of perchlorate exposure caused decreased thyroid function in women. The study also found a "widespread presence of perchlorate in the environment." Yet the Environmental Protection Agency (EPA) didn't act to label perchlorate a contaminant — and they *still* haven't issued any regulations concerning its presence in public water systems. I know the EPA has an impossible job, but come on, folks! We can do better than *that*.

When she learned about perchlorate, Jenny grimaced. "I'm starting to see why you want me to buy organic!" she said ruefully. "And why you want me to install a water filter on my sinks and shower. Message received!"

The iodine look-alikes

We've seen how mercury and perchlorate fool your thyroid into thinking they are iodine. Three more chemicals do the same: fluorine, chlorine, and bromine, all of which are in the halogen family of chemicals along with iodine. Accordingly, your thyroid will absorb these three chemicals and store them in place of iodine, effectively displacing iodine. And the result — you guessed it — is that your thyroid is short of the iodine it needs to make T3 and T4.

Unfortunately, these three chemicals are now frequently added to our water, foods, and household products. Again, no wonder we have a virtual thyroid-dysfunction epidemic! Luckily, your toxin defense plan will protect you against most of the potential damage, so let's take a closer look.

Fluorine, in the form of fluoride, has been added to public water systems in the United States since the 1950s — supposedly to promote dental health. However, recent research has shown that fluoride does not actually decrease the risk of cavities in adults at any significant level. What fluoride *does* do is disrupt your endocrine system, to the point where, like perchlorate, it was once used as a treatment for hyperthyroidism. A recent, large-scale study confirms the connection: areas where fluoride is added to the water system have rates of hypothyroidism that are twice as high as non-fluoride areas. Fluoride disrupts other aspects of your endocrine system as well, including your stress hormones and your sex hormones, which is why keeping the toxins out and detoxing them once they're in is going to do wonders for your overall health.

Chlorine is also added to our water supply, as a disinfectant. Yes, this is the same chlorine that's used in bleach, because it has an oxidizing effect that kills organic molecules. That might be good for making things clean, but why would you want it in your body? Chlorine is also used in a number of industrial processes to make plastics, dyes, insecticides, paper products, and other goods, which means that even when it's not deliberately added to our water supply, it's getting into our water and ground soil along with other industrial runoff.

Bromine is used as a flame retardant in furniture and upholstery and as a sanitizer in hot tubs, whose high temperatures make chlorine ineffective. It's also found in pesticides and in our old friend plastics. Bromine is even frequently added to foods such as citrus-flavored soft drinks, baked goods, and — wait for it — flour (commonly labeled *enriched flour*). Are you starting to feel iodine-challenged? Even worse, bromine can be found in many gluten-free products, another reason to avoid them completely for your first twenty-eight days on The Myers Way Thyroid Connection Plan and to use them only sparingly after that.

Luckily, your diet on The Myers Way Thyroid Connection Plan is rich in iodine. I also recommend you take a comprehensive multivitamin that contains iodine as well. That's a good way to compensate for this toxin-induced depletion. But you also want to keep this terrible trio as far away from your body as possible.

One way to protect yourself is with a good water filter, ideally on your shower and tub as well as your sink, since exposure comes through the skin as well as through the mouth. If possible, choose saltwater rather than chlorine pools for swimming, or at least, keep your chlorine exposure to a minimum, showering afterward with filtered water.

You can also avoid the fluoride by cutting out processed beverages, using fluoride-free toothpaste (see my website for how to make your own), and finding alternatives for medications like Cipro, which contains fluoride. (Talk to your doctor about substitutions, and ask your pharmacist about possible additives in your medications.)

On The Myers Way, you're already avoiding gluten in the form of breads and baked goods, but the added bromine gives you yet another reason to skip the pastry aisle. Since both chlorine and bromine are commonly found in insecticides, you can avoid them by choosing organic produce and meats. Since they are also added to plastic, please avoid storing food in plastic bags or containers. And *please* avoid plastic water bottles, which transfer those iodine thieves right into your water. A stainless-steel or glass thermos works just as well—and is much cheaper.

The Iodine Controversy

In the past few years, there has been quite a bit of controversy over whether thyroid and autoimmune patients need to supplement with iodine. Some researchers advocate megadoses of iodine, which they say helps to prevent thyroid disease and breast cancer. Conventional physicians argue against iodine supplements at any dosage if you have Hashimoto's or Graves' because they think your system already has too much iodine and that more will only make your condition worse.

However, the experts I trust most have come to a different conclusion: We need to strike a balance. No, we don't need megadoses. But we often *do* need to supplement with iodine, even those of us who are autoimmune.

Why? Because, as you've just seen, our exposure to iodine-depleting chemicals is so great. To compensate, our bodies often need some extra iodine—but not too much. That's why I recommend iodine supplements for virtually all of my thyroid patients, including the ones with autoimmune conditions.

Now, at this point you might be wondering how much iodine you should take. I'll be straight with you again: There is no definitive way to know exactly how much you need. I do make a recommendation that is part of The Myers Way Thyroid Connection Plan. But it's possible that your body needs more—or less.

Why can't I be more specific? Because, as I explained on page 126, there is no reliable way to test your body's iodine levels. If you've had a lot of toxic exposure, you probably need more iodine than most. But you won't necessarily know what your level of exposure has been, so that isn't very helpful. I can say that going forward, you will be significantly reducing your toxic exposure because you will be following The Myers Way, which is terrific. Still, a lifetime of exposure, which basically all of us have had, has affected your thyroid's relationship to iodine.

Best advice? Start with the dosages I recommend as part of The Myers Way Thyroid Connection Plan. If you aren't getting the results you want, you can work with a functional medicine physician to adjust the dose as needed.

Nasty nitrates

Nitrates are various combinations of nitrogen and oxygen that you can find in both fertilizer and foods. Spinach and celery naturally contain nitrates, as do some other foods, but nitrates are also used as preservatives in many processed and cured meats, notably hot dogs, cold cuts, and bacon.

And, as you've probably guessed by now, nitrates also resemble iodine enough to competitively block its absorption. As a result, consuming nitrates can reduce your thyroid function.

A 2010 study also linked nitrates to thyroid cancer. Women whose water was more contaminated with nitrates were more likely to develop thyroid cancer. Yet the level of contamination was so low that it didn't even come close to what the EPA permits! Likewise, women whose food was more contaminated with nitrates were more likely to develop thyroid cancer and hypothyroidism. It seems clear to me that nitrate contamination is a problem.

I don't want you to worry about natural nitrates — feel free to make spinach and celery a part of your diet, because their concentration of nitrates isn't high enough to cause concern and those foods are full of nutritional benefits. I do, however, want you to avoid the processed meats that contain artificial nitrates as well as do everything you can to protect your water supply (more about this below). Don't worry, you can enjoy nitrate-free bacon, which you'll find in some mouth-watering recipes in The Myers Way Thyroid Connection Plan.

...And the kitchen sink

I could easily fill this entire book with information about environmental toxins. After all, a whopping eighty thousand chemicals are registered for use in the United States, and every year, another seventeen hundred are added to the list. Even the ones that *are* studied — and, as you can see on pages 180–181, most of them aren't — are researched over only short periods, in isolation. We don't know what happens to our bodies when these hundreds of thousands of chemicals start to interact, let alone what happens after they've all been in our bodies for decade after decade.

I tell my patients that your body is like a cup, and each toxin you're exposed to is like another drop of liquid filling that cup. The plastic dish that you microwave your lunch in — *drip.* Your plastic water bottle — *drip.* Those dry-cleaned clothes you just put on ... the conventional cleaning products that you use ... the fluoride-laden toothpaste you put in your mouth — *drip, drip, drip.* Your cup can handle *some* toxins ... a few more ... a few more ... But sooner or later, if you're not careful, your cup will overflow, and you'll develop a thyroid condition or an autoimmune disease or any one of a number of disorders, potentially even cancer.

But as you've seen, we have a two-step plan to combat this danger. I follow it, my patients follow it, and now you will follow it too.

- *Step 1 — Prevention:* We're going to keep as many toxins as possible from dripping into your cup.
- *Step 2 — Detoxification:* We're going to empty your cup every day, every week, and every month, so it never gets too full.

These two strategies will make all the difference in your thyroid, immune, and overall health — so let's get started.

Whose Fault Is This?

Gosh, this is a tough one. On the one hand, the EPA and the Food and Drug Administration (FDA) are supposed to keep us safe, right? And on the face of it, they don't seem to be doing a very good job.

For example, in 2003, the Environmental Working Group (EWG) in collaboration with the Mount Sinai School of Medicine in New York City tested nine people living in apparently clean areas for 210 different industrial chemicals. They found that each person's body contained an average *of 91 toxins,* including industrial chemicals, heavy metals, and other significant toxins. And of those 91, at least 53 were known to suppress the immune system—I can only imagine the damage they did to thyroid function. In 2004, the Centers for Disease Control and Prevention (CDC) tested 2,500 people for 116 industrial chemicals—and found evidence of all 116. In 2005, a similar study found evidence of 287 industrial chemicals. And that's just the chemicals they were looking for. What about the ones they weren't?

I used to think that the burden of proof was on corporations to show that each new industrial chemical was safe. Nope. In order to get the EPA or FDA to issue a regulation on any one of the thousands of industrial chemicals in our environment, someone has to show that a particular chemical is unsafe. You might as well ban a few snowflakes in the midst of an avalanche.

That being the case, what are the EPA and FDA supposed to do? The EPA alone is deluged with forty to fifty applications each week for permission to use new industrial chemicals. As corporations wait impatiently for a response, an underfunded and understaffed EPA rushes to comply, approving some 80 percent of those applications in three weeks or less—often without a single piece of data!

It's not really the government making these decisions. It's the industry lobbyists, the ones hired by corporations to get those approvals through as quickly as possible so all the money spent on research and development can start paying off. Our health isn't their concern. So whose concern is it?

I don't like this, and you shouldn't either. If we want cleaner food, water, and air, we're going to have to figure out another way to get there. The current system isn't working for us—that's for sure.

YOUR TOXIN DEFENSE PLAN IN DETAIL

Step 1: Prevention

Don't fill up your cup! These suggestions will help keep toxins out of your body so that your thyroid and immune system can function at their peak.

Clean Your Air

Mercury can be found in the air near coal-burning plants, so your first move is to get a HEPA filter for your home and office. (I make some recommendations in Resources.) *HEPA* stands for "high-efficiency particulate air," which is another way of saying that HEPA filters trap dust, dirt, and other particles, including toxins. If you're looking for some extra motivation, check out the Center for Media and Democracy's interactive map, which allows you to see if there are any coal-burning

power plants in your area: http://www.sourcewatch.org/index.php/
Existing_U.S._Coal_Plants.

Ideally, you want a whole-house HEPA filter. If that is not practical
or affordable for you, start with your bedroom. You spend at least eight
hours a day there, and you detox primarily while you sleep, making it
even more important not to be flooding your body with new toxins
while the old ones are being removed. Next priority is your living
room, since, after the bedroom, that's probably where you spend most
of your time.

If you work for yourself, getting a HEPA filter for your office space
is another priority. If you work for someone else, ask your employer if
you may have a HEPA filter by your desk.

Jenny didn't understand why she needed to purify the air *indoors.*
Then I told her that indoor air can be up to *one hundred times more toxic*
than outdoor air. Not a typo, folks—one hundred times. At home,
toxic chemical fumes waft out of your cabinetry, wood floors, mattresses,
carpets, and pieces of furniture, not to mention your home-cleaning
products. At work, cabinetry, carpets, furniture, industrial-strength
cleaners, photocopying chemicals, and a number of other toxins get into
the mix. In the words of the EPA:

> Most people are aware that outdoor air pollution can damage
> their health but may not know that indoor air pollution can also
> have significant effects. EPA studies of human exposure to air
> pollutants indicate that indoor air levels of many pollutants may
> be 2–5 times, and on occasion more than 100 times, higher than
> outdoor levels. These levels of indoor air pollutants are of par-
> ticular concern because it is estimated that most people spend as
> much as 90 percent of their time indoors. In recent years, com-
> parative risk studies performed by the EPA and its Science Advi-
> sory Board (SAB) *have consistently ranked indoor air pollution among
> the top five environmental risks to public health* [emphasis mine].

Now, this information can be daunting, but don't panic—arm
yourself! Get the HEPA filters that you need and move on to cleaning

up your water supply. And if you want to take it all a step further, check out appendix B for more information on a toxin-free home.

Purify Your Water

Jenny told me proudly that she already drank only bottled water purchased from the health-food store. I was not so happy to hear that; toxic molecules from plastic bottles can migrate into the water. Besides, bottled water isn't regulated; despite the pretty pictures of springs and glades on the label, the water can be even more contaminated than water from your faucet. And plastic bottles have to go somewhere—usually into landfills. There, the toxins leach into the groundwater and rise up into the rain, ultimately affecting our water and food supply again and again and again.

Stop the madness! Get yourself a home water filter and buy a glass or stainless-steel water bottle so you can make your own bottled water. Problem solved for Jenny *and* the environment!

Now, let's take it a step further: I want you to shower, bathe, and wash in filtered water as well. You don't really want the toxins soaking into your skin, do you? Among other industrial chemicals, a contaminant known as trichloroethylene (TCE) makes its way from industrial runoff into the groundwater, with possibly disastrous consequences for your immune system. Experiments suggest that TCEs might cause you to produce antibodies against your own tissue, drive up inflammation, and otherwise disrupt immune function. I don't want you soaking your skin in TCE-laden water while breathing in the contaminated steam.

Many water supplies contain *fluoride*. Besides depleting your iodine supply, the fluoride itself is rather nasty. Yes, it's supposed to combat tooth decay, but what they use is not the natural calcium fluoride that was first proposed for that purpose but rather sodium fluoride, a toxic waste product that results from the manufacture of aluminum. Yuck. Last but sadly not least, most public water supplies also contain chlorine and bromine, which, as you now know, compete with iodine.

So please, put water filters on every tap in your living space or, if you live in a house, get a whole-house water filtration system (see Resources for suggestions for both). Your thyroid, your immune system, your whole body, and your family deserve nothing less.

Filter Finesse

Unfortunately, most water-filtration systems do not remove fluoride from your water unless they use reverse osmosis. And while reverse osmosis does get rid of fluoride, it also removes essential minerals found in water, minerals that your body needs, including calcium and magnesium. Cooking with reverse-osmosis water can actually deplete these minerals in your food.

I negotiate this little dilemma by using a water-filtration system that does not utilize reverse osmosis. Then I focus on minimizing my exposure to fluoride from all other sources. For more on finding a water filter, see Resources.

Eat Clean Food

Okay, folks, in an ideal world, we'd all eat 100 percent organic, because that is definitely the best choice for our health. But we *don't* live in an ideal world, and even I can't eat organic 100 percent of the time, if only because I travel and because I love to socialize with my friends. If someone invites me over to dinner, I'm sure not giving him or her a shopping list! And I want to be able to go to restaurants with my friends, and that means making compromises.

Jenny had another concern, which I know a lot of you share: organic food is expensive, and your budget just might not stretch that far. That's okay—stressing over your food is bad for your health too, so please don't stress! Instead, let me tell you what I told Jenny about how to prioritize.

Your top priority should be organic and pasture-raised animal products. I strongly recommend you buy 100 percent organic meat and animal products that have been pasture-raised, because those animals are not fed GMO corn and soy. Equally important, animals sit at the top of the food chain, which means that all the toxins at the water or soil level and all the toxins and GMOs in conventional feed will be concentrated in your beef, chicken, and pork. Focus on organic, grass-fed, and pasture-raised meat and poultry.

As you know, *GMO* stands for "genetically modified organism," and it mainly refers to foods that have been genetically modified. I want you to avoid GMO foods, because they are not good for your immune system and they don't do your thyroid any favors either.

- They contain more pesticides than non-GMO foods, since many of them were developed precisely so that they could be sprayed and sprayed and sprayed some more.
- They frequently cause leaky gut, especially the ones engineered to contain Bt toxins, which kill insects by destroying the lining of their digestive tracts; guess what they do to yours.
- They disrupt your gut balance through glyphosate, the herbicide frequently used on genetically modified crops to kill weeds; it doubles as an antibiotic.

To make matters worse, most conventional meat and dairy are loaded with antibiotics too, because the unhealthy conditions in which those poor animals are raised mean that they are always getting sick. It's bad enough when you have to take antibiotics for a medical reason, but to get them because some company wanted to save money while growing crops...words fail me. As you already know, antibiotics set you up for leaky gut, yeast (Candida), and SIBO, as well as disrupt your microbiome, further weakening your immune system and undermining your overall health.

Plus, antibiotics fatten you up—by disrupting your gut bacteria, among other reasons—so farmers use them to make their animals fat too. Yes, you read that right—farmers give their cattle antibiotics to make them fat. Draw your own conclusions about what those very same medications are doing to you. (And remember to take your probiotics, which help counteract their effect!)

GMOs, antibiotics, insecticides, herbicides—you don't need any of that burdening your body, disrupting your gut, and stressing your immune system. Buy organic, be sure to eat only grass-fed meat, and check out the EWG guide to help you further (http://www.ewg.org/research/shoppers-guide-to-avoiding-gmos).

For fruits and vegetables, I've got another helpful tip: take a look at the Dirty Dozen and Clean Fifteen lists kept by the Environmental Working Group on its website (www.ewg.org). The dirty list steers you away from the most heavily pesticide-laden fruits and vegetables, while the clean list tells you which conventionally grown ones are less contaminated and safer to consume. Check every couple of months or so, because the lists tend to change.

The EWG also has a great chart to advise you on which types of fish are lowest in mercury. You don't have to avoid fish altogether, but do steer clear of the ones that are high in mercury.

Reduce your nitrate exposure by buying nitrate-free cured and processed meats—or, even better, avoid those products altogether.

What I like about this whole approach to clean eating is that it eliminates so many of the toxins that you would otherwise be getting hit with every day. Until our society makes sweeping changes, industrial runoff will affect even organic food through the mercury and perchlorate in our public water sources, leaving trace amounts. But you can rest assured that your own toxin defense plan will keep out so many toxins that your thyroid and immune function will be well supported. I've seen the exciting results that many of my patients have achieved with just a few simple changes, and I was eager to see how much Jenny's health would likewise improve.

The Problem with Plastics

Hey, I get it. Plastics are everywhere—from the receipt you get when you buy your produce to the container you use to take your healthy salad to work. Some people distinguish between BPA and non-BPA plastics. Honestly, I'm not sure that even matters, because so many health hazards are now starting to be linked to non-BPA plastics as well.

Avoiding plastics isn't easy, and you've got to come to your own decision about how far you're willing to go. You know as well as I do that the world doesn't make it easy for us to initiate healthy changes, and we each have to do our best.

So here's how I negotiate this complicated and frustrating dance. I avoid plastic water bottles (except in foreign countries where bottled water is my safest option). I don't own any plastic bags or containers; I use glass. But sometimes, if I haven't had time to make my lunch, I pick up something from the local health-food store, which offers only plastic containers for their prepared food and salad bar. Yes, I'd like to refuse to take that BPA-coated receipt, and sometimes I do—but sometimes I need it for my records.

For those of you who aren't yet ready to do the full Monty, here are a few guidelines to start. You get double benefits from these; they're fairly easy to follow, and by sticking to them, you eliminate a lot of the worst risks, giving your thyroid and immune function an immediate and much-appreciated boost.

- Replace plastic containers for food storage with glass or stainless steel.
- If you must use a microwave, make sure to use only glass containers for heating.

- Use a stainless-steel or glass thermos instead of a water bottle.

- Toss the Teflon.

Why no Teflon? Because a biochemical known as perfluorooctanoic acid (PFOA) has been found to potentially disrupt the immune system. Unfortunately, we come into contact with PFOA quite often. It rubs up against our food in nonstick cookware, disposable coffee cups, and grease-resistant boxes, including pizza boxes and those cardboard boxes you get at salad bars and from some restaurants. It's also found in clothing, Stainmaster carpet guard, computer chips, phone cables, car parts, and flooring.

We're not happy about any of this, right? But nonstick cookware's effects on food are especially nasty, so when you switch to cleaner cookware, your thyroid and immune system will breathe a sigh of relief and reward you with better energy, weight loss, and, as a bonus, great hair. Altogether a win-win-win!

Protect Your Body

As I always say, you aren't just what you eat, you're also what you apply to your skin! Some foreign-produced skin-lightening cosmetics, including products that claim to lighten age spots and freckles, were found by the Food and Drug Administration to have dangerous levels of mercury. Although American-made products have more stringent regulations, they can still be full of harmful chemicals, many of which mimic hormones in your body and disrupt the endocrine system, including your thyroid and adrenals.

Check out your own personal body-care products at Skin Deep (www.Ewg.org/skindeep), which ranks the risk level of various products and their ingredients. Teensturninggreen.org put together a Dirty Thirty list of chemicals that affect your thyroid and other hormones.

I know it's daunting—and expensive—to throw out all your personal-care products at once, so, luckily, you've got a kinder, gentler option: as each problematic product is used up, replace it with a cleaner one. Problem solved, and it will take you only about three months.

When you go to buy new products, read the labels carefully and stay away from any of the following ingredients:

• *Parabens.* These mimic the effects of estrogen and disrupt the hormonal system of both men and women. Sometimes *paraben* appears as part of a word, such as *methylparaben.* Same difference—avoid it!

• *Phthalates.* Another estrogen mimic—avoid it too.

• *Dyes and artificial colors.* Why do you want more industrial chemicals in your body?

• *Fragrance.* Ditto. It can be anything, and it's almost certainly chemical. Stay away.

• *Gluten and wheat.* You find these ingredients even in organic products. I don't want you eating them, and I don't want you rubbing them into your face, scalp, or skin. Avoid, avoid, avoid.

• *Oats, soy, and dairy products.* You're either avoiding these food groups or eating minimal, occasional amounts. You are *not* rubbing them into your skin multiple times each week—right?

I wish I could tell you that *organic* or *all-natural* means a product is safe—but I can't. You just have to read the ingredients or check out the safer options in the Resources section. Once you figure out which products work for you, you're done. Buying clean, healthy products becomes routine, and you can just relax and enjoy your good health.

Phthalates in Your Food

For years when I warned my patients about the dangers of phthalates, I focused on personal-care products. Now it turns out that phthalates are in fast foods also. A study conducted by the Centers for Disease Control and Prevention that included nearly nine thousand people over seven years found that levels of phthalates were up to 39 percent higher in the urine of people who had gotten 35 percent of a day's calories from fast foods and up to 25 percent higher for people who had eaten smaller amounts of fast food. Grain-based foods and fast foods containing meat seemed to be the worst culprits, either because of the way they were processed and packaged or because of the way their fats bind phthalates.

Significantly, the high phthalate content in fast food came primarily from the higher degree of handling and packaging. All processed foods travel along conveyor belts and through tubing, whose phthalates leach into the food. Fast food is also handled by people wearing gloves, which contaminate the food with even more chemicals.

As you saw in chapter 7, I'm not thrilled about the idea of you eating fast food or processed foods anyway. Now you've got another reason to avoid fake food!

Care for Your Mouth

Your mouth harbors many sources of inflammation that your immune system will thank you to avoid. Root canals can become inflamed or infected, as can the hole in the bone below wisdom teeth you have had removed. Bridges, posts, and porcelain crowns are potential occasions for toxins, heavy metals, and inflammation.

Most concerning, however, are those silver-colored mercury fillings, which are made from an amalgam of copper, silver, and mercury. The quickest way to know if you have them: open your mouth, look in the mirror, and see if you notice any silver. Because of the potentially toxic results, I recommend that all my patients have their metal fillings replaced with white resin or zirconium. I'm not crazy about the resin, honestly, because it contains plastic, but it is sooooo much better than the alternative, so make the change and feel terrific about what a big boost you have just given to your health.

Please make sure to use a biological dentist—a dentist who is committed to holistic, organic, and natural practices. A conventional dentist might switch out your mercury fillings, but he or she won't necessarily know how to keep the mercury from spilling into your mouth or how to prevent you from breathing in the vapors while the amalgams are being removed. (For more information on dental issues and your immune system, see appendix B. For help finding a biological dentist, see Resources.)

Step 2: Detoxification

You can't keep every single toxin out of your system—but you *can* keep emptying your cup so it doesn't overflow. Your body has natural detox pathways, so our goal is to give them all the support we can. Here's how.

Know Your SNP Status

SNPs are types of common genetic mutations. Their full name is single-nucleotide polymorphisms, but you can just say "snips."

SNPs are a problem because they interfere with your detox pathways. Specifically, they make it harder for your body to absorb the vitamins it needs to complete the detox process. If you've got a SNP—and a surprising number of people have one or more of them—you'll want to take extra supplements to compensate for it, especially since SNPs keep you from detoxing heavy metals, including mercury.

There are two potential SNPs in the MTHFR gene and one in the GSTM1 gene. You can ask your doctor to test for them or, if necessary, get an at-home kit sold online by 23andMe.com. (See Resources.) It costs $199, which I realize is not cheap. However, you get an amazing amount of information and since your SNPs don't change, you need to test only once. It's really worth it, because if you do have SNPs, you'll need to take supplements to ensure that your body can rid itself of toxins.

- For the MTHFR SNP, you need pre-methylated B_6, B_{12}, and folinic acid.
- For GSTM1, you need glutathione. Be careful—not all glutathione is created equal! Many available glutathione supplements are nearly impossible for your body to absorb, so you're basically wasting your money on a pill that won't do you any good. See Resources for my recommended form of glutathione, which is a fabulous detox aid.

Love Your Liver

Your liver is your body's chief detox organ, so supporting it is crucial for optimal detox. There are two phases to the detox process, and in order to complete both of them, your liver needs specific chemicals known as *cofactors*. Detoxification also requires a lot of energy. Accordingly, you want a nutrient-rich diet that is high in protein—which is exactly what you get on The Myers Way Thyroid Connection Plan.

Please don't ever detox with a total fast or juice fast—that actually *deprives* your liver of the nutrients and protein it needs to complete a full detox. And if your liver starts detoxing but doesn't complete the whole process, the toxins that were trapped in your fat end up flowing through your body, and you're much worse off than you were before. Instead, detox on The Myers Way by eating healthy foods, avoiding inflammatory foods, reducing toxic exposure, and taking the supplements your body needs for healthy liver function and to compensate for any SNPs.

Heal Your Gut

Gut healing is also a crucial part of detox. If your gut is leaky, toxins pass through into your bloodstream, which your immune system is definitely not happy about. A healthy gut processes toxins without letting them enter the rest of your body. You'll be able to heal your gut on The Myers Way.

Cleanse Your Body

The body is meant to expel toxins through the natural trio of pee, poop, and sweat. Drinking plenty of filtered water will help with the pee, while eating whole fruits and vegetables aids with the poop. In the next chapter, we'll talk about thyroid-friendly exercise, which helps with the sweat.

Infrared saunas are also a great sweat option, especially for those days when you just can't exercise. You can find infrared saunas and even collapsible solo saunas that will fit in your house or apartment. (See Resources.) I love my infrared sauna for both detox and stress relief, especially after work. Nothing helps me make the transition like a nice relaxing sauna in my own living room—mmm!

Do You Need Chelation?

Chelation is a process used to rid your body of heavy metals. Some of my patients have done it, with good results, but it's not something I necessarily advise for everyone. My suggestion is to start with my recommendations in this chapter and see how you feel. If you want to take things a step further, check out appendix C to find out more.

Supplements and Detox

I don't want you thinking of detox as a sometime thing—I want your detox pathways working to the max every single day. That's why you'll take supplements to support your detox pathways. And believe me, with hundreds of thousands of toxic chemicals in our environment, your detox pathways need all the help they can get, especially if you have an autoimmune condition or a SNP. Because our soil is so nutrient-depleted—even for organic produce—you also need supplements to make up for what your food isn't giving you.

I'm a big believer in supplements, but I know that the industry isn't regulated, so buyer beware! *You* don't have to beware, though, because I've suggested my own favorite supplements companies in the Resources section, listing only places I've researched myself. If you want to go another way, make sure your company is third-party-tested, follows good manufacturing practices, and produces only high-quality gluten-, dairy-, and soy-free products.

ONE MORE POTENTIAL THREAT: TOXIC MOLD

For most of you, the toxin defense plan I've outlined in this chapter should be enough. But you can always do more, especially if you are still feeling less than optimal after a few months. Go further in cleaning up your house (appendix B), take it to the next level with your dental work (appendix C), or find out if chelation is right for you (appendix D). One more frontier: toxic mold, aka *mycotoxins*.

Mycotoxins are volatile organic compounds (VOCs) that are given off by certain types of molds. Only about one-quarter of the population is vulnerable to these toxic chemicals, which means that you might be suffering while your family sails along without incident. You might be exposed to mycotoxins at home, at work, or at school—all places where you spend a lot of time, maximizing your exposure.

Unfortunately, even most functional medicine physicians know very little about molds and mycotoxins. I *wish* I didn't know about them, but unfortunately, I'm in the 25 percent of the population who is vulnerable, so I've become a reluctant expert. So far I've had two significant exposures, including one while I was working on this book— can you say stressful?

If you are in that 25 percent along with me, you should know that mycotoxins can suppress your immune system. Hence, they have been linked to various autoimmune diseases as well as non-autoimmune thyroid dysfunction. If you are not getting the results you want, toxic mold could be a factor. Check out appendix D to learn more.

JENNY'S DETOX

Jenny and I talked quite a bit about how she should approach her detox project, as she called it. Eventually, she understood that toxins were a significant factor in both aspects of her Hashimoto's—her thyroid and her immune system. On the one hand, the toxins created inflammation, which revved up her immune system, making it more likely to attack her own cells. On the other hand, the toxins signaled *danger* to the body, leading her thyroid to slow down and conserve energy—its typical response to any potential danger. This double whammy made taming the toxins doubly important.

"I feel so overwhelmed," Jenny confessed. "It just seems that the toxins are everywhere and that I should be changing everything at once!"

"You might get further by taking just a few steps at a time," I suggested. I shared with her my favorite motto: *Control what you can, and let go of what you can't.*

As I told Jenny, we each need to come up with our own personal decisions about what we can control and how much effort it makes sense for us to expend. Since I work for myself, I've chosen to keep my home and office as toxin-free as possible, using nontoxic building materials and furniture as well as water filters and HEPA air filters. When I cook at home, I stick strictly to organic food and nontoxic cookware, with no plastics anywhere in sight. That makes me feel as though I've got some leeway when I eat in restaurants, join friends in their homes, or buy takeout. I also feel free to travel, which I love; in the last couple of years, I've been to Europe, Mexico, Nicaragua, Argentina, Paraguay, Brazil, and India. So you know I'm not staying cooped up, afraid to enjoy this amazing world! You'll find your own way, but, like me, you can definitely protect your health while also living a full, adventurous life.

Jenny was inspired by the possibilities, and she came up with her own compromise while still making sure to *prevent* and *detoxify*. First, she made sure to get HEPA air filters and water filters on her tap and showers. She bought two lightweight stainless-steel thermoses, one for work and one for her car, so she'd never find herself without. She used glass containers for food storage at home and to take her healthy lunch and snacks to work.

It wasn't in Jenny's budget to make a clean sweep of her personal-care products, so she decided that she would simply replace each product with a nontoxic one as soon as she ran out. When she traveled, she brought her own products with her so she didn't have to rely on hotels or her hosts for clean shampoo or soap. (Her hostess gifts often included toxin-free bath products, which, she told me, were very popular!)

At home, Jenny decided to focus on organic, pasture-raised choices for meats, and to follow the Dirty Dozen and Clean Fifteen lists for produce. She was completely dedicated to avoiding high-mercury fish and made sure to check the EWG website every few months so she wouldn't mistakenly end up with a thyroid-unfriendly choice. She also made sure to replace her home-cleaning products with nontoxic choices. "I don't want my home full of chemicals that can undermine me," she told me.

Jenny managed to track down an ecofriendly dry cleaner, but then she realized that doing so would add a two-hour drive to her weekends. She decided that conventional dry cleaning was a compromise she could live with, but she told me, "If I start going backwards or feel even a little less than a hundred percent, I'll reconsider." I recommended that she remove the plastic bags and hang her clothes on the porch for an hour or so to let the chemicals air out. That way, they wouldn't linger in her closet. Jenny was excited to find yet another doable way to reduce the toxins in her life.

Jenny realized she had six mercury fillings, so she made arrangements with a biological dentist to have them gradually replaced. Because this was a challenging and time-consuming procedure, she spaced out the appointments. I also tested her for SNPs, and we discovered that she needed to supplement with glutathione. Finally, Jenny bought a small, portable solo infrared sauna and organized her time to take a half-hour home sauna at least three times a week.

Following The Myers Way made such a difference that we didn't even need to change Jenny's Synthroid prescription. The last time I saw her, she was at her target weight, glowing, energized, and content. "I am now at my full one hundred percent!" she informed me. "And with The Myers Way, I intend to stay there!"

CHAPTER 9

The Infection Connection

My patient Bernadette came to me with two autoimmune conditions—Hashimoto's thyroiditis and rheumatoid arthritis (RA). Bernadette had read my book *The Autoimmune Solution* and followed its recommendations for diet and lifestyle. She had basically cut out gluten, grains, legumes, and dairy, and she took the supplements that I recommended.

Bernadette was well educated about the toxins that pervade our food, air, and water. She had done a great job of gradually taming the toxins in her life: choosing clean personal-care items, filtering her air and water, avoiding plastic containers, and generally living clean.

In addition, Bernadette's prescription for supplemental thyroid hormone was fairly close to what I would consider optimal, although I did want to adjust it slightly. And her rheumatoid arthritis symptoms seemed to be in remission—so much so that she had stopped taking any medications for that condition.

Yet periodically, Bernadette would struggle with joint pain, brain fog, and fatigue. These symptoms could have been either the Hashimoto's or the RA flaring up—but why?

Then I took Bernadette's complete history, and I noticed two interesting points:

- As a teenager, Bernadette had suffered a bout of mononucleosis.
- Two years earlier—six months before she was diagnosed with Hashimoto's—she had been laid up for nearly a week with a

severe case of food poisoning, which she believed had come from eating food at a seafood festival.

Bernadette's mono led me to suspect that her flares might be due to a lingering infection from the Epstein-Barr virus, a member of the herpes family that causes mono and perhaps chronic fatigue syndrome too. I also wondered whether her apparent food poisoning was actually a sign of yersinia, a bacteria that can linger in the body after an initial bout of flulike symptoms. Significantly, due to molecular mimicry, yersinia infections can trigger Hashimoto's (and Graves'). Yersinia might also have been a factor in her flares of thyroid dysfunction.

"Bernadette," I told her, "you've done a terrific job of addressing diet, nutrition, and toxins. Now there's one more area we need to look at—infections."

HOW LINGERING INFECTIONS CHALLENGE YOUR IMMUNE SYSTEM

Most conventional MDs ignore the role of infections in autoimmune conditions. In my practice, however, I've seen many patients like Bernadette whose symptoms were triggered by an underlying infection caused by a bacterium, virus, or parasite. We tend to think of an infection as an active condition with lots of symptoms, and often that *is* the case. But many infections are silent—either they have no symptoms or they linger in your body for years in a dormant state before flaring up. These infections can become the straw that breaks the camel's back for your immune system, bringing on an autoimmune disorder or triggering a flare-up of an existing autoimmune condition.

Significantly, stress—whether physical, mental, or emotional—can retrigger infections as well. And indeed, when Bernadette and I talked further, we discovered that she had been undergoing a stressful time at home, as she and her husband had just lost the lease on their apartment and were trying to find a new place they could afford. I thought Bernadette's high stress levels might be activating these latent infections, burdening both her thyroid gland and her immune system.

HOW INFECTIONS TRIGGER
AUTOIMMUNE CONDITIONS

Our immune system is supercomplex, and each infection is unique. As a result, we don't know exactly how infections trigger autoimmune diseases, especially because multiple factors are usually involved and scientists are still trying to figure the whole thing out. Here is our latest thinking about three possible ways infections trigger autoimmune disorders, any or all of which might be in play at the same time:

- *Molecular mimicry.* As you saw in chapter 4, gluten and sometimes dairy (casein) can trigger thyroid dysfunction by molecular mimicry, the mistaken identity in which your immune system wants to attack gluten and dairy but gets confused and attacks your thyroid gland instead. In the same way, your immune system might try to attack an infectious agent—a virus or bacteria—but then get confused and attack your thyroid gland.
- *Bystander activation.* In this case, a bacteria or virus invades your thyroid gland, and your immune system mobilizes to respond. It sends immune cells to your thyroid to kill the infection—just as it's supposed to—but while the killer cells are attacking the invader, they accidentally injure some of the surrounding thyroid tissue, creating inflammation. The inflammation signals more immune cells to rush to the thyroid, where they then attack the thyroid gland.
- *The hijacking effect.* The technical term is *cryptic antigens,* but do what I do and just call it hijacking, because it helps you visualize what is going on. An infection—usually a virus such as herpes simplex or Epstein-Barr—hijacks your thyroid cells' DNA, masquerading as thyroid tissue in order to hide from your immune system. Your immune system is smart enough to detect the virus anyway. But when it attacks the hijacker virus, it also attacks the thyroid cells that the virus has hijacked.

You can see why we want to heal any infections that might be lingering in your body—if we don't, they can trigger one or more of these types of autoimmune attacks on your thyroid. Luckily, we've got a number of ways to deal with these infections; we'll get to them in a moment.

But first, you might be wondering if this information even applies to you. After all, you might be thinking that you don't *have* any infections. And maybe you don't. But quite possibly, you do, so read on.

DO I HAVE AN INFECTION?

Here's the problem: Many infections are very subtle, and you might have one or more of them without even realizing it. And if you do, your thyroid and your immune system are *not* going to be happy about it. Any type of viral infection, including the flu or the stomach flu, can potentially trigger *thyroiditis*—inflammation of the thyroid, with symptoms of either hypo- or hyperthyroidism. Usually this condition goes away within a few weeks of the infection clearing up. For some people, however, this infection can trigger autoimmune thyroid dysfunction.

For still others, one or more infections might linger in the body. If your immune system can hold it at bay, you won't notice any symptoms or other problems. But if leaky gut, an inflammatory food, stress, increased toxic exposure, or some other factor overburdens your immune system, the infection might become stronger and trigger problems for both your immune system and your thyroid.

Following are the most common infections implicated in causing autoimmune thyroid disease, either at the time of infection or through a dormant infection.

Herpes

There's a whole family of herpes infections, and researchers believe that all of them can play a role in autoimmune disorders. The ones we've studied most thoroughly are herpes simplex type 1 and type 2— yep, the very same ones that cause oral and genital herpes, giving you cold sores and herpes sores. Human herpesvirus 6 (HHV-6) is another type of herpes implicated in thyroid/autoimmune conditions.

Once you've been infected with viruses in the herpes family, they stay in your body for life. They're not always active, of course—some of them flare up only now and then, and some, like HHV-6, don't flare up at all. However, the virus can still be active, and when it is—which can happen without you really being aware of it—it can trigger an autoimmune response in your thyroid via either bystander activation or the hijacking effect.

Significantly, stress—whether physical, mental, or emotional—can incite a herpes virus to become active. That's because, as we've seen, stress hormones suppress your immune system, making your body a more welcoming environment for viruses. So, over the millennia, viruses have evolved to become active whenever they detect the presence of enough stress hormones. As you can see, stress and infections are interrelated, so if we want your thyroid and immune system to be functioning optimally, we have to address both of them.

Epstein-Barr

Epstein-Barr is actually part of the herpes family. It's the virus that causes mononucleosis, which is why hearing about Bernadette's youthful bout of the kissing disease made me think infections were likely a factor in her condition. By the way, that's kind of a misleading nickname, because you don't get mononucleosis just from kissing. Like many other viruses—the flu, the common cold—you get it from contact with another person's saliva, which can happen if you're near an infected person who coughs or sneezes or if you share a glass, drinking straw, or utensil with him or her.

So here's the thing: Even if you don't *think* you've had mono, you might very well have had it anyway; a whopping 95 percent of U.S. adults have picked it up by age forty, and it can present without any symptoms. Moreover, Epstein-Barr has been linked to both Hashimoto's and Graves' disease, just as it seemed to be in Bernadette's case.

I myself had mono as a teenager, which I now realize was one factor—along with my diet, leaky gut, mercury exposure, and stress—that likely contributed to my Graves'. Epstein-Barr has also been linked to other autoimmune diseases, most notably multiple sclerosis and lupus, as well as chronic fatigue syndrome, fibromyalgia, and Sjögren's syndrome.

Hepatitis C

Nearly three million Americans have hepatitis C. But 70 to 80 percent of them don't even know it because they have no symptoms. The hepatitis C virus attacks the liver, but research has found that chronic untreated hepatitis C patients have a higher rate of autoimmune thyroid dysfunction, suggesting that when the virus is active, it can trigger your immune system to attack your thyroid.

Unfortunately, hepatitis C patients who have been treated *also* have high rates of autoimmune thyroid disease. That's because interferon—the primary treatment—is an antiviral drug that can suppress your immune system, sometimes with the result of triggering autoimmune conditions. So both the virus and its treatment are potential risk factors.

Yersinia enterocolitica

This bacterium is typically transmitted via undercooked pork or in contaminated water, meat, or milk. If you're infected with yersinia, your symptoms will resemble food poisoning. When I heard about Bernadette's bout with food poisoning, I wondered whether she had been exposed to yersinia—and whether it and the stress of house-hunting were the final drops of water that caused her cup to finally overflow.

Most people overcome yersinia infections on their own, but sometimes the bacteria take up residence in your gut lining and continue to multiply. This is yet another case of molecular mimicry; yersinia so resembles your thyroid receptors that the antibodies targeting yersinia attack your thyroid as well. Yersinia is linked to both Hashimoto's and Graves'.

Small Intestine Bacterial Overgrowth (SIBO)

SIBO is what results when your gut bacteria go out of balance, with too many unfriendly bacteria proliferating in your intestinal tract. SIBO has been linked to hypothyroidism—in fact, some studies have found that up to half of hypothyroid patients suffer from it. In addition, any gut infection challenges your immune system, making SIBO a special challenge for people with Hashimoto's.

Helicobacter pylori

Also known as *H. pylori,* this bacterium causes ulcers by attacking the stomach lining, allowing your stomach acid to seep in and eat away at your gut wall. Like the other infections we've reviewed, *H. pylori* is very common—and, like the others, it often fails to cause symptoms, leaving people unaware that they've been infected.

A significant study found that 40 percent of non-autoimmune thyroid patients tested positive for *H. pylori,* as well as 45 percent of autoimmune patients with no thyroid condition. And if someone had *both* an autoimmune *and* a thyroid dysfunction? A whopping 86 percent of that group tested positive for the bacterium. So if you've got any type of thyroid dysfunction—but especially if you have Hashimoto's or Graves'—*H. pylori* is very likely a factor, and you want to address it, which you'll learn how to do below.

Toxoplasmosis

Another potential trigger for autoimmune thyroid dysfunction is toxoplasmosis, a disease caused by a parasite found in undercooked pork and infected cat feces. If you've been infected, you might not have any symptoms, or you might experience mild flulike symptoms such as tender lymph nodes and achy muscles. For pregnant women, toxoplasmosis poses a risk to the fetus. In most people, the parasite passes, but sometimes, it can linger in your system, eventually triggering Hashimoto's or Graves'.

Blastocystis hominis

This parasite has been linked to Hashimoto's thyroiditis. *Blastocystis hominis* is common in developing countries, so if you've traveled to the developing world, you might well have picked it up. The Centers for Disease Control says that this parasite doesn't really cause any harm; however, I've seen case reports in which people are treated for this parasite—and then their Hashimoto's resolves. I also see this in my clinic all the time, and I know how effective treating this parasite can be. So if you think you might have acquired it, please do get tested and treated.

TESTING FOR INFECTIONS

As I told Bernadette, testing is the first step. You can't just wonder if you've got an infection—you need to find out for sure.

For SIBO and *Blastocystis hominis*, you can complete the questionnaires on pages 260 and 261, which will then help you to create your individualized supplement plan. There are also laboratory tests for these infections:

- Herpes, Epstein-Barr, toxoplasmosis, and hepatitis C can all be found in blood tests that can be run by any doctor.
- *H. pylori* is identified using a breath test, stool test, or blood test, all of which your doctor can run for you. Please note that the blood test will tell you only whether you've had *H. pylori,* not whether it's still active.
- SIBO is detected through a breath test, which your doctor can order.
- For *Blastocystis hominis,* you need a stool test, though these are not infallible, so if you test negative and you think you've still got something, you might consider seeing a functional medicine practitioner for a more specialized stool test.
- Although there isn't a good conventional test for yersinia, a functional medicine doctor can run a specialized stool test for it.

TREATING YOUR INFECTIONS

Okay, suppose you test positive for one or more infections. What's your next move?

Your specific treatment then depends on whether your infection is caused by a virus, bacteria, or parasite. However, I want to emphasize that whatever treatments you rely on, you also need to follow The Myers Way

Thyroid Connection Plan. Why? Because if you don't remove inflammatory foods from your diet, heal your gut, and support your immune system, your chances of winning the battle against an infection—and your chances of preventing a recurrence of it—go way down. Give yourself the best shot at defeating infections by combining the following treatments with the right diet, supplements, and gut healing.

Treating viral infections: Herpes and Epstein-Barr

For these, I recommend Lauricidin, a nonprescription supplement. Lauricidin is an acid derived from coconut oil and humic acid. Coconut oil has been shown to act as a natural antiviral by enveloping infected cells and destroying their cell walls. Humic acid is very helpful for latent infections because it prevents a reactivated virus from entering your cells and reproducing, which eventually reduces your viral load.

Treating bacterial infections: Yersinia and H. pylori

For *H. pylori,* you can use a natural treatment that combines mastic gum, zinc, berberine, and bismuth citrate. Several companies make this product.

For yersinia, my first line of defense is a combination herbal formula composed of berberine, sweet wormwood, grapefruit seed extract, black walnut, and uva ursi (see Resources). If those don't work, antibiotics should do the trick. I don't normally recommend antibiotics became of the serious damage they do to your microbiome and therefore to your digestive and immune systems. However, in this case, I think they are warranted. You should be taking probiotics anyway, but you especially need to take them when you're taking antibiotics. Otherwise, the disruption to your gut bacteria can undermine digestion, sabotage your immune system, and generally wreak havoc with your health. (Plus, you're likely to gain weight.)

For SIBO, you will be taking the supplements listed on pages 260–261 as part of your individualized supplement plan. You can also get a prescription from your doctor for Xifaxan, a gut-specific antibiotic—but if you do, *please* remember to take probiotics, as you should also do whenever taking antibiotics.

Treating parasites: Toxoplasmosis and Blastocystis hominis

For toxoplasmosis, you need to see your doctor, who will probably suggest antibiotics. Again, make sure you take probiotics too or your gut bacteria—and therefore your digestive and immune systems—will really suffer.

To treat *Blastocystis hominis*, you will be taking the supplements listed on page 262 as part of your individualized supplement plan. You can also get a prescription from your doctor for Flagyl, an antibiotic—but if you do, *please* remember to take probiotics, as you should whenever taking antibiotics.

Whenever You Take Antibiotics, Take Probiotics!

This is beyond critical—make *sure* you support your gut while you're on antibiotics. As the name suggests, antibiotics kills biota—that is, gut bacteria. Sure, some of that bacteria is out to do you harm, but a lot of it wants to keep your gut and your whole body in optimal shape. You want to replenish the friendly bacteria while you're trying to kill off the bad guys—via *probiotics,* pills, powders, or capsules that contain billions of friendly bacteria. You'll be taking probiotics on The Myers Way Thyroid Connection Plan, but going forward, whenever you are taking antibiotics, make sure you're balancing their effects with daily probiotics.

In addition to probiotics, it's often useful to take a type of yeast called *Saccharomyces boulardii,* commonly known as *S. boulardii.* This fabulous friendly yeast helps counter the effects of unfriendly yeast and is known to help prevent antibiotic-associated diarrhea as well as the infection *C. difficile,* another common result of taking antibiotics. It's amazing how powerful *S. boulardii* can be, and I can't think why doctors don't commonly prescribe it whenever they prescribe antibiotics. However, some people do find that it makes their yeast issues worse, so if you notice unwanted symptoms, stop taking it.

You're also taking L-glutamine during The Myers Way, but if you have to take antibiotics after your twenty-eight days, please take L-glutamine then too. That will protect your gut lining and help it rejuvenate from any of the antibiotics' effects, thereby preventing leaky gut.

HOW BERNADETTE HEALED HER INFECTIONS

As Bernadette continued with The Myers Way Thyroid Connection Plan, we also had her follow the 4R gut-healing program that I described on page 154. She took L-glutamine to heal her gut lining, digestive enzymes and Betaine HCl to improve digestion, and probiotics to replenish her friendly gut bacteria. Fixing her gut gave a huge boost to her immune system, which helped her defeat the lingering Epstein-Barr and yersinia.

I also gave her the herbal formula to counteract yersinia, and I gave her Lauricidin and humic acid for her Epstein-Barr. If the herbal preparation hadn't worked, I would have prescribed antibiotics (with probiotics!), but, fortunately, Bernadette responded well and her infections cleared up.

I explained to Bernadette that stress can also trigger infections, so I urged her to try the stress-relief suggestions that you will read about in the next chapter. Alleviating stress every day, rather than allowing it to build up, can be a huge support to every aspect of your health.

Bernadette was relieved to have solved the final piece of her healing puzzle. With the infections gone, her symptoms resolved and her energy levels bounced back. No more brain fog or fatigue—just optimal, glowing health.

CHAPTER 10

The Stress Solution

My patient Laila had a complicated, interesting life as an international business consultant. She was often crossing time zones as she flew to China, Japan, and other locations in South Asia. When she wasn't traveling to Asia, she was on the phone at odd hours speaking with colleagues in those far-flung time zones. To make her life even more interesting, her boyfriend was in the foreign service in Europe, adding another set of time zones and travel destinations into the mix. As you might imagine, this schedule played havoc with Laila's sleep patterns.

Laila's job was quite challenging in any case, especially since she had begun working for her latest department head. The man who'd hired Laila had been warm and understanding, and Laila had always felt highly motivated in working for him. The new woman who had taken over Laila's division seemed to be far more demanding, and Laila never knew whether her boss would be pleased with her work or not. As a result, she was often worried about work.

Laila had always been physically active, and even with her demanding work schedule, she managed to make time for CrossFit several days a week. When she traveled, she went running. She told me that this vigorous exercise schedule helped her blow off steam, and if she had to sacrifice sleep or socializing to keep to her regimen, she always did.

When Laila came to me, she had all the signs of hyperthyroidism: racing heart, insomnia, trembling muscles, frequent panic attacks. I thought she might well have Graves' disease, which would mean that both her thyroid and her immune system were functioning poorly, and

I ordered a complete panel of thyroid blood work to see exactly what was going on. Meanwhile, when I took Laila's detailed history, I learned about her demanding schedule.

Although I wouldn't have an exact diagnosis until the labs came back, I did pick up a few red flags in Laila's story — factors that were almost certainly disrupting the effective functioning of both her thyroid and her immune system:

- *Her lack of regular, restful sleep.* While her recent symptoms included insomnia and other sleep disturbances, Laila admitted that ever since she had started her internationally focused job, her sleep had been irregular and often insufficient. Lack of sleep disrupts thyroid function, partly by raising stress levels. As we saw in chapter 3, stress is not just psychological — it's also physical. Not giving your body the sleep it needs is a huge — and very common — stressor.
- *Her intense exercise schedule.* Like many of my patients, Laila was probably exercising too intensely for the needs of her body, and this too disrupted thyroid function. A lot of my thyroid patients do extreme forms of exercise that push their bodies to the max — CrossFit, marathon training, Ironman, boot camps. For some people, these are great, but for most, these types of exercise are more physically demanding than their bodies can handle, especially after they reach their thirties or forties. If intense exercise is not right for your body, your stress hormones and thyroid gland will protest.
- *Her psychological stress.* Laila's anxiety about her boss's responses kept her stress levels perpetually high. Even with more sleep and healthier exercise choices, Laila would need to find ways to relieve this stress if her thyroid and immune system were to achieve optimal function. While Laila may not have had control over this stressful aspect of her life, she could find ways in the evenings, on weekends, and even during the day to relieve the stress, bringing her stress hormones down and engaging the relaxation response.

I explained to Laila that if she did indeed have Graves' disease, these factors were playing a significant role, as they do in all forms of thyroid and autoimmune dysfunction. (So whatever your condition, this all applies to you too!) And in fact, her lab work came back positive for Graves'. For Laila to get well, we would need to relieve her stress. She would need to get regular, restful sleep, exercise in ways that better suited her body, and alleviate the stress she felt about her job and her boss.

Stress is a very common factor in thyroid dysfunction and autoimmune conditions, but perhaps at this point it will not surprise you to learn that most conventional practitioners basically ignore it in treating both types of dysfunction. Well, we are *not* going to ignore it. So let's take a closer look.

HOW STRESS MESSES WITH YOUR THYROID AND IMMUNE SYSTEM

As we saw in chapters 3 and 4, stress of all types disrupts thyroid and immune function in a number of ways.

• Your body redirects its resources *toward* coping with the stressor ("Danger! Danger!") and *away* from business as usual, including thyroid and immune function.

• Stress suppresses your gut function, leading to leaky gut, a major factor in autoimmune disorders. If you have an autoimmune condition, leaky gut will make it worse. If you don't have one, leaky gut could help bring one on. Because the vast majority of serotonin is made in your gut, leaky gut (which depletes serotonin) can also contribute to depression, anxiety, and insomnia.

• Excess cortisol cues your body to slow its production of thyroid hormone.

• Stress hormones reduce the conversion of T4 to T3, making less of the active form of the hormone available to you. They also increase the conversion of T4 and free T3 into reverse T3, effectively putting the brakes on your metabolism.

• Excess cortisol engenders excess estrogen. Estrogen promotes thyroxine-binding globulin, causing more thyroid hormone to *bind* so that your body has less free T4 and free T3 to work with.

• Inflammatory immune cells known as *cytokines* are also part of the stress response, and they create thyroid hormone resistance, making your thyroid receptors less sensitive to thyroid hormone. As a result, even if blood tests show that you have enough thyroid hormone—and even if you're taking supplemental hormone—your cells can't absorb the hormone properly, and you still end up with symptoms.

Unfortunately, there isn't nearly as much research into the effects of stress as there should be. Perhaps because you can't exactly medicate stress, conventional medicine has tended to ignore it. I do want to tell you about two studies that really gave me pause, though. In one, researchers found that stress increased the occurrence of Graves' eightfold. In the other, severe emotional stress was seen to be the primary precipitating factor in 14 percent of those studied with Graves'.

When I think of my own stressors before I developed Graves'—the relatively sudden death of my mother and the challenges of being a second-year medical student—I wish I'd known about those studies. At least I know about them now, though, so I can recognize similar factors in the lives of patients like Laila. And now I've got way more resources to *relieve* stress, all of which you'll learn about later in this chapter.

First, though, I want you to be able to test your own adrenal function so you'll have some data on the role that physical, mental, and emotional stress might be playing in your body.

DO I HAVE ADRENAL DYSFUNCTION?

Ask just about any conventional doctor, and he or she will tell you that there are only two types of adrenal dysfunction worth mentioning: Addison's disease, in which the adrenals are seriously underproducing, and Cushing's syndrome, in which they are seriously overproducing. These two ends of the spectrum are the result of various structural problems; in Addison's, the adrenals are not capable of producing enough stress hormones; in Cushing's, the adrenal glands are forced to produce too much. This can be caused by steroids—a common treatment for many conditions, including autoimmune disorders—or by an adrenal or a pituitary tumor.

These diseases are relatively rare, though, while adrenal dysfunction—the middle of the spectrum—is incredibly common. The vast majority of my patients have it when they first come in, and I'm sorry to say that most of the people I meet outside my clinic seem to have it too. Read just about any blog or Facebook page, and you'll hear people talking about feeling stressed, overwhelmed, on edge, burned out, "no good till I have my coffee," "ready for a nap by midafternoon," and "snapping at my spouse and my kids, even though they don't deserve it." Those are the symptoms of adrenal dysfunction, folks, and we could probably call it our national disease.

What's going on in your body when you feel tired, wired, edgy, foggy, and frequently dependent on caffeine? Basically, your adrenals are producing either not enough stress hormones, too much, or both; too much during some parts of the day and not enough during others. And as we saw in chapter 3, this type of dysfunction has a huge impact on your thyroid, your immune system, and your overall health and well-being.

This is another one of those "which came first, the chicken or the egg" scenarios. Sometimes an underperforming thyroid causes your adrenals to go into overdrive so that instead of being powered by thyroid hormone, your body is relying on stress hormones for energy, motivation, and focus. Then, when you finally start taking supplemental thyroid hormone, you end up with symptoms like shaking hands or a racing heart because you've now got the right amount of thyroid hormone but too much stress hormones.

Malfunctioning adrenals also stress out your thyroid, as your thyroid tries to compensate for those missing stress hormones. Eventually, you have dysfunction in two systems instead of one—and each dysfunction keeps making the other one worse.

How do we break this vicious cycle? Often, we begin by testing to find out whether you actually have adrenal dysfunction, because with a malfunctioning thyroid, it can be hard to tell. Conventional doctors typically rely on a blood test to measure cortisol levels, but I don't find that very useful. After all, your stress hormone levels fluctuate significantly throughout the day. In a healthy body, they will be highest in the morning and lowest as you prepare to fall asleep, with small spikes along the way as you encounter and respond to challenges.

So, if you're struggling with adrenal dysfunction, you might feel sleepy and foggy in the morning because stress hormone levels are too low and then perhaps feel wired and edgy at night when they begin to rise and keep you awake. You might also respond with huge surges of stress hormones throughout the day as you face various challenges, or, like Laila, you might be at a continually high level for most of the day as you anxiously cope with a hard-to-please boss, a sick child, or some other upsetting situation.

So I begin with giving my patients the questionnaire on pages 265–266. If, based on your results, you need adrenal support, I've made some suggestions to include in your Myers Way Thyroid Connection Plan. There is a more accurate saliva test you can take, but you will need a functional medicine practitioner to order and interpret it for you.

Treating adrenal dysfunction: Herbs and supplements

When I told Laila that we could help address her adrenal dysfunction with herbs and supplements, her eyes lit up. I could see exactly what was going through her mind.

"You're thinking that if you take these herbs and supplements, you won't have to make other changes," I said. "You think you can keep skimping on sleep, pushing your body too hard with CrossFit and running, and ignoring your work stress as though it weren't a genuine problem."

Laila nodded guiltily. I sighed.

"Look," I told her, "the herbs and supplements are going to make a difference, and I want you to benefit from them. But it's like I'm handing you a bigger bucket so you can bail water out of your leaky boat faster—you still need to plug the leaks. Otherwise, you're setting yourself up for more thyroid dysfunction and more immune issues— maybe even for another autoimmune condition. Sleep, exercise, and psychological stress relief aren't 'extras,' and they can't be fixed by taking a pill. Let's use the herbs and supplements to give you a jump start— but we still have to get to the root of the problem."

What I told her, I'm telling you. In a moment, you'll learn about several herbs and supplements that can make a big difference in your adrenal health (again, see pages 267–269 to find out if you need them). That will give you a fabulous feel-good boost, and within a few weeks, you should notice that you feel calmer, more energized, and more optimistic. I'm happy for you just thinking about it!

But however well the adrenal supplements work, please don't make the mistake of ignoring the other types of physical, mental, and emotional stress in your life. If you do, you're setting yourself up for failure—and I want you to set yourself up for success!

As a starting point, first I recommend the following vitamins and minerals, which you are already going to take as part of The Myers Way:

- *Magnesium.* If you're stressed, you tend to excrete extra magnesium through your urine, so you want to supplement, especially since magnesium deficiency can make you anxious or depressed. Magnesium gives you a buffer against stress by raising the point at which your adrenals trigger the fight-or-flight response so that little things don't set off your anger, frustration, or despair quite so quickly. This is also a great supplement for sleep problems.

- *Vitamin B complex* is crucial—that's what your adrenals use to make stress hormones, and that's why stress depletes vitamin B. When your adrenals are deprived of B vitamins, they start working less well and—you get the picture. Interrupt the stress cycle with some Bs, and breathe a sigh of relief.

- *Vitamin C.* Many parts of your body use vitamin C, of course, but the highest concentration of this fabulous antioxidant is in our adrenals, which use it to make cortisol and other stress hormones. Stress depletes your store of vitamin C too, so make sure to replenish, especially since a shortage of vitamin C is itself a trigger for excess cortisol.

You most likely want to supplement with magnesium, B vitamins, and vitamin C for life.

Second, for an additional short-term boost when you have adrenal dysfunction, I recommend *adaptogenic herbs*. These wonder herbs have two different effects. If your adrenal hormones are too low, the herbs will boost them. If your adrenal hormones are too high, they will lower them. Amazing, but true—they are self-adjusting!

Third, I recommend a hormone known as dehydroepiandrosterone (DHEA), one of the most abundant compounds produced by the adrenal glands. Your body converts it into androgens and estrogens, which affect multiple metabolic processes. If you're past the age of twenty-five, you have been experiencing a natural decline in DHEA since then— which is normal, but sometimes your DHEA drops *too* low, and then we want to give it a little boost. In people whose levels are low, supplemental DHEA has been shown to increase emotional well-being and immune function.

Autoimmune dysfunction is associated with low levels of DHEA, and even people without autoimmune disorders are often running low. So here's what I want you to do—get your doctor to test your levels. If they are below 100, work with your doctor to get your levels to 100 or above. Whatever you do, *please* don't self-medicate with DHEA. I know it's available over the counter, but it is a hormone that converts to testosterone, and, ultimately, estrogen, so you really need to take it under the care of someone who knows what he or she is doing.

Self-Help—or Getting Help?

I've given you a lot of tools and resources to help bring your stress hormones into balance while supporting your adrenals, thyroid, and immune system. In many cases, a do-it-yourself approach is all you need. But if you don't notice a marked improvement after twenty-eight days of following The Myers Way Thyroid Connection Plan, you might want to find a functional medicine practitioner. The thyroid-adrenal relationship is a delicate balance, and it sometimes takes several months of testing and tinkering with doses before you can get the balance exactly right. You *can* achieve optimal health—but you might need some extra patience and help in getting there.

SLEEP YOUR WAY TO HEALTH

One of the keys to getting deep, regular sleep is to maintain a good *circadian rhythm*. That's a term for your body's regular daily rhythms. Many of your hormone receptors are geared to these rhythms, which may be governed by clock genes that evolved to keep your body adjusted to the daily, seasonal, and annual rhythms of the planet. A whole body of new research has found that metabolism and weight are very profoundly interconnected with circadian rhythms, as explained in a May 2014 article in the journal *Advances in Nutrition*. I conclude that your thyroid's optimal function depends on this daily cycle, which is why sleep is so important.

One of the major cues that your body uses to regulate its activity is the amount of light in your surroundings. Not surprisingly, we evolved to be awake when it is light and asleep when it is dark, with numerous hormonal and metabolic cues linked to those primal patterns. When we don't follow them, our thyroid and metabolism suffer.

You can see from this explanation why Laila's irregular sleep schedule might have been causing problems for her. Her frequent shifts in time zone and schedule made it hard for her to sleep, while her insufficient, irregular sleep kept boosting her stress hormones. Then, feeling stressed, she had even more difficulty sleeping.

Laila and I talked about how she could try to arrange her work and travel schedule to minimize disruption as far as possible. We also went over the following suggestions that she could follow to improve the quality of her sleep:

• Get as much natural light as possible during the day, and get outside as close to first thing in the morning as you can. Being in natural light cues your circadian rhythms that you are awake. Ideally, you'll be outside within thirty minutes of waking up.

• Determine the number of hours of sleep you need—and then make sure you get them! Give yourself a couple of weekend days when you can sleep uninterrupted, without an alarm to wake you up. That's how you'll know how much sleep you really need. Then count backward from the time you need to wake up to make sure you get the right amount of sleep.

• As far as you can, go to bed and wake up at the same times every day. For Laila, this was often challenging—hopefully, for you, it will be less so. Ideally, early to bed and early to rise is healthier for you than late and late—10:00 p.m. to 6:00 a.m. is probably optimal, but many of us have lives that simply don't accommodate that schedule. Or you may find that your optimal sleep time is nine or ten hours. Just do the best you can! If you have children, you know how important it is to get them on a schedule. Guess what—your body needs that too!

• Progress slowly through the evening with amber light. After sundown, you want to replace your bright white lights with amber bulbs or wear amber glasses (see Resources) to cue your body toward nighttime. I recommend getting the f.lux program for your computer—it's free, and it will shift the color of your computer's light from blue to orange as the sun goes down. Most smartphones and iPads now have a night-shift setting that will change the lighting on your device to an amber color based on the time of day.

• Keep your sleep space as dark as possible. Your body needs to believe that it is surrounded by complete darkness to enter into the deepest, most restful sleep. You especially want to block out the blue light emitted by electronic screens and many types of lightbulbs, as these mimic most closely the effects of daylight, altering your circadian clock. Sleep masks and blackout curtains are very helpful. Keep electronics out of the bedroom, turn off electronic devices, or at least thoroughly cover their screens with red sheets that block out blue and green light (see Resources).

• Sleep cool, not warm. Your body temperature needs to drop to maintain a healthy circadian rhythm. Make sure your bedroom is cool or even cold.

• Institute an electronic sundown. At least one hour before bed, turn off all screens: phone, computer, television. Your goal is to minimize your exposure to blue light as your body prepares itself for sleep.

- You also want to keep electronics out of the bedroom to minimize your exposure to the electromagnetic fields (EMFs) that they emit. While we don't yet know all the effects of EMFs, they're just another exposure that your body doesn't need.

I told Laila that the nutrients and supplements on The Myers Way Thyroid Connection Plan would make a big difference in her sleep quality. For example, selenium, which your thyroid needs, is also crucial to good sleep. Bringing down your inflammation will also support your sleep, as will getting the right type of exercise (next section) and practicing stress relief (the section after that).

FINDING THE RIGHT EXERCISE: THE GOLDILOCKS APPROACH

Here's the challenge when it comes to exercise: You want enough difficulty to stress your muscles a *little* but not too much—that is, like Goldilocks, you want the level of stress that is *just right*. Sure, pushing yourself to the limit can sometimes feel terrific because of the endorphin rush that your body generates in response. But that rush can mask an underlying problem as your adrenals and thyroid struggle with what they perceive as danger rather than an invigorating workout.

How can you find your perfect balance? The first step is to take the questionnaire on pages 265–266. If you are suffering from adrenal dysfunction, there's only one healthy response: cut back on any intense exercise, at least until your adrenals and thyroid are in better shape. If you have the energy, by all means, get some exercise, but don't overdo it. If you push yourself too hard, you are likely to feel fatigued, stressed, and foggy, and you put yourself at risk of gaining weight rather than achieving a healthy weight.

Here are some ways to keep your body moving during The Myers Way Thyroid Connection Plan. Pick the level of energy that fits where you are now—not where you'd like to be or used to be. You can always work up gradually to a more vigorous schedule when your body has had time to heal.

Low intensity

- Walking
- Stretching
- Restorative yoga

Medium intensity

- Pilates
- Playing with your kids
- Swimming
- Dancing
- Jogging

High intensity

- Cycling
- Running
- Tennis
- Weight lifting
- Hot yoga
- Interval training
- CrossFit

A NEW APPROACH TO STRESS RELIEF

When Laila and I began to talk about stress relief, I could see that the very idea was making her anxious.

"Dr. Myers," she said, "people have been telling me to relax and calm down my entire life! Believe me, I would if I could, but it's just really hard for me to wind down. I've tried yoga, I've tried meditation, but they just don't work for me. Everyone else in the class is blissing out, and I'm sitting there trying to remember if I took the chicken out of the freezer for dinner or whether I have time to run to the dry cleaner's on the way home. And my job just *is* really stressful, especially with this new boss. I just don't see what I can do about it."

I also have a highly demanding job that is frequently stressful, and I too have a mind that likes to keep working even when my body is at rest. Yet I know too much now about how stress disrupts thyroid and immune function—I can't just leave stress relief off the list because it's hard!

Fortunately, there is a way that Laila and I—and you too—can have it both ways. We don't have to become entirely different people, and we don't have to back off from our commitments. This is true for you too, whether the stress in your life comes from work, family issues, personal concerns, or some of each. The goal here is not to *eliminate* stress but to *relieve* it—to balance the hours of being alert, focused, and active with thirty to sixty minutes of being calm, relaxed, and at rest. Remember, your autonomic nervous system has two halves: a sympathetic nervous system to gear you up and a parasympathetic nervous system to bring you down. You just need to make sure that every single day you engage the parasympathetic nervous system for a while so that your revved-up stress can be balanced with a wind-down hour.

Yoga is terrific, of course, and if it works for you, I'm all for it. Its health benefits have been documented in multiple studies, and it will do wonders for your thyroid and immune system as well as for your entire body and overall well-being. Go, yoga!

But if you're looking for other ways to de-stress, you're in luck, because I have spent quite a bit of time pulling together a long list of delicious, relaxing options. Here are a few of my favorite tools—I'd love for you to do one or two of these once or twice a day.

Binaural beats

In the mid-1800s, the physicist Heinrich Wilhelm Dove discovered that when your brain receives two different frequencies—one in each ear—it creates a third frequency in an effort to synchronize them. This third frequency can be used to guide your mind into a more relaxed state that helps you disconnect from your anxiety and enables you to relax and feel more positive. It's basically an aid to achieving the state of mind that experienced meditators attain. You can also use this technique for even deeper relaxation, similar to the state you experience during a profound sleep.

There are many different types of binaural beats albums, so you just need to determine the right one for you. Many can easily be found on iTunes and played directly from your smartphone. For more information on how to use binaural beats, see Resources.

HeartMath

Here's a fascinating fact: When you're stressed, your heart rate is more regular; when you're relaxed, the intervals between heartbeats vary. So if you've been told that your pulse is 60 beats per minute, it's actually more like 55 beats one minute and 65 the next. Also, when you inhale, your heart rate speeds up; when you exhale, it slows down. This is known as *heart-rate variability (HRV),* and the lack of it has been linked to a number of disorders, including heart disease, diabetes, and post-traumatic stress disorder (PTSD).

Although we don't yet know how to measure a person's stress levels, heart-rate variability is probably a good benchmark. If your HRV is high, you're less stressed and more resilient. If your HRV is low, you're more stressed and less resilient. Accordingly, if you can increase your HRV, you can bring your stress levels down.

How can you increase something as automatic as your heart rate? Ah, that's where HeartMath comes in (see Resources for where to buy)—a wonderful feedback mechanism that lets you know when your HRV is up and when it's down. It turns out that simply getting the feedback helps you learn to adjust your HRV more consciously.

If you've got a smartphone, you can get a HeartMath Inner Balance app, which uses an external sensor on your earlobe to help you synchronize your heart rate, breath, and mind. It's super-easy to use as well as convenient. Plus, as a very goal-oriented person (yes, even in my stress reduction!), I love that the app lets you set goals and track your progress. You can also find a wide range of inexpensive monitors to use in the form of ear clips, finger clips, chest straps, and even "smart" clothing.

When you start to monitor your own HRV, a wonderful thing begins to happen. First, you notice when you're stressed—something that many of us aren't aware of. Second, you can take tiny but effective means to de-stress. Say you've just come out of an important meeting and are rushing to the bathroom before your next phone call. Or perhaps you've just dropped off one of your kids at school and are dashing to the grocery store before it's time to put your second child down for her nap. Either way, you're stressed and rushed—but you probably don't even realize it. Check your HRV, though, and you'll see it's down. And if you can pause for just the space of ten deep breaths—not even a minute!—you can immediately boost your HRV. Your stress releases, your body says, "Thanks!," and you go on to your next task. What a fabulous invention!

Biofeedback

Like HeartMath, this approach gives you feedback on what's happening within your body—feedback that you can then use to let go of stress. Biofeedback has been used to treat stress as well as a number of other conditions, including asthma, chronic pain, constipation, high blood pressure, incontinence, irritable bowel syndrome, migraine, and stress headaches. People also use it to cope with the side effects of chemotherapy. In all these cases, you have more control over your body's responses than you think. Biofeedback empowers you to become aware of how your thoughts and actions affect your body so that you can induce the effects you want.

Usually, you sign up for a few sessions at a clinic, where you are connected to a variety of electrical sensors that measure heart rate, skin temperature, brain waves, and muscle function. If you're getting biofeedback for stress, you might see that the machine beeps or a red light flashes as your body tenses up. By using various relaxation techniques, you can make the beeps or the flashing stop. In this way, you become more aware of your body's responses and you gain the power to direct them, shifting from a tense state into a relaxed one. By enabling you to increase your awareness of your own body, biofeedback is remarkably effective.

Biofeedback is a growing field that offers a wide variety of approaches.

- Electromyography gives you feedback on muscle tension.
- Thermal biofeedback measures your skin temperature, since that usually drops under stress.

- Galvanic skin response training measures the amount of sweat produced by your sweat glands — a key indicator of anxiety.
- Heart-rate variability biofeedback is basically HeartMath.

You can also buy biofeedback devices. Some are handheld, others connect to your computer, and still others are apps, like the HeartMath monitor. Check with your doctor to see what's available, or check out the Resource section of this book.

Audio-Visual entrainment (brain-wave entrainment)

This is a technique that involves using visual patterns plus sounds to induce a hypnotic state of relaxation: you look at the waves on eyeglasses while listening to the sounds (like binaural beats) through headphones. I've been using it during the time I was working on this book, and it's been fantastic! It's an initial investment of about three hundred dollars — but I promise you, the emotional and mental de-stressing is worth it. The brain boost you get not only can relax you; it also helps with academic and sports performance, anxiety, depression, ADHD, pain, and seasonal affective disorder (SAD). (See Resources for one I use.)

Infrared sauna therapy

Gosh, I love this one! I have an infrared sauna at home that I use most nights. As you might remember from chapter 8, you can get your own infrared sauna — they even make portable ones for apartments — or find a spa or gym that has one. In my sauna (see Resources for the brand I use) I often use the time to meditate, do HeartMath, or listen to binaural beats. I also edited much of this book and *The Autoimmune Solution* while detoxing and relaxing in my sauna.

Relaxing hot bath

It's a classic for a reason! I love winding down my evening with a relaxing hot bath with Epsom salts and essential oils. Epsom salts are full of magnesium, which helps to relieve tension and relax your muscles. A few drops of your favorite organic essential oil can create a relaxing environment as well. I like to make my own bath salts because they are so easy and much cheaper that way. I personally enjoy the silence, but music has been known to lower cortisol levels, so feel free to listen to your favorite tunes or binaural beats in the tub. Turning off the overhead and relying on candlelight or an amber light can help cue your body toward restful sleep. Making your bath a nightly ritual can also help with sleep rhythms. But you know what? There is just about *no* way to do this wrong, so please—enjoy!

Nature walks

Please add these to your prescriptions for good health! As we have seen, getting out into natural light during the day is good for your circadian rhythms, while some gentle walking—or, if you're able, a not-too-challenging hike—is a great way to let go of physical stress. (Serious hiking and climbing go under the heading of exercise, so make sure you're not stressing your body too greatly, especially if you're struggling with adrenal dysfunction.)

Nature walks also put you in touch with the awe-inspiring qualities of our natural world, and that is great for your immune system as well as your state of mind. I personally find that when I'm out walking, I'm able to marvel at the beauties of the world around me, so my list-making mind gives way to my sense of wonder and appreciation. If you can build some nature walks into your day, your week, or your month, your thyroid and immune system will be grateful.

Here's an extremely cool new idea that brings us back to the way our ancestors used to live: *earthing,* in which you walk barefoot on the soil. This is relaxing for many reasons, not least of which being that the bacteria in the soil are very friendly—the kind you want in your gut—and they help your body produce serotonin, a natural antidepressant that assists in regulating sleep. Proponents of earthing also claim that it provides you with a mixture of ions that help balance your electrical charge. Whatever the reason, we can all agree that feeling the cool grass or the warm sand under your feet is a great way to relieve stress.

Time with loved ones

Have you ever noticed how much better you feel when you get off the phone with a dear friend or after you've spent an evening with your partner? That's not just psychological — your cortisol levels have dropped and your whole body feels better. Many of us have trouble making time for our loved ones; something always seems to be more important. But your health really will benefit from having fun and feeling connected, so do what you can to make that a regular part of your life.

Breathing, prayer, and meditation

There are so many ways in which you can benefit from these approaches to stress relief. One of the most exciting — which I have been using while writing this book — is known as Muse (see Resources), a head-band that measures your brain's response to meditation and gives you feedback in real time. This helps you achieve deeper and move effective meditation.

Just breathing deep-belly breaths can shift you from sympathetic stress to parasympathetic relaxation mode. Here's one deep-belly breathing exercise that I use when I am stressed or anxious:

- With one hand on the chest and the other on the belly, take a deep breath in through the nose, ensuring the diaphragm (not the chest) inflates with enough air to create a stretch in the lungs.
- Inhale over a count of 6.
- Exhale over a count of 6.

If someone is getting on your last nerve, if you doubt your own ability to make it to the end of the day, if you just feel the tension mounting — *stop,* do ten cycles, and then go on about your business. Once you start noticing your own stress levels and relieving them even in this tiny way, you'll be amazed at how much better you (and your thyroid!) feel.

WEEKLY STRESS RELIEF

The stress-relief techniques I've just listed are all practices that you can do at home, at your convenience—which is what makes them so useful. But once a week I would like you to step it up a bit. Try one of the relaxation techniques I describe below. Once you find a technique that works for you, enjoy it as often as your schedule and budget permit.

Acupuncture

This is one of my biggest go-tos for stress relief. I try to go every Friday—it's my happy hour!

Acupuncture feels so good, I honestly don't care why, but the scientist in me was pleased to read a 2013 study that was published in the *Journal of Endocrinology*. Researchers at Georgetown University School of Nursing and Health Studies found that acupuncture seemed to relieve stress by blocking the HPA release of stress hormones along with the peptide involved in the fight-or-flight response. Pretty cool, huh? If you need to release stress at the end of *your* week, I urge you to find your own healthy happy hour!

Float tank

This is like a warm Epsom-salts bath on steroids! Basically, you float in salt water, at skin temperature, inside a soundproof tank with no light—that is, you've got absolutely no stimulation whatsoever, and you're not making any effort to do anything; you're just simply floating, resting, relieved of absolutely all responsibility for the duration of your float. The technical name for this approach is restricted environmental stimulation therapy, or REST, which suits it very well.

Local float-tank centers are popping up all over the place—a simple Google search can help you find one. You'll usually have your choice of either an hour or ninety minutes. You can even buy a float tank for your home, although they are quite expensive.

As I told Laila, float tanks are especially good for sleep disturbances and insomnia, and also for recovering from jet lag. I encouraged her to use them while she traveled, if possible, and as a sort of time-zone detox every time she came home. Float tanks are terrific for stress relief—your cortisol levels drop, which is great for your adrenals, thyroid, and immune system. They're also good for pain relief—the relaxation cues your body to release endorphins and remove the lactic acid that causes muscle pain. A number of studies confirm that flotation tanks relieve stress, anxiety, depression, and fibromyalgia while improving blood circulation, your body's self-healing abilities, and immune function. They also seem to enhance scientific creativity as well as performance in a number of sports. One study even found that it improves your ability at the piano!

Massage

When I shared this stress-relief approach with Laila, she was skeptical at first. How could the luxurious experience of getting a massage be good for her health? But massages are not only one of life's greatest treats, they are also absolutely wonderful for lowering your cortisol levels and letting go of stress. They're good for sleep problems too, and I promise your brain will work better once you've been getting regular massages.

If you can manage it, I urge you to make a massage part of your weekly routine—or at least, get one once a month. Even better, learn to notice when you are feeling especially stressed and, if you can, book a massage to help you release the extra layers of tension. If price is a concern, see if there's a massage school in your area. Often, the students will offer massages at lower rates.

Neurofeedback

A subcategory of biofeedback, and one that I personally have gotten a lot of benefit from, is known as *neurofeedback*. Basically, you get feedback on how your brain is operating so that you can modulate processes that usually happen subconsciously. For example, your brain needs to be in a specific state to fall asleep. So you might wear a cap with electrodes that measures brain-wave activity, and when your brain is in the proper state of relaxation or readiness for sleep, you see a green circle become larger on the screen.

I know it seems mysterious, but somehow, just by getting that visual feedback, you become able to put your brain into the state that affects the circle — and that enables you to sleep and/or relax. My own experience is that you begin to recognize what relaxation feels like, and that recognition enables you to re-create it. It all happens remarkably quickly, a testament to the power of your brain!

Neurofeedback has been found to be especially useful for treating such neurological issues as ADHD, epilepsy, traumatic brain injury, and other related conditions. It's also super-useful for stress, anxiety, and sleep disorders.

...And more!

Here are some other stress-relieving strategies that my patients and I have found useful:

- Art: You can relieve stress both by making art and looking at art.
- Counseling: Psychodynamic therapy, cognitive-behavioral therapy, or art or music therapy are all options that can be helpful.
- Dance it out: Put on a favorite song and dance your stress away.
- Eye movement desensitization and reprocessing (EMDR): This form of therapy focuses on letting go of traumatic events or upsetting feelings.
- Hot tub, whirlpool, or Jacuzzi: All are super-relaxing, even if you go in for just a ten-minute soak.
- Martial arts: These incorporate relaxation and stress relief in their vigorous workouts.
- Music: Studies show that just half an hour's worth of listening can cause your cortisol levels to drop.
- Passion: Make some time for whatever you're passionate about.
- Pets: This one is huge for me; just looking at my dog, Mocha, makes me happy.
- Play: Whatever makes you happy will relieve your stress. Go for it!
- Sex: Nature's own stress reliever, in all its forms. Highly recommended.
- Shake it off: Literally, shake your arm, leg, or head and envision shaking off the worry or stress, especially after having an upsetting conversation or receiving a difficult piece of news.

- Tai chi: There are many forms of tai chi, from the martial-artist version to a far less demanding approach, but all involve breathing, relaxation, and stress relief.
- Tapping: This practice is an integral part of Emotional Freedom Technique (EFT), a way of letting go of stressful thoughts or emotions.
- Tea: Take even five minutes to sit quietly with a fragrant cup of caffeine-free herbal tea, focusing on the smell, the warmth, and the taste.

HOW LAILA SOLVED HER STRESS PROBLEM

Laila had already committed to the diet portion of The Myers Way Thyroid Connection Plan. She found ways to bring her own Laila-friendly foods with her on the long plane rides, and she found her own go-to restaurants in each of her frequent destinations.

Beyond diet, however, Laila realized how much sleep, exercise, and stress were exacerbating her Graves' disease, and she decided that she had to make some changes. As she and I began to work with the thyroid-calming herbs and supplements, Laila addressed these other areas of her life.

Although she had really enjoyed her extreme exercise routines, we agreed that until her thyroid had fully healed, the best exercise for her was to focus on stress reduction with no exercise more intense than gentle walking.

For stress relief, Laila originally tried neurofeedback, but she found it was just too time-consuming for her busy schedule. HeartMath worked better because she could do it at odd moments on her phone, which of course she always had with her. She discovered that she really enjoyed making time to talk with loved ones, which she had been neglecting in favor of work and exercise. She also came to love a nightly ritual of a warm, scented bath under the glow of amber lights with her favorite music playing in the background.

Laila's favorite stress-release tool, though, turned out to be the flotation tank. I was delighted, because they are terrific for helping you reset your sleep schedule. We agreed that she was not going to be able to keep to an ideal circadian rhythm but that she would find flotation tanks on her trips abroad as well as make regular visits to one in her neighborhood. Blackout curtains, an electronic sundown, and amber lightbulbs also made a significant difference in her sleep patterns. Laila even carried amber eyeglasses and a sleep mask with her when she traveled so she could make her hotel room more conducive to sleep.

Over the next six months, as her stress reduced and her thyroid responded to the calming herbs and supportive supplements, she began to add in a few sessions of swimming. She found that she loved the quiet, thoughtful time she spent in the water. For Laila, swimming was the best of both worlds: a vigorous workout *and* a way to give her thyroid and adrenals a break.

As I met with Laila over several months, we kept coming back to the idea that her responses were a work in progress. I told her that she didn't have to find the perfect stress-relief program right away, that she could be gentle with herself and give herself time to work out the lifestyle that was right for her. The important thing was to be aware of how her choices affected her body, so she could choose the strategies that would leave her calm yet energized throughout a long and satisfying life.

After several months, Laila's Graves' symptoms subsided, her antibodies disappeared, and she no longer needed any form of medication. Although if she didn't follow The Myers Way Thyroid Connection Plan, her Graves' might come back, the right diet and lifestyle could keep her thyroid, immune system, and gut all functioning at peak condition. Effectively, we had reversed her Graves', and she could enjoy a sense of well-being along with vibrant, glowing health. As Laila told me, the stress relief made a big difference in her condition—and her outlook.

"The really exciting thing is how *empowered* I feel," she told me. "If something stops working, I know I have the power to create a new solution. Knowing that, for me, is the best stress relief of all!"

Part Five

THE MYERS WAY STEP BY STEP

CHAPTER 11

The Myers Way Thyroid Connection Plan

Hey, this is the most exciting moment in this book, because you are about to begin my twenty-eight-day plan to support your thyroid and immune system and jump-start your health. I'm so thrilled for you! This is where the rubber meets the road as you begin your journey to optimal health through a four-part approach:

- Engage the power of food while healing your gut
- Tame the toxins
- Treat your infections
- Relieve your stress

So, how is this all going to work?

STEP 1: FOLLOW THE TWENTY-EIGHT-DAY PLAN THAT BEGINS ON PAGE 270

This plan tells you exactly what to do from the moment you wake up to the moment you go to bed. It includes all the foods and supplements you need for optimal support while keeping you away from inflammatory and thyroid-suppressing foods that will prevent your body from healing. I've built stress relief into the plan as well, including exercise (see page 219 for your list of healthy choices).

Develop your own personalized supplement plan

As part of your twenty-eight-day plan, you'll be taking supplements—but which ones? That depends on your own personal situation—what type of thyroid dysfunction you have, whether or not you are autoimmune, whether you have SNPs, and whether you suffer from gut infections, other infections, or adrenal dysfunction. If you were my patient, I'd do a complete workup and come up with a specific, detailed plan based on your health history and your test results. In this book, we're going to do the next best thing. Starting on page 246, I'm going to walk you through your individual situation. You'll use that information to complete your own personal supplement plan. Then you'll take those supplements for twenty-eight days and, in some cases, beyond.

Begin your toxin defense plan

As we saw in chapter 8, this is going to be a personalized plan that fits your own individual lifestyle, budget, and health conditions. Check out page 268 for a reminder of the basics, and get started on taming the toxins in *your* life.

STEP 2: AFTER TWENTY-EIGHT DAYS, CONSULT WITH YOUR DOCTOR AND POSSIBLY ADD SOME FOODS BACK IN

See pages 124–125 for a list of all the tests you need, and review chapter 6 for suggestions on working with your doctor. See page 316 to find out how to add some foods back in, including small amounts of sugar, caffeine, and alcohol if you desire.

I know that for some of you, this might seem daunting. You might have been looking for a simple diet and maybe a supplement or two, something that resembles more closely the plans you've seen in other diet and health books. But as you have learned throughout this book, your body works as a whole. You can't just pull out a couple of foods and add in a few vitamins—not if you want terrific results! I want you to benefit in every possible way: diet, supplements, gut healing, toxin taming, infection healing, and stress relief.

Don't worry, though. Once you have completed your supplement plan, pretty much all you need to do is follow the daily steps beginning on page 270. And once you've done that for a day or two, it's going to become your new normal. Go check it out now to see how simple it's going to be!

WHAT TO EAT

Okay, I'll be honest with you. If someone told me every single thing I had to eat for the next twenty-eight days, I flat-out wouldn't do it. I'd want to substitute chicken for salmon, or basil for cilantro, or have an apple instead of a pear. Sure, I'd want all my choices to be healthy. But I'd want them to be *mine*.

However, I know plenty of folks who like to have all the choices laid out for them so they just don't have to think about it. I get it—you've got plenty of other things going on; you don't want to have to worry about what kind of protein to prepare for dinner.

Well, you know what? Whichever way you like it, that's the way you'll have it. I've worked with my registered dietician, Brianne Williams, to prepare three meals plus a snack each day for twenty-eight days. And starting on page 236, I lay out all the basics of what you can eat and what you can't so that if you *do* want to substitute something, you'll know how. Switching fish for chicken is just fine. Adding in eggs or dairy is not—at least, not for the next twenty-eight days. So if you just want to follow the meal plans we've put together, terrific! And if you want to play around with them, that's also great. We couldn't possibly include every single food that's okay to eat—there are just too many. Just make sure you don't include *any* food on the Foods to Toss list. Otherwise, you risk inflaming your immune system and undermining your thyroid—and why sabotage your chance to jump-start your health?

I'd really like all your meals to be home-cooked and organic for the twenty-eight days so that you can make absolutely sure you're getting all nutrients you need and none of the inflammatory, toxic, or thyroid-suppressing foods that will disrupt your thyroid, gut, or immune system. After this month, you'll be able to broaden your diet and enjoy eating in restaurants—I certainly do! But to give your thyroid health the best possible foundation, you'll do best by following this plan.

I've made cooking at home as easy as possible for you, which is why each of these amazingly delicious and nutritious recipes will take you no more than half an hour to prepare. We have arranged the plan so that you'll pretty much always have enough for leftovers, which will cut down your cooking time even more. I can guarantee that you will not feel deprived while on the plan because the recipes are yummy as well as filling. In addition, you'll be getting your thyroid back in balance and gaining energy, feeling more clearheaded, and enjoying a calm, optimistic, balanced mood.

You'll avoid a lot of potentially inflammatory foods for the next four weeks to give your thyroid and immune system the best possible chance of recovering. Then, as you'll see on pages 313–317, you'll find out how to add some foods back into your diet, including small amounts of caffeine, sugar, and alcohol—but please continue to eat organic.

I am thrilled you have decided to embark on this twenty-eight-day journey. I can't wait for you to experience more energy, less brain fog, and more vitality and to be at your ideal weight. So let's get going!

Approved foods: The overview

- *Quality proteins:* organic grass-fed and pasture-raised meats or wild meats and game, including beef, bison, pork, lamb, chicken, duck, turkey, and wild-caught seafood
- *Complex carbohydrates:* fruits and vegetables, including sweet potatoes and winter squashes
- *Healthy fats:* avocado, coconut, coconut oil, extra-virgin olive oil, full-fat coconut milk, olives, and animal fat
- *Flavorful spices:* cinnamon, garlic, ginger, and turmeric are among your healthiest choices
- *Refreshing beverages:* filtered water, herbal teas (caffeine-free), homemade vegetable juices, mineral water, seltzer, and some organic green tea if desired

Foods to Enjoy

Quality Proteins

1. To save time and energy, consider cooking your meat and poultry at the beginning of the week — perhaps on Sunday evening — to use for the week's meals.

2. Focus on lean organic, grass-fed, pasture-raised, or wild meats. Avoid processed products like cold cuts, which may contain gluten, sugar, soy, and corn and are generally lower-quality meats.

3. Consider buying organic, free-range, pasture-raised, or wild meat in bulk from a local farmer or hunter.

4. See Resources for my recommendations of where to buy quality meats.

5. Before buying fish and seafood, be sure to check out this resource from the Natural Resources Defense Council to avoid those that are high in mercury (see http://www.nrdc.org/health/effects/mercury/guide.asp), and check out Resources for my recommendations of where to buy healthy fish and seafood online.

Enjoy:

- Free range organic pasture-raised poultry
  - Chicken
  - Turkey
  - Duck
- Organic grass-fed lamb
- Wild game
- Wild-caught fresh fish
  - Pacific salmon
  - Halibut
  - Haddock
  - Cod
  - Snapper
  - Sole
  - Pollock

- ○ Trout
- Water or oil-packed fish
  - ○ Sardines
  - ○ Wild-caught salmon
- Organic lean grass-fed beef or bison
- Organic pork or bacon

The Myers Way Paleo Protein Powder

You'll see that I've included The Myers Way Paleo Protein powder in some recipes because it's important for your thyroid and immune system to get all the amino acids and protein they need. Most protein powders are made from dairy, grain, seeds, eggs, or legumes, all of which can be potentially inflammatory to your thyroid and, in some cases, trigger molecular mimicry (see page 94). I'm delighted to share with you a better option: paleo protein, which is made from beef raised without hormones, antibiotics, or GMO feed.

The Myers Way Paleo Protein powder is dairy-free, grain-free, seed-free, egg-free, and legume-free, so it's perfect for your Thyroid Connection Plan. It's a quick and easy source of the complete amino acids needed to support your thyroid and immune system. Even more important, it tastes great!

Fruits

1. Choose from organic fresh fruit or frozen fruits with no additives. Whole, fresh fruit will help you feel full (the technical term is "promote satiety") more than any other kind.
2. Please avoid fruits that have been sweetened or dried. They feed unhealthy bacteria, as well as Candida, other types of yeast overgrowth, and SIBO. They also promote blood-sugar spikes and crashes, leaving you ravenous as a result.
3. A great way to enjoy your daily fruit is in your morning smoothie. Berries add some extra fiber, so they're a terrific choice.

4. Rather than buying processed lemon juice, squeeze some fresh lemon into your water or onto your salad.

Enjoy:
- Apples
- Applesauce, unsweetened
- Apricots — fresh only unless otherwise specified in a recipe
- Bananas
- Berries: blueberries, blackberries, raspberries, strawberries
- Cherries
- Cranberries
- Figs — fresh only
- Grapefruit
- Grapes
- Kiwi
- Kumquats
- Lemons
- Limes
- Mangoes
- Melons: cantaloupe, honeydew, watermelon
- Nectarines
- Oranges
- Peaches
- Pears
- Plantains
- Plums

Vegetables

1. You can enjoy your organic vegetables raw (except the cruciferous ones), steamed, sautéed, baked, juiced, or roasted — any way but deep-fried.
2. A great time-saving tip is to get your vegetables ready to cook as soon as you get them home: wash them, chop them, and then store them in glass or ceramic containers (no plastic, please!).

You'll be amazed how much easier it is to cook when the veggies are all ready for you.

3. Pack your snacking veggies into small glass or stainless-steel containers that you can just grab and go.

4. Dip vegetables into guacamole for some healthy fats.

5. If you have more fresh vegetables than you can eat before they go bad, whip up a stir-fry and store it in the freezer for the next time you're too busy to cook.

Note: Cruciferous vegetables are potential *goitrogens*—foods that can disrupt thyroid function. They have loads of important nutrients, so I don't want you to omit them from your diet—quite the contrary! Cooking reduces their goitrogenic properties, so make sure you cook them. Fermenting does the same thing. If you must go raw, consume only very small amounts. I've put an asterisk beside each cruciferous vegetable in the list.

Enjoy:

- Artichokes
- Arugula*
- Asparagus
- Bamboo shoots
- Beets
- Bok choy*
- Broccoli*
- Broccolini*
- Brussels sprouts*
- Cabbage*
- Collard greens*
- Carrots
- Cauliflower*
- Celery
- Chives
- Cucumbers

- Kale*
- Leeks
- Lettuce
- Mustard greens*
- Parsnips
- Radishes*
- Spinach
- Turnips*
- Yellow summer squash
- Zucchini

Starchy Vegetables

Feel free to include these organic vegetables on your Thyroid Connection Plan, but be aware that they are somewhat less healthy than the nonstarchy vegetables, so enjoy them in moderation. If you are on the SIBO or anti-yeast protocol, only one serving each day; otherwise up to two servings each day.

Enjoy:

- Acorn squash
- Butternut squash
- Kabocha squash
- Pumpkin
- Spaghetti squash
- Sweet potatoes

Healthy Oils and Fats

1. To avoid the heat and chemicals used to produced most oils, choose organic cold-pressed or expeller-pressed oils (read the label).
2. You want to avoid butter, but coconut oil and bacon fat are great substitutes.
3. For a little sweetness, coconut butter/manna is a terrific choice.
4. All forms of canola oil are GMO, so avoid them, please.

Note: Avocados are technically fruits, but they are low in sugar and very high in healthy fat, so I want you to think of them as healthy fats instead.

Enjoy:

- Animal fat, from beef, pork, or poultry
- Avocado
- Avocado oil
- Coconut
- Coconut oil
- Grape-seed oil
- Olive oil

Spices and Flavorings

1. The label *spices* is a catchall that might even mean gluten. Avoid anything with this ingredient.
2. You can enjoy stevia but only in small amounts. If you can go without, even better!

Enjoy:

- Apple cider vinegar
- Basil
- Bay leaf
- Black pepper
- Cardamom
- Carob
- Cilantro
- Cinnamon
- Clove
- Cumin
- Dandelion
- Dill
- Fennel
- Garlic
- Ginger

- Mustard
- Nutmeg
- Oregano
- Parsley
- Rosemary
- Sea salt
- Stevia
- Tarragon
- Thyme
- Turmeric

Beverages

1. Our planet provides us with water, and you know what? It's the healthiest drink of all! See Resources for water filters.
2. Flavor your water with cucumber, lemon, or a few berries.
3. Seltzer is *almost* as good as water. Add a slice of lemon or lime for extra zest.
4. Generally avoid coconut water, which is naturally high in sugar. However, if you need a sports drink, coconut water is high in electrolytes.
5. I don't recommend 100 percent fruit juices—even natural or homemade—because they're so high in sugar and lack the fiber that makes fresh fruit so healthy and satisfying. Juicing with lots of vegetables and no more than half a piece of fruit or half a cup of berries per serving of juice is a great alternative to high-sugar fruit juices and can be very cleansing.

Enjoy:

- Filtered water—far and away your best choice
- Organic coconut milk, in moderation because of the high sugar content
- Organic herbal tea—caffeine-free
- Pure, unsweetened organic vegetable juice with no more than half a piece of fruit or half a cup of berries in any serving of juice
- Sparkling water or seltzer

Gut-Healing Collagen

Collagen is a protein—actually, the most abundant protein in your body—and the substance that holds your body together, supporting your bones, muscles, skin, and tendons. It's also a vital element in gut healing, used to repair your intestinal wall. By now you know just how important it is to heal your leaky gut, and collagen will do just that.

Because collagen is so important, I've included it both as a supplement and as an ingredient in some of your smoothies and The Myers Way Gut-Healing Tea (page 322), a delicious recipe that will do wonders for your intestinal and immune health. See Resources for some online sources of collagen.

Foods to toss

Remember, some of these foods will stay out of your diet permanently. However, you might be able to add many of them back in after twenty-eight days. On pages 166–167, I explain which foods you might be able to reintroduce and tell you how to test them.

Toxic Foods to Toss

- Alcohol
- Fast foods, junk foods, processed foods
- Food additives: any foods that contain artificial colors, flavors, or preservatives
- Genetically modified foods (GMOs), including canola oil and beet sugar
- Processed meats: canned meats (such as Spam; canned fish is okay), cold cuts, hot dogs; sausage is okay, but make sure it's gluten-free
- Processed and refined oils: hydrogenated fats, margarine, mayonnaise, salad dressings, shortening, spreads, trans fats
- Stimulants and caffeine: caffeinated tea, chocolate, coffee

- Sweeteners: sugar, sugar alcohols, natural sweeteners (such as honey, agave, maple syrup, molasses, and coconut palm sugar), sweetened juices, high-fructose corn syrup; stevia in moderation is okay

Condiment and Spices to Toss

- Barbecue sauce
- Cayenne pepper (black pepper is okay)
- Chocolate in any form that is less than 90 percent cacao
- Ketchup
- Paprika
- Red pepper flakes
- Relish
- Soy sauce
- Tamari
- Teriyaki sauce

Inflammatory Foods to Toss

- Corn and anything made from corn (corn flour, cornmeal, grits) or containing high-fructose corn syrup
- Dairy: butter, casein, cheese, cottage cheese, cream, frozen yogurt, ghee, goat cheese, ice cream, milk, nondairy creamer, whey protein, yogurt
- Eggs
- Gluten: anything that contains barley, rye, or wheat
- Gluten-free grains and pseudograins: amaranth, millet, oats, quinoa, rice
- Legumes: beans, garbanzos, lentils, peas (dried and fresh), snow peas
- Nightshades: eggplant, peppers, potatoes, tomatoes; sweet potatoes are okay
- Nuts, including nut butters
- Peanuts
- Seeds, including seed butters
- Soy
- Sweetened fruit juices

Remember: During your twenty-eight days, you can choose any food you like, just as long as it's not on the Foods to Toss list. The foods on pages 236–243 are just examples of the kinds of healthy foods you can choose.

WHICH SUPPLEMENTS TO TAKE

As you've seen, which supplements you need depends on your individual situation. So what I want you to do is read through this section very carefully. Each time you discover a supplement that you need, add it to your personalized supplement plan on pages 268–269. Then, throughout the twenty-eight days, you can consult your plan for a reminder of which supplements you need to take and when you should take them.

As I said above, it can seem complicated. I wish I could have you in my office right now — I'd be the one to prepare this list and hand it over to you, and then you'd know exactly what to do. Since we can't do that, I'm going to talk you through preparing your own list. Once you've got the list, everything gets easy, so let's just take it step by step.

Preparing your individualized supplement plan

There is a complete multivitamin, omega-3 fish oils, and probiotic that I want everyone to take, so I've just written them in for you on pages 268–269. The rest of the supplements you take will depend on which conditions you have:

If you are hyperthyroid
If you are autoimmune, including Hashimoto's and Graves'
If you have intestinel yeast overgrowth
If you have small intestine bacterial overgrowth (SIBO)
If you have parasites
If you have leaky gut
If you have systemic infections
If you have adrenal dysfunction
If you have SNPs or high homocysteine levels

You already know whether you have some conditions—such as hyperthyroidism or autoimmune dysfunction. For others—such as gut infections and adrenal dysfunction—you'll need to complete the questionnaires I have included; you'll see them as you go through pages 253–269 to complete your plan. And for still others, such as infections and SNPs, you'll need to check with your doctor.

When It Comes to Supplements, Buyer Beware!

The supplement industry is unregulated, so you need to be very careful where you buy your supplements. Please make sure to get a high-quality, pharmaceutical-grade multivitamin, one that is free of soy, corn, gluten, and dairy, that has been manufactured according to good manufacturing practices (GMP), and that has been third-party-tested to ensure that it is what it says it is.

I know it's tempting to save money on bargain products and sales at the local vitamin store. But please resist the temptation, because the products you find at your local drugstore or even at most health-food stores will *not* give you the same quality.

Instead, you can get most of the supplements I recommend at my online store (store.amymyersmd.com). See Resources for the other brands I recommend and where to purchase them. High-quality supplements are one of the best investments in your health that you can possibly make.

Thyroid Support—for Everyone

Omega-3 Fish Oils: 1,000 mg twice a day with food

- I've already filled this in for you on pages 268–269, so you don't have to!

Fresh fish is great, and you'll be eating some this coming month. But I also want to make sure you supplement with omega-3 fatty acids, which help decrease inflammation while supporting your immune system. Some studies have even indicated that omega-3 fatty acids can increase thyroid hormone uptake. In a study published in the *Journal of*

Nutritional Biochemistry in 2010, rats received diets containing either soybean oil or fish oil; the fish-oil group was found to have higher levels of the receptors that cells use to take in thyroid hormone as well as high levels of the enzymes involved in thyroid hormone uptake.

Probiotics: 30 billion to 100 billion units/day taken with food

- I've already filled this in for you on page 268, so you don't have to!

Your gut is full of friendly bacteria that help you digest your food and prevent the unfriendly bacteria from moving in. Unfortunately, these friendly bacteria can be depleted by antibiotics, steroids, or acid-blocking medications, by a poor diet, by stress, and by many other factors. Taking a highly concentrated dose of probiotics each day can help you regain a healthy balance of bacteria in your gut. Be sure not to take it within two hours of taking the supplements for yeast and SIBO. Although I've just noted one probiotic per day, if you end up with pills that contain smaller amounts, feel free to spread your dose over more than one meal.

Note: If you have small intestine bacterial overgrowth (SIBO), I recommend taking the probiotic found on page 260.

The Myers Way Multivitamin Complete, with or without iron as needed (see page 253): Three pills with lunch and three pills with dinner. (If you choose to substitute a different multivitamin, use the guidelines below to choose an alternative brand and then follow the directions on the bottle.)

- I've already filled this in for you on pages 268–269, so you don't have to!

A multivitamin is the most efficient way to ensure that you get the full spectrum of nutrients that your body needs. However, all multivitamins are *not* created equal. To ensure that you get everything you need for optimal thyroid function, I have specially formulated my own complete multivitamin. You don't have to buy it from me (see Resources), but I highly recommend it. Take it with food because it includes several fat-soluble vitamins. However, don't take it at breakfast because it contains calcium, which can interfere with the absorption of supplemental thyroid hormone. (If you're not taking supplemental thyroid hormone, you can take it at breakfast if you prefer.)

Of course, you don't have to buy the specific multivitamin I recommend—but I do want you to make sure that your multi contains all the essential ingredients in all the right amounts:

Vitamin A: 5,000–10,000 IU per day

Without sufficient quantities of vitamin A, your body can't move free T3 into your cells. Vitamin A also supports your immune system. Because vitamin A is a fat-soluble vitamin, you want to take it with food. Most multivitamins have a mix of vitamin A in the form of retinyl acetate or retinyl palmitate (preformed vitamin A) plus some beta-carotenes, which your body can convert into vitamin A. Be careful: vitamin A is stored in the liver and can be toxic if taken too much. I would prefer you get a multivitamin that contains about 75 percent of its vitamin A in the form of mixed beta-carotenes and 25 percent as actual vitamin A to prevent any toxicity issues.

B Vitamins:

> **Riboflavin: 50 mg per day**
> **Niacin: 200 mg per day**
> **Vitamin B_6: 50 mg per day**
> **Folate: 800 mcg per day**
> **Vitamin B_{12}: 1,000 mcg per day**

Your thyroid gland needs iodine to make thyroid hormone, and it needs vitamin B_2 to bring it the iodine. B_2 also helps to activate other vitamins and to increase the absorption of other B vitamins.

You also need B_{12} to produce TSH, as well as for red blood cell formation, neurological function, and a host of other functions. It's hard to get all the B_{12} your body needs just from food alone, especially if you have leaky gut, SIBO, or yeast overgrowth. And it's even harder if you don't eat meat. So make sure your multivitamin includes enough B_{12}, or else take some extra to make sure you are getting 1,000 mcg per day (see "Is Your Multivitamin Enough?" on page 252). The type of B_{12} is important, too. Most multivitamins contain B_{12} in the form of cyano-cobalamin, which is actually synthetic and which your body must convert to the usable form of B_{12}, methylcobalamin. Please make sure your multivitamin has methylcobalamin, especially if you have one or two of the SNPs known as at MTHFR (see page 191).

The rest of the B vitamins are important supports for immune function, stress relief, and many other bodily processes. They work synergistically with one another as well as with other key nutrients in your body. So either take the multivitamin I recommend or read labels very carefully to make sure you're getting all of the B vitamins you need—and in the form you need. I recommend finding a brand that has the B vitamins in their coenzymated forms (check the label!) and that has a blend of active isomer naturally occurring folates as well as TMG, choline, and methylcobalamin to support methylation, especially if you have one of the SNPs that affect methylation (MTHFR, see page 191). (I know that list reads like a foreign language, but check out the labels—or just buy one of the brands I recommend.)

Vitamin C: 1,000 mg per day

This is another vitamin that you need to bring iodine into your thyroid gland. Vitamin C is also one of those miracle antioxidants that seems to help just about every process in your body. It helps protect you from free-radical damage; it is a key to making collagen (which you'll also be taking as a supplement); it helps your body absorb iron (which you also need for thyroid function); and it's a terrific support for your immune system. Take a moment to cheer for fabulous vitamin C!

Vitamin D₃: 1,000 IU per day

Vitamin D deficiency might increase your risk of autoimmune thyroid disease. A study conducted in New Delhi, India, found that when the numbers were adjusted for age, the higher the vitamin D levels, the fewer thyroid antibodies. Other evidence suggests that vitamin D deficiency is more common among people with thyroid cancer or thyroid nodules, further pointing to the importance of vitamin D in thyroid health.

Iodine: 150–300 mcg per day

As you know by now, your thyroid gland needs iodine to make T4 and T3. Although you can—and should!—get iodine from your diet, I want to be sure you supplement too, just to be absolutely sure you get enough. For more on iodine and why you need it, check out pages 177–178 in chapter 8.

Magnesium: 50 mg per day

You need magnesium to produce sufficient levels of TSH, an integral part of the thyroid signaling system. Your body uses magnesium to synthesize glutathione, which, as we just saw, is a crucial support for your detox pathways. You also need this amazing mineral for the function of more than three hundred enzyme systems, including protein synthesis, muscle and nerve function, blood-glucose control, and blood pressure regulation. Last but not least, magnesium is also crucial for nerve impulses, muscle contraction, and normal heart rhythms.

Selenium: 200 mcg per day

After iodine, selenium is probably the next most important mineral affecting your thyroid function. Your body needs selenium to convert T4 to T3. Significantly, people who live in areas where the soil is low in selenium are more likely to develop Hashimoto's. An exciting study published in 2002 affirms the value of supplementing with selenium. In a placebo-controlled study, German researchers gave 200 mcg of sodium selenite daily to patients with Hashimoto's disease and high levels of thyroid peroxidase (TPO) antibodies. After three months, the people taking selenium saw a huge drop in antibodies—66.4 percent—and in a few people, TPO antibodies even returned to normal. So if you want to reverse your Hashimoto's, selenium is key.

Zinc: 25 mg per day

Zinc is another metal your body needs to make TSH. It plays a role in immune function, protein synthesis, wound healing, and cell division. Your body has no way to store zinc, so you need to get some every day. Because zinc is so vital to thyroid function, I want you to have enough of it in your multivitamin so you can be 100 percent sure of getting as much as you need.

Iron: 25 mg per day (if you're a woman who is still menstruating)

If you want to convert T4 into T3—and you do!—you need iron. Iron is also crucial for forming hemoglobin, which enables your cells to carry oxygen.

Is Your Multivitamin Enough?

In most cases, a high-quality multivitamin as recommended above gives you all the nutrients you need—but there are some exceptions. I recommend you start by taking your multi for thirty to sixty days and then have your doctor test your blood levels of various nutrients, as described on pages 124–125. Depending on your results, you might need to add individual nutrients on top of the multi. Work with your doctor to figure out what you need and how much. Everyone's body is different. Make sure to support *your* unique body through testing and supplementation.

Here are some of the most common examples of nutrients that you might need on top of your multivitamin. Take them with food, either as single dose (if that's how you buy them) or, if possible, in divided doses.

Vitamin B_{12}

Depending on your SNP status, you might need even more B_{12} than you can get from any multivitamin, including mine (see pages 249–250 for guidelines).

Vitamin D_3

Most people are deficient in vitamin D and it is likely that you will need to take an additional vitamin D supplement in order to get your levels into the optimal range of 60 to 80 ng/mL. Most of my patients need to take at least 1,000 IU a day. I suggest you have your doctor test you and then work with you to determine how much supplemental vitamin D you need to take.

If you do supplement with vitamin D$_3$, remember that it's a fat-soluble vitamin that is best taken with food, with calcium, and with vitamin K. Work with your doctor to get the right amounts.

Be careful: Vitamin D$_3$ is stored in the liver and can be toxic if your levels are too high. Make sure to work with your doctor to recheck your levels every few months.

Iron

If you're a man who eats meat, you probably don't need any extra iron. However, if you are a woman who has not yet started menopause, and especially if you don't eat meat, you most assuredly do. As I explain on page 125, you should work with your doctor to test your ferritin levels and then figure out with him or her how to supplement until you have reached a level between 50 to 100 ng/mL.

For some people, iron supplements can be constipating. When I hear this, I think they are taking a poor-quality supplement or taking it in a form that is not well absorbed. I believe iron glycinate usually labeled as ferrous bisglycinate chelate is the best tolerated and most absorbable form.

If You Are Hyperthyroid

Supplements to Help Your Entire Body

When you're hyperthyroid, your whole body is in overdrive. Your overactive thyroid is pushing your body as if you were running on a treadmill 24/7. As you saw in chapter 6, your body needs a lot of extra support to cope with the wear and tear.

L-Carnitine: 2,000 mg per day, working up to 4,000 mg per day as needed. (If you have mild hyperthyroidism, 2,000 mg per day should be enough; if your hyperthyroidism is more severe, add 1,000 mg after 3 days and, if needed, an additional 1,000 mg after another 3 days.)

- If you need this, please add it to your personalized supplement plan on pages 268–269.

L–carnitine seems to help prevent thyroid hormone from getting into at least some of your cells, which mitigates the muscle weakness associated with hyperthyroidism as well as reduces insomnia, heart palpitations, tremors, and nervousness. A hyperactive thyroid causes you to lose this crucial mineral through your urine, so please supplement.

CoQ10: 100 mg per day to 400 mg per day, taken with a meal containing fat. The more severe your hyperthyroidism, the more CoQ10 you should take, within the range given above. As your condition improves, you can slowly decrease the dose.

- If you need this, please add it to your personalized supplement plan on pages 268–269.

I want all my hyperthyroid patients to take CoQ10. First, research links hyperthyroidism to low levels of this powerful antioxidant. Second, CoQ10 helps protect cell integrity. It also helps convert food into energy. Finally, both beta-blockers and cholesterol-lowering medications inhibit mitochondrial CoQ10 enzyme, so you absolutely need to supplement if you are taking either.

Glucomannan: Start with 1.5 gm twice daily for 7 days, then take 3.0 gm twice daily until your hyperthyroidism resolves.

- If you need this, please add it to your personalized supplement plan on pages 268–269.

This fiber affects the way your liver metabolizes thyroid hormone, thereby decreasing levels of circulating thyroid hormone in your body. It can be very useful in calming an overactive thyroid gland. This supplement can be helpful for a wide range of issues—it can lower blood pressure, reduce cholesterol, and control appetite by promoting fullness—so you can certainly continue to take it if you want to, or you can stop taking it when your thyroid symptoms abate.

Herbs to Calm Your Thyroid

You have two choices: thyroid-calming formula or bugleweed, motherwort, and lemon balm. Either way, please check with your doctor and continue to work with him or her.

OPTION 1: THYROID-CALMING FORMULA (40 DROPS IN 2 OUNCES OF WATER 2 TO 4 TIMES A DAY, BETWEEN MEALS)

- If you need this, please add it to your personalized supplement plan on pages 268–269.

My online store carries a product that conveniently combines bugleweed, motherwort, and lemon balm into one product: Thyroid-Calming Formula. As far as I know, it's the only such product, though there may be others I'm not aware of.

OPTION 2: BUGLEWEED, MOTHERWORT, AND LEMON BALM, ALL TAKEN BETWEEN MEALS

- If you need these, please add them to your personalized supplement plan on pages 268–269.

- *Bugleweed* (Lycopus virginicus)*:* In a liquid extract in the ratio of 1 part herb and 2 parts water, take a daily dose of 2mL and gradually increase to 6mL as needed. Bugleweed decreases your TSH and T4 levels, helps keep your body from synthesizing thyroid hormone, and helps keep antibodies from binding to your thyroid gland.

- *Motherwort* (Leonurus cardiaca)*:* In a liquid extract in the ratio of 1 part herb to 2 parts water, take a daily dose of 2 mL and gradually increase to 4 mL as needed. This herb doesn't actually affect your thyroid itself, but it does mitigate such symptoms as heart palpitations, anxiety, sleep problems, and, occasionally, loss of appetite. Don't take it with any type of sedating medication, including antihistamines. Potential side effects include miscarriage, increased uterine bleeding, and negative interactions with many cardiac medications. Be sure to check with your doctor before taking it.

- *Lemon balm* (Melissa officinalis)*:* Start with 300 mg and gradually increase to 600 mg as needed. This member of the mint family seems to block hormone receptors. As a result, TSH is less able to bind to your thyroid tissue, and your antibodies are less able to attach to your thyroid. Lemon balm will help you reduce anxiety, improve sleep, and ease pain, as well as decrease digestive symptoms and restore appetite.

Good for lowering stress and boosting mood, lemon balm can also help with migraine and hypertension.

If you are autoimmune

Acetyl Glutathione: 300 mg one to two times a day on an empty stomach *or* each of the following, taken all together, one to two times a day on an empty stomach:

- N-acetylcysteine: 1,000 mg
- Vitamin C: 1,000 mg
- Milk thistle: 250 mg
- Alpha-lipoic acid: 200 mg
- If you need these, please add them to your personalized supplement plan on pages 268–269.

You live in a toxic world, so you can't afford to detox just once or twice a year: You need to support your detox pathways every single day. Glutathione is the mother of all antioxidants naturally produced in your body—that is, glutathione converts to all the other antioxidants. Studies show that people with chronic illness have lower levels of glutathione, so I want you to get those levels up! You're already boosting your glutathione by eating cooked crucifers and sulfur-containing vegetables such as garlic and onions. However, I want to be sure you get all the detox support you need. Many of you could take the three supplements listed above, which your body converts to glutathione. However, as you saw on pages 190–191, some people have SNPs that interfere with the conversion process. That's why taking glutathione directly is a good option.

I need to caution you that most brands of glutathione are virtually useless, because your body has a hard time absorbing it. To avoid this problem, I recommend a brand that is specially designed to maximize glutathione absorption.

Curcumin Phytosome: 500 mg twice a day with glutathione, with meals

- If you need this, please add it to your personalized supplement plan on pages 268–269.

Curcumin is the orange pigment in turmeric, a potent antioxidant that offers numerous health benefits. It supports joint health and cardiovascular function, modulates inflammation, promotes the body's natural antioxidant system, protects the liver, and supports detox. I highly recommend this brand, which offers a time-release capsule so that you can maintain optimal levels all day long. (See Resources.)

Be aware: High doses of curcumin can increase the risk of bleeding, especially if you also take blood thinners such as warfarin (Coumadin), clopidogrel (Plavix), or aspirin, so check with your doctor before taking it.

Resveratrol: 25 mg under tongue taken twice a day with curcumin and glutathione, with meals

- If you need this, please add it to your personalized supplement plan on pages 268–269.

You might have heard about the resveratrol in red wine, but I'd rather you take it as a supplement to avoid the sugar and alcohol! The many benefits of resveratrol include decreased inflammation, balanced blood sugar, improved athletic endurance, and increased blood flow to the heart, arteries, and brain. When you take resveratrol, curcumin, and glutathione together, they all enhance one another's antioxidant effects.

Here's how to take it: Dissolve a lozenge under the tongue, where there is a permeable rich blood supply. This introduces the resveratrol directly into the bloodstream and bypasses the liver and digestive tract, making a lower dose more effective.

Immune Booster: two capsules twice a day with or without food

- If you need this, please add it to your personalized supplement plan on pages 268–269.

Immune Booster capsules are immunoglobulin concentrates derived from colostral whey peptides, which are also found in the breast milk that supports a baby's immune system. This supplement supports *your* immune system and promotes gut repair and healthy microbial balance while eliminating all of the dairy proteins. Although it does contain trace amounts of lactose, it's not enough to cause an immune reaction in most people. (See Resources.)

If You Have Intestinal Yeast Overgrowth

Complete the following questionnaire to see whether you have intestinal yeast overgrowth. Check every box that applies to you. Then see below for your score.

- ☐ I have an autoimmune disease, such as Hashimoto's thyroiditis, Graves' disease, rheumatoid arthritis, ulcerative colitis, lupus, psoriasis, scleroderma, or multiple sclerosis.
- ☐ I have skin or nail fungal infections, such as athlete's foot, ringworm, or toenail fungus.
- ☐ I suffer from chronic fatigue or fibromyalgia, or I am tired all the time.
- ☐ I have digestive issues, such as bloating, constipation, or diarrhea.
- ☐ I have difficulty concentrating, poor memory, lack of focus, ADD, ADHD, or brain fog.
- ☐ I have skin issues, such as eczema, psoriasis, hives, rosacea, or an unexplained rash.
- ☐ I am easily irritated and/or have frequent mood swings, anxiety, or depression.
- ☐ I get vaginal yeast infections, have rectal itching, or have vaginal itching.
- ☐ I suffer from seasonal allergies or itchy ears.
- ☐ I have cravings for sugar and refined carbohydrate.

If you checked three or more items, you have tested positive for yeast overgrowth. I recommend you take the following supplements for at least twenty-eight days and continue as long as you have any of the above symptoms. (For more information about yeast overgrowth, check out my website: www.amymyersmd.com.)

Caprylic Acid: two pills upon waking and two pills before bed, at least two hours before or after probiotics

- If you need this, please add it to your personalized supplement plan on pages 268–269.

Also known as *octanoic acid,* this is a naturally occurring fatty acid that comes from coconut oil, known for its antiviral and antifungal activity. You will be taking this supplement on an empty stomach when you wake up and before you go to bed. Make sure to take it at least two hours before or after your probiotics. This product contains a small amount of calcium, which in theory means you shouldn't take it with your supplemental thyroid hormone. However, the amount is so small that I believe you can take the two products together with no concerns. Due to its anti-yeast activity, you may experience slight die-off symptoms—headache, digestive issues, fatigue, or other symptoms that result from the yeast dying off. If that happens to you, back down to one pill a day and gradually over the next week increase to two pills twice a day.

Candisol: two pills upon waking and two pills before bed, at least two hours before or after your probiotics

- If you need this, please add it to your personalized supplement plan on pages 268–269.

This substance contains a combination of plant-based enzymes that break down the cell walls of Candida and other species of yeast. Due to its anti-yeast activity, you may experience slight die-off symptoms— headache, digestive issues, fatigue, or other symptoms that result from the yeast dying off. If that happens to you, back down to one pill a day and gradually over the next week increase to two pills twice a day. Take this supplement for thirty to sixty days, using the questionnaire on page 258 to monitor your progress.

If You Have Small Intestine Bacterial Overgrowth (SIBO)

Complete the following questionnaire to see whether you have small intestine bacterial overgrowth. Check every box that applies to you. Then see below for your score.

- ☐ I have been diagnosed with hypothyroidism —either Hashimoto's or non-autoimmune.
- ☐ I have been diagnosed with irritable bowel syndrome or inflammatory bowel disease.
- ☐ I get bloated after meals or feel bloated a lot of the time.
- ☐ I have gas, abdominal pain, or cramping.
- ☐ I have odorous, loose stools.
- ☐ I have food intolerances, such as gluten, dairy, soy, or corn.
- ☐ I have histamine intolerance.
- ☐ My joints ache.
- ☐ I feel tired all the time.
- ☐ I have skin issues, such as eczema, psoriasis, hives, rosacea, or an unexplained rash.
- ☐ I have asthma or other respiratory problems.
- ☐ I feel depressed and hopeless.
- ☐ I have been diagnosed with a vitamin B_{12} deficiency.

If you checked three or more items above, you have tested positive for SIBO. I recommend you take the following supplements for at least thirty days and continue as long as you still have any of the above symptoms.

Prescript-Assist Soil-Based Probiotic, taken with meals

- If you need this, please note the change on your personalized supplement plan on pages 268–269.

Instead of the complete probiotic recommended on page 268, take the Prescript-Assist Soil-Based Probiotic. (See Resources.) This probiotic contains twenty-nine strains of bacteria designed to mimic the composition of your gut microbiome. I've found it to be helpful in promoting healthy gut bacteria while not supporting the unfriendly bacteria that predominate if you have SIBO.

Microb-Clear: Take one pill upon waking and one pill before bed two hours away from probiotics

- If you need this, please add it to your personalized supplement plan on pages 268–269.

This broad-spectrum antimicrobial supplement contains a blend of botanicals that fight against bacterial overgrowth in the intestines. Due to its antimicrobial activity, you may experience slight die-off symptoms— headache, digestive issues, fatigue, or other symptoms that result from the unfriendly bacteria dying off. If this happens to you, back down to one pill a day and gradually over the next week increase to two pills. (See Resources.)

If You Have Parasites

Complete the following questionnaire to see whether you have parasites. Check every box that applies to you. Then see below for your score.

- ☐ I have been diagnosed with hypothyroidism—either Hashimoto's or non-autoimmune.
- ☐ I have constipation, diarrhea, or gas.
- ☐ I have traveled internationally.
- ☐ I remember getting traveler's diarrhea while outside the country.
- ☐ I have had what I believe was food poisoning and my digestion has not been the same since.
- ☐ I have trouble falling asleep and I wake up multiple times during the night.
- ☐ I have skin issues, such as eczema, psoriasis, hives, rosacea, or an unexplained rash.
- ☐ I grind my teeth in my sleep.
- ☐ I have pain or aching in my muscles or joints.
- ☐ I feel exhausted, depressed, or apathetic almost all the time.
- ☐ I never feel satisfied after I eat.

☐   I have iron-deficiency anemia.

☐   I have been diagnosed with irritable bowel syndrome, ulcerative colitis, or Crohn's disease.

If you checked three or more items above, you have tested positive for parasites. I recommend you take the following supplements for at least twenty-eight days and continue as long as you still have the above symptoms.

Microb-Clear: Take one pill upon waking and one pill before bed two hours away from probiotics

• If you need this, please add it to your personalized supplement plan on pages 268–269.

This broad-spectrum antimicrobial supplement contains a blend of botanicals that fight against bacterial overgrowth in the intestines. Due to its antimicrobial activity, you may experience slight die-off symptoms—headache, digestive issues, fatigue, or other symptoms that result from the unfriendly bacteria dying off. If this happens to you, back down to taking one pill a day and over the next week gradually increase to two pills. (See Resources.)

If You Have Leaky Gut

Complete the following questionnaire to see whether you have leaky gut. Check every box that applies to you. Then see below for your score.

Digestion

☐   I see undigested food in my stool.

☐   I have gas and/or bloating after eating meals.

☐   I have reflux, burning in my chest, or burping after meals.

☐   My stomach feels heavy after eating.

☐   I do not have at least one bowel movement a day.

☐   I have frequent loose stools.

☐   My stools are small and poorly formed or they are very hard.

Health

☐ I have food sensitivities or intolerances.

☐ I have yeast overgrowth or SIBO (see pages 258–259 and 260–261)

☐ I have an autoimmune disease (including Hashimoto's or Graves')

☐ I am under chronic stress.

☐ I have trouble getting 7½ to 9 hours of good-quality sleep.

If you checked two or more under Digestion, I recommend taking GI Repair Powder or L-glutamine, digestive enzymes, and Betaine HCl (see below). *If you checked zero or one under Digestion but two or more under Health,* I recommend taking GI Repair Powder or L-glutamine only.

In both cases, take the supplements for at least twenty-eight days and continue as long as you have the above symptoms.

GI Repair Powder: one scoop per day, taken on an empty stomach *or* L-glutamine: 3.5 grams per day, taken on an empty stomach

• If you need this, please add it to your personalized supplement plan on pages 268–269.

L-glutamine is an amino acid that is fundamental to the well-being of the digestive and immune systems. It aids in producing the mucosal lining of the gastrointestinal tract.

In my clinic, I use a combination product called GI Repair Powder, which contains licorice and aloe vera, plant extracts that work with the L-glutamine to support the mucosal lining and heal the gut. The product also contains arabinogalactan, a prebiotic that feeds your gut bacteria and has many other beneficial effects. (See Resources.)

Digestive Enzymes: You can either buy The Myers Way Digestive Enzymes or look at its label on my website to match ingredients and amounts through another product; take them with at least two of your daily meals (follow instructions on the product).

• If you need this, please add it to your personalized supplement plan on pages 268–269.

As your gut is healing, you want to restore all the enzymes that you need to break down your food so that you can absorb it properly. You need to make sure you are getting a broad-spectrum combination of enzymes to maximize the breakdown, absorption, and utilization of macronutrients from proteins, carbohydrates, lipids/fats, and vegetable fibers. For twenty-eight days, take these enzymes with your meals. Depending on how you're doing, you can either stop taking them then or continue until you no longer have digestive symptoms such as gas, bloating, indigestion, constipation, or diarrhea.

Betaine Hydrochloride (HCl) with Pepsin: up to two capsules with each meal (see below)

- If you need this, please add it to your personalized supplement plan on pages 268–269.

Just as many people need digestive-enzyme support, many benefit from restoring stomach acid, or hydrochloric acid (HCl), for optimal digestion. You want your stomach to be an acidic environment to break down nutrients, particularly proteins. Here's a simple, at-home test you can do to see whether you have low stomach acid and need to replace some HCl. Start to eat a meal, take 650 mg of HCl, and then finish your meal. If you experience heartburn or warmth in your stomach, you have enough HCl. If you don't feel any burning, take two capsules of HCl at each meal. If that causes burning, reduce your dose to one capsule. Continue to take HCl until the supplement causes burning— which means that you have enough acid without it.

If you have infections

If your doctor has found that you have Epstein-Barr (EBV) or herpes simplex 1 or 2 (see chapter 9), here are some natural remedies you can take in response.

Lauricidin: one teaspoon three times a day with food

- If you need this, please add it to your personalized supplement plan on pages 268–269.

Lauricidin is made from a combination of lauric acid (obtained from coconut oil) and a plant-based glycerol (non-soy), creating a compound known as monolaurin, a monoglyceride. It can help to reduce your viral load if you've been infected with viruses in the herpes family.

Humic Acid: two pills twice a day, with food

- If you need this, please add it to your personalized supplement plan on pages 268–269.

Humic acid is a powerful free-radical scavenger and natural immune support. Although infections from Epstein-Barr and herpes simplex stay in the body, humic acid can help decrease your body's viral load, making reactivation less likely.

L-Lysine (for Herpes Simplex Virus only): 500 mg daily for prevention; 1 to 4 grams daily during an outbreak, with food

- If you need this, please add it to your personalized supplement plan on pages 268–269.

This amino acid can help prevent a herpes outbreak or make an outbreak less severe and easier to heal.

If You Have Adrenal Dysfunction

Complete the following questionnaire to see whether you have adrenal dysfunction. Check every box that applies to you. Then see below for your score.

- ☐ I am frequently tired.
- ☐ I feel tired even after 8 to 10 hours of sleep.
- ☐ I am chronically stressed.
- ☐ It is difficult for me to handle stress.
- ☐ I am a night-shift worker.
- ☐ I work long hours.
- ☐ I have little relaxation in my days.
- ☐ I get headaches frequently.

☐ I don't exercise consistently.

☐ I am or have been an endurance athlete, or I participate in CrossFit.

☐ I have erratic sleeping patterns.

☐ I wake up in the middle of the night.

☐ I crave salt.

☐ I crave sugar.

☐ I have high sugar intake.

☐ I have difficulty concentrating.

☐ I carry weight in my midsection (apple body shape).

☐ I have blood-sugar issues (hypoglycemia).

☐ I have irregular periods.

☐ I have low libido.

☐ I have PMS or perimenopausal/menopausal symptoms.

☐ I get sick frequently.

☐ I have low blood pressure.

☐ I have muscle fatigue or weakness.

☐ I rely on caffeine for energy (coffee, energy shots, etc.).

Scoring

<2   Great! Continue to manage your stress (the stress relief in your twenty-eight-day plan will help).

2–5 Good. No additional supplementation needed, but make sure to include stress relief every day as outlined in your twenty-eight-day plan.

6–10 Take the adaptogenic herbs recommended below and make sure to include stress relief every day as outlined in your twenty-eight-day plan.

>10 Take adaptogenic herbs recommended below and make sure to include stress relief every day as outlined in your twenty-eight-day plan. See a functional medicine practitioner (see Resources) if your symptoms don't resolve in twenty-eight days.

Adrenal Support: Start with one capsule twice daily and work up to two capsules twice daily; take your full dose in the morning

- If you need this, please add it to your personalized supplement plan on pages 268–269.

This product (see Resources) contains adaptogenic herbs, including *Rhodiola rosea* and *Panax ginseng*, to help your body adapt and cope with stress. This is my go-to treatment to support the adrenal gland while you also work to alleviate stress.

Vitamin B Complex: One pill a day with food

- If you need this, please add it to your personalized supplement plan on pages 268–269.

You'll get B vitamins in your multivitamin, but if you have adrenal dysfunction, you may need a dedicated supplement of complete B vitamins, including B_1, B_2, B_3, B_5, B_6, B_7, B_{12}, and folinic acid. As I explained earlier, I recommend finding a brand that has the B vitamins in their coenzymated forms (check the label!) and a blend of active isomer naturally occurring folates, as well as TMG, choline, and methyl-cobalamin to support methylation, especially if you have one of the SNPs that affect methylation (on MTHFR, see page 191). (I know that list can be tough to get through, but please do read the label very carefully—or just buy one of the brands I recommend.) By the way, caffeine depletes your stores of vitamin B, so if you've been living on coffee and caffeinated soda, you're likely going to need some replenishment to feel really well.

Magnesium: 500 to 1,000 mg/day with or without food

Magnesium is so fabulous for stress, I've included 50 mg in my multivitamin just as a daily support. If you're dealing with excessive stress, you can take more, which will be good for your mood and cognitive function as well as for your adrenals, thyroid, and immune system. There are lots of different types of magnesium for sale. We offer one called NeuroCalm Mag, which is able to cross the blood-brain barrier for enhanced stress reduction, but any high-quality brand will do. (See Resources for recommended brands.)

MY PERSONALIZED TWENTY-EIGHT-DAY SUPPLEMENT PLAN

I've filled in the supplements that all of you will be taking. Please add the others based on your individual condition.

Upon Waking:

_____

_____

_____

_____

Breakfast:

- Probiotics: 50 to 100 billion units

_____

_____

_____

_____

Lunch:

- The Myers Way Multivitamin Complete: 3 capsules
- Omega-3 fish oil: 2 capsules

_____

_____

_____

_____

Dinner:

- The Myers Way Multivitamin Complete: 3 capsules
- Omega-3 fish oil: 2 capsules

_____

_____

_____

_____

Bedtime:

_____

_____

_____

CHAPTER 12

The Myers Way Thyroid Connection Twenty-Eight-Day Plan

Each day, please wake up with plenty of time to make sure that you are not stressed. For some of you, that's one hour before you have to leave the house. For others, it might be up to two hours. The important thing is not to start your day already feeling rushed and overwhelmed— that puts a lot of pressure on your thyroid, your adrenal glands, and your immune system, depriving you of the energy and calm you need to handle whatever challenges come up!

For the twenty-eight-day plan, the meals are designed to serve two people and in most cases include enough for leftovers. So here's what I suggest:

- **If you're cooking for two,** just follow the recipes regardless of the amount of servings they make. You'll get leftovers only for the food that keeps well.
- **If you're cooking for one,** cut every recipe in half. That leaves you one portion of leftovers for the recipes where the food keeps and no leftovers for the food that doesn't keep.
- **If you're cooking for four,** double the recipes. Again, you'll get leftovers when you need them, and not when you don't.

Enjoy!

DAY 1

Morning

- Take your supplemental thyroid hormone, if applicable.
- If you are following the SIBO, yeast-overgrowth, or parasite protocol, take your upon-waking supplements.
- Drink one to two cups filtered water with juice from ½ lemon.
- Go outside for at least five minutes within twenty minutes of waking to let the natural daylight hit your eyes and skin.
- Relax with HeartMath, Muse, binaural beats, brain-wave entrainment, meditation, prayer, breath work for ten to thirty minutes.
- Enjoy one cup of *The Myers Way Gut-Healing Collagen Tea (page 322).*

Breakfast

- *Sweet Potato and Greens Breakfast Hash (page 322)* with *Cinnamon Apple Breakfast Sausages (page 324)*
- Take your breakfast supplements (page 268).

One daily snack (enjoyed either before lunch or before dinner)

- ½ cup mixed berries

Lunch

- *Citrus Shrimp over Red Leaf Lettuce Salad (pages 329–330)*
- Take your lunchtime supplements (pages 268–269).

After your workday is done

- Choose your thyroid- and adrenal-friendly exercise: walk, yoga, cardio, light weights, Pilates, dancing, playing actively with your kids.

Before dinner

- Use lamps with amber lightbulbs exclusively or put on amber eyeglasses.
- Make sure your phone and computer are set to f.lux app or nighttime settings.

Dinner

- *Apricot Chicken Salad (page 334)*
- Put *Gut-Healing Bone Broth (page 331)* in crockpot overnight.
- Take your dinnertime supplements (page 269).

After dinner

- Spend at least thirty minutes doing something that brings you joy: socializing, reading, crafting, yoga, writing/journaling, taking a walk.

Before bed

- Relax with HeartMath, Muse, binaural beats, brain-wave entrainment, meditation, prayer, breath work for ten to thirty minutes.
- Enjoy a warm bath with epsom salt and your favorite essential oils.
- Drink your bedtime herbal tea.
- If you are following the SIBO, yeast overgrowth, or parasite protocol, take your bedtime supplements.

Bedtime

- Turn off all electronics.
- Make sure your room is dark or use an eye mask.
- Lower your thermostat to a cool and relaxing temperature.
- Enjoy seven and a half to nine hours of deep, restful sleep.

Once a week I would love you to try a new relaxation technique—for example, acupuncture, float tank, massage, or neurofeedback (see pages 226–228). Once you find one or more techniques that work for you, enjoy them as often as your schedule and budget permit.

DAY 2

Morning

- Take your supplemental thyroid hormone, if applicable.
- If you are following the SIBO, yeast overgrowth, or parasite protocol, take your upon-waking supplements.
- Drink one to two cups filtered water with juice from ½ lemon.
- Go outside for at least five minutes within twenty minutes of waking to let the natural daylight hit your eyes and skin.
- Relax with HeartMath, Muse, binaural beats, brain-wave entrainment, meditation, prayer, breath work for ten to thirty minutes.
- Enjoy one cup of leftover *Gut-Healing Bone Broth* or *The Myers Way Gut-Healing Collagen Tea (page 322).*

Breakfast

- *Cinnamon Cocoa Smoothie (page 319)*
- Take your breakfast supplements (page 268).

One daily snack—enjoyed either before lunch or before dinner

- *Classic Green Juice (page 321)*

Lunch

- Leftover *Citrus Shrimp over Red Leaf Lettuce Salad*
- Take your lunchtime supplements (pages 268–269).

After your workday is done

- Choose your thyroid- and adrenal-friendly exercise: walk, yoga, cardio, light weights, Pilates, dancing, playing actively with your kids.

Before dinner

- Use lamps with amber lightbulbs exclusively or put on amber eyeglasses.
- Make sure your phone and computer are set to "f.lux app" or nighttime settings.

Dinner

- *Pineapple Taco Salad with Grass-Fed Beef (page 325)*
- Take your dinnertime supplements (page 269).

After dinner

- Spend at least thirty minutes doing something that brings you joy: socializing, reading, crafting, yoga, writing/journaling, taking a walk.

Before bed

- Relax with HeartMath, Muse, binaural beats, brain-wave entrainment, meditation, prayer, breath work for ten to thirty minutes.
- Enjoy a warm bath with epsom salt and your favorite essential oils.
- Drink your bedtime herbal tea.
- If you are following the SIBO, yeast overgrowth, or parasite protocol, take your bedtime supplements.

Bedtime

- Turn off all electronics.
- Make sure your room is dark or use an eye mask.
- Lower your thermostat to a cool and relaxing temperature.
- Enjoy seven and a half to nine hours of deep, restful sleep.

DAY 3

Morning

- Take your supplemental thyroid hormone, if applicable.
- If you are following the SIBO, yeast overgrowth, or parasite protocol, take your upon-waking supplements.
- Drink one to two cups filtered water with juice from ½ lemon.
- Go outside for at least five minutes within twenty minutes of waking to let the natural daylight hit your eyes and skin.
- Relax with HeartMath, Muse, binaural beats, brain-wave entrainment, meditation, prayer, breath work for ten to thirty minutes.
- Enjoy one cup of leftover *Gut-Healing Bone Broth* or *The Myers Way Gut-Healing Collagen Tea (page 322)*.

Breakfast

- Leftover *Sweet Potato and Greens Breakfast Hash* with *Cinnamon Apple Breakfast Sausages*
- Take your breakfast supplements (page 268).

One daily snack (enjoyed either before lunch or before dinner)

- Avocado with mixed raw veggies: cucumbers, carrots, celery, zucchini

Lunch

- Leftover *Apricot Chicken Salad*
- Take your lunchtime supplements (pages 268–269).

After your workday is done

- Choose your thyroid- and adrenal-friendly exercise: walk, yoga, cardio, light weights, Pilates, dancing, playing actively with your kids.

Before dinner

- Use lamps with amber lightbulbs exclusively or put on amber eyeglasses.
- Make sure your phone and computer are set to "f.lux app" or nighttime settings.

Dinner

- *Wild-Caught Cod with Sage Parsnip Mash and Asparagus (pages 342–343)*
- Prepare *Gut-Healing Bone Broth (page 331)* in crockpot overnight.
- Take your dinnertime supplements (page 269).

After dinner

- Spend at least thirty minutes doing something that brings you joy: socializing, reading, crafting, yoga, writing/journaling, taking a walk.

Before bed

- Relax with HeartMath, Muse, binaural beats, brain-wave entrainment, meditation, prayer, breath work for ten to thirty minutes.
- Enjoy a warm bath with epsom salt and your favorite essential oils.
- Drink your bedtime herbal tea.
- If you are following the SIBO, yeast overgrowth, or parasite protocol, take your bedtime supplements.

Bedtime

- Turn off all electronics.
- Make sure your room is dark or use an eye mask.
- Lower your thermostat to a cool and relaxing temperature.
- Enjoy seven and a half to nine hours of deep, restful sleep.

DAY 4

Morning

- Take your supplemental thyroid hormone, if applicable.
- If you are following the SIBO, yeast overgrowth, or parasite protocol, take your upon-waking supplements.
- Drink one to two cups filtered water with juice from ½ lemon.
- Go outside for at least five minutes within twenty minutes to let the natural daylight hit your eyes and skin.
- Relax with HeartMath, Muse, binaural beats, brain-wave entrainment meditation, prayer, breath work for 10 to 30 minutes.
- Enjoy one cup of leftover *Gut-Healing Bone Broth* or *The Myers Way Gut-Healing Collagen Tea (page 322)*.

Breakfast

- *Pear and Parsley Smoothie (page 319)*
- Take your breakfast supplements (page 268).

One daily snack (enjoyed either before lunch or before dinner)

- Leftover *Apricot Chicken Salad*

Lunch

- Leftover *Pineapple Taco Salad with Grass-Fed Beef*
- Take your lunchtime supplements (pages 268–269).

After your workday is done

- Choose your thyroid- and adrenal-friendly exercise: walk, yoga, cardio, light weights, Pilates, dancing, playing actively with your kids.

Before dinner

- Use lamps with amber lightbulbs exclusively or put on amber eyeglasses.
- Make sure your phone and computer are set to "f.lux app" or nighttime settings.

Dinner

- *Wild-Caught Salmon with Zucchini Noodle Pesto and Garlic Butternut Squash (pages 340–341)*
- Take your dinnertime supplements (page 269).

After dinner

- Spend at least thirty minutes doing something that brings you joy: socializing, reading, crafting, yoga, writing/journaling, taking a walk.

Before bed

- Relax with HeartMath, Muse, binaural beats, brain-wave entrainment, meditation, prayer, breath work for ten to thirty minutes.
- Enjoy a warm bath with epsom salt and your favorite essential oils.
- Drink your bedtime herbal tea.
- If you are following the SIBO, yeast overgrowth, or parasite protocol, take your bedtime supplements.

Bedtime

- Turn off all electronics.
- Make sure your room is dark or use an eye mask.
- Lower your thermostat to a cool and restful temperature.
- Enjoy seven and a half to nine hours of deep, restful sleep.

DAY 5

Morning

- Take your supplemental thyroid hormone, if applicable.
- If you are following the SIBO, yeast overgrowth, or parasite protocol, take your upon-waking supplements.
- Drink one to two cups filtered water with juice from ½ lemon.
- Go outside for at least five minutes within twenty minutes of waking to let the natural daylight hit your eyes and skin.
- Relax with HeartMath, Muse, binaural beats, brain-wave entrainment, meditation, prayer, breath work for ten to thirty minutes.
- Enjoy one cup of leftover *Gut-Healing Bone Broth* or *The Myers Way Gut-Healing Collagen Tea (page 322)*.

Breakfast

- Breakfast: *Grass-Fed Beef and Veggie Breakfast Scramble (page 323)*
- Take your breakfast supplements (page 268).

One daily snack (enjoyed either before lunch or before dinner)

- ½ cup mixed berries

Lunch

- Leftover *Wild-Caught Cod with Sage Parsnip Mash and Asparagus*
- Take your lunchtime supplements (pages 268–269).

After your workday is done

- Choose your thyroid- and adrenal-friendly exercise: walk, yoga, cardio, light weights, Pilates, dancing, playing actively with your kids.

Before dinner

- Use lamps with amber lightbulbs exclusively or put on amber eyeglasses.
- Make sure your phone and computer are set to "f.lux app" or nighttime settings.

Dinner

- *Turkey Meatballs over Spaghetti Squash with Tuscan Kale Pesto (pages 337–338)* with *Spinach Salad with Outstanding Dressing (page 330)*
- Take your dinnertime supplements (page 269).

After dinner

- Spend at least thirty minutes doing something that brings you joy: socializing, reading, crafting, yoga, writing/journaling, taking a walk.

Before bed

- Relax with HeartMath, Muse, binaural beats, brain-wave entrainment, meditation, prayer, breath work for ten to thirty minutes.
- Enjoy a warm bath with epsom salt and your favorite essential oils.
- Drink your bedtime herbal tea.
- If you are following the SIBO, yeast overgrowth, or parasite protocol, take your bedtime supplements.

Bedtime

- Turn off all electronics.
- Make sure your room is dark or use an eye mask.
- Lower your thermostat to a cool and relaxing temperature.
- Enjoy seven and a half to nine hours of deep, restful sleep.

DAY 6

Morning

- Take your supplemental thyroid hormone, if applicable.
- If you are following the SIBO, yeast overgrowth, or parasite protocol, take your upon-waking supplements.
- Drink one to two cups filtered water with juice from ½ lemon.
- Go outside for at least five minutes within twenty minutes of waking to let the natural daylight hit your eyes and skin.
- Relax with HeartMath, Muse, binaural beats, brain-wave entrainment, meditation, prayer, breath work for ten to thirty minutes.
- Enjoy one cup of leftover *Gut-Healing Bone Broth* or *The Myers Way Gut-Healing Collagen Tea (page 322)*. Freeze leftover bone broth.

Breakfast

- *Berry Coconut Breakfast Parfait with Cocoa Dust and Orange Zest (pages 324–325)*
- Take your breakfast supplements (page 268).

One daily snack (enjoyed either before lunch or before dinner)

- *Cucumber Seaweed Salad (page 350)*

Lunch

- Leftover *Wild-Caught Salmon with Zucchini Noodle Pesto and Garlic Butternut Squash*
- Take your lunchtime supplements (pages 268–269).

After your workday is done

- Choose your thyroid- and adrenal-friendly exercise: walk, yoga, cardio, light weights, Pilates, dancing, playing actively with your kids.

Before dinner

- Use lamps with amber lightbulbs exclusively or put on amber eyeglasses.
- Make sure your phone and computer are set to "f.lux app" or nighttime settings.

Dinner

- *Coconut Chicken Curry (pages 335–336)*
- Take your dinnertime supplements (page 269).

After dinner

- Spend at least thirty minutes doing something that brings you joy: socializing, reading, crafting, yoga, writing/journaling, taking a walk.

Before bed

- Relax with HeartMath, Muse, binaural beats, brain-wave entrainment, meditation, prayer, breath work for ten to thirty minutes.
- Enjoy a warm bath with epsom salt and your favorite essential oils.
- Drink your bedtime herbal tea.
- If you are following the SIBO, yeast overgrowth, or parasite protocol, take your bedtime supplements.

Bedtime

- Turn off all electronics.
- Make sure your room is dark or use an eye mask.
- Lower your thermostat to a cool and relaxing temperature.
- Enjoy seven and a half to nine hours of deep, restful sleep.

DAY 7

Morning

- Take your supplemental thyroid hormone, if applicable.
- If you are following the SIBO, yeast overgrowth, or parasite protocol, take your upon-waking supplements.
- Drink one to two cups filtered water with juice from ½ lemon.
- Go outside for at least five minutes within twenty minutes of waking to let the natural daylight hit your eyes and skin.
- Relax with HeartMath, Muse, binaural beats, brain-wave entrainment, meditation, prayer, breath work for ten to thirty minutes.
- Enjoy one cup of *The Myers Way "Spa" Water (pages 321–322)*

Breakfast

- Leftover *Grass-Fed Beef and Veggie Breakfast Scramble*
- Take your breakfast supplements (page 268).

One daily snack (enjoyed either before lunch or before dinner)

- Leftover *Cucumber Seaweed Salad*

Lunch

- Leftover *Organic Turkey Meatballs over Spaghetti Squash with Tuscan Kale Pesto* with *Spinach Salad with Outstanding Dressing*
- Take your lunchtime supplements (pages 268–269).

After your workday is done

- Choose your thyroid- and adrenal-friendly exercise: walk, yoga, cardio, light weights, Pilates, dancing, playing actively with your kids.

Before dinner

- Use lamps with amber lightbulbs or put on amber eyeglasses.
- Make sure your phone and computer are set to "f.lux app" or nighttime settings.

Dinner

- *Greek Lamb Burger with Coconut Tzatziki and Zucchini Half-Moons (pages 346–348)*
- Dessert: *Lemon Coconut Macaroons with Dark Chocolate Drizzle (pages 352–353)*
- Take your dinnertime supplements (page 269).

After dinner

- Spend at least thirty minutes doing something that brings you joy: socializing, reading, crafting, yoga, writing/journaling, taking a walk.

Before bed

- Relax with HeartMath, Muse, binaural beats, brain-wave entrainment, meditation, prayer, breath work for ten to thirty minutes.
- Enjoy a warm bath with epsom salt and your favorite essential oils.
- Drink your bedtime herbal tea.
- If you are following the SIBO, yeast overgrowth, or parasite protocol, take your bedtime supplements.

Bedtime

- Turn off all electronics.
- Make sure your room is dark or use an eye mask.
- Lower your thermostat to a cool and relaxing temperature.
- Enjoy seven and a half to nine hours of deep, restful sleep.

DAY 8

Morning

- Take your supplemental thyroid hormone, if applicable.
- If you are following the SIBO, yeast overgrowth, or parasite protocol, take your upon-waking supplements.
- Drink one to two cups filtered water with juice from ½ lemon.
- Go outside for at least five minutes within twenty minutes of waking to let the natural daylight hit your eyes and skin.
- Relax with HeartMath, Muse, binaural beats, brain-wave entrainment, meditation, prayer, breath work for ten to thirty minutes.
- Enjoy one cup of caffeine-free herbal tea or herbal coffee

Breakfast

- *Blueberries and Cream Smoothie (pages 318–319)*
- Take your breakfast supplements (page 268).

One daily snack (enjoyed either before lunch or before dinner)

- Avocado with mixed raw veggies: cucumbers, carrots, celery, zucchini

Lunch

- Leftover *Coconut Chicken Curry*
- Take your lunchtime supplements (pages 268–269).

After your workday is done

- Choose your thyroid- and adrenal-friendly exercise: walk, yoga, cardio, light weights, Pilates, dancing, playing actively with your kids.

Before dinner

- Use lamps with amber lightbulbs exclusively or put on amber eyeglasses.
- Make sure your phone and computer are set to "f.lux app" or nighttime settings.

Dinner

- *Wild-Caught Scallop Spinach Salad with Pomegranate Vinaigrette (page 327)*
- Take your dinnertime supplements (page 269).

After dinner

- Spend at least thirty minutes doing something that brings you joy: socializing, reading, crafting, yoga, writing/journaling, taking a walk.

Before bed

- Relax with HeartMath, Muse, binaural beats, brain-wave entrainment, meditation, prayer, breath work for ten to thirty minutes.
- Enjoy a warm bath with epsom salt and your favorite essential oils.
- Drink your bedtime herbal tea.
- If you are following the SIBO, yeast overgrowth, or parasite protocol, take your bedtime supplements

Bedtime

- Turn off all electronics.
- Make sure your room is dark or use an eye mask.
- Lower your thermostat to a cool and relaxing temperature.
- Enjoy seven and a half to nine hours of deep, restful sleep.

Once a week I would love you to try a new relaxation technique, for example acupuncture, float tank, massage, or neurofeedback (see pages 226–228). Once you find one or more techniques that work for you, enjoy them as often as your schedule and budget permit.

DAY 9

Morning
- Take your supplemental thyroid hormone, if applicable.
- If you are following the SIBO, yeast overgrowth, or parasite protocol, take your upon-waking supplements.
- Drink one to two cups filtered water with juice from ½ lemon.
- Go outside for at least five minutes within twenty minutes of waking to let the natural daylight hit your eyes and skin.
- Relax with HeartMath, Muse, binaural beats, brain-wave entrainment, meditation, prayer, breath work for ten to thirty minutes.
- Enjoy one cup of leftover *The Myers Way "Spa" Water*

Breakfast
- *Ginger Avocado Green Smoothie (page 320)*
- Take your breakfast supplements (page 268).

One daily snack (enjoyed either before lunch or before dinner)
- *Beet Fennel Juice (pages 320–321)*

Lunch
- Leftover *Greek Lamb Burger with Coconut Tzatziki and Zucchini Half-Moons*
- Take your lunchtime supplements (pages 268–269).

After your workday is done
- Choose your thyroid- and adrenal-friendly exercise: walk, yoga, cardio, light weights, Pilates, dancing, playing actively with your kids.

Before dinner
- Use lamps with amber lightbulbs exclusively or put on amber eyeglasses.
- Make sure your phone and computer are set to "f.lux app" or nighttime settings.

Dinner
- *Chimichurri Grass-Fed Skirt Steak Salad with Garlic Lime Asparagus (pages 328–329)*
- Take your dinnertime supplements (page 269).

After dinner

- Spend at least thirty minutes doing something that brings you joy: socializing, reading, crafting, yoga, writing/journaling, taking a walk.

Before bed

- Relax with HeartMath, Muse, binaural beats, brain-wave entrainment, meditation, prayer, breath work for ten to thirty minutes.
- Enjoy a warm bath with epsom salt and your favorite essential oils.
- Drink your bedtime herbal tea.
- If you are following the SIBO, yeast overgrowth, or parasite protocol, take your bedtime supplements.

Bedtime

- Turn off all electronics.
- Make sure your room is dark or use an eye mask.
- Lower your thermostat to a cool and relaxing temperature.
- Enjoy seven and a half to nine hours of deep, restful sleep.

DAY 10

Morning

- Take your supplemental thyroid hormone, if applicable.
- If you are following the SIBO, yeast overgrowth, or parasite protocol, take your upon-waking supplements.
- Drink one to two cups filtered water with juice from ½ lemon.
- Go outside for at least five minutes within twenty minutes of waking to let the natural daylight hit your eyes and skin.
- Relax with HeartMath, Muse, binaural beats, brain-wave entrainment, meditation, prayer, breath work for ten to thirty minutes.
- Enjoy one cup of caffeine-free herbal tea or herbal coffee.

Breakfast

- *Sweet Potato and Greens Breakfast Hash (pages 322–323)* with *Cinnamon Apple Breakfast Sausages (pages 324)*
- Take your breakfast supplements (page 268).

One daily snack (enjoyed either before lunch or before dinner)

- ½ cup mixed berries

Lunch

- Leftover *Wild-Caught Scallop Spinach Salad with Pomegranate Vinaigrette*
- Take your lunchtime supplements (pages 268–269).

After your workday is done

- Choose your thyroid- and adrenal-friendly exercise: walk, yoga, cardio, light weights, Pilates, dancing, playing actively with your kids.

Before dinner

- Use lamps with amber lightbulbs exclusively or put on amber eyeglasses.
- Make sure your phone and computer are set to "f.lux app" or nighttime settings.

Dinner

- *Kelp Noodle Stir-Fry with Chicken and Veggies (page 335)*
- Put *Gut-Healing Bone Broth (page 331)* in crockpot overnight.
- Take your dinnertime supplements (page 269).

After dinner

- Spend at least thirty minutes doing something that brings you joy: socializing, reading, crafting, yoga, writing/journaling, taking a walk.

Before bed

- Relax with HeartMath, Muse, binaural beats, brain-wave entrainment, meditation, prayer, breath work for ten to thirty minutes.
- Enjoy a warm bath with epsom salt and your favorite essential oils.
- Drink your bedtime herbal tea.
- If you are following the SIBO, yeast overgrowth, or parasite protocol, take your bedtime supplements.

Bedtime

- Turn off all electronics.
- Make sure your room is dark or use an eye mask.
- Lower your thermostat to a cool and relaxing temperature.
- Enjoy seven and a half to nine hours of deep, restful sleep.

DAY 11

Morning

- Take your supplemental thyroid hormone, if applicable.
- If you are following the SIBO, yeast overgrowth, or parasite protocol, take your upon-waking supplements.
- Drink one to two cups filtered water with juice from ½ lemon.
- Go outside for at least five minutes within twenty minutes of waking to let the natural daylight hit your eyes and skin.
- Relax with HeartMath, Muse, binaural beats, brain-wave entrainment, meditation, prayer, breath work for ten to thirty minutes.
- Enjoy one cup of leftover *Gut-Healing Bone Broth* or *The Myers Way Gut-Healing Collagen Tea (page 322)*.

Breakfast

- *Berry Coconut Breakfast Parfait with Cocoa Dust and Orange Zest (pages 324–325)*
- Take your breakfast supplements (page 268).
- One daily snack (enjoyed either before lunch or before dinner)
- *Cranberry Ginger Juice (page 321)*

Lunch

- Leftover *Chimichurri Grass-Fed Skirt Steak Salad with Garlic Lime Asparagus*
- Take your lunchtime supplements (pages 268–269).

After your workday is done

- Choose your thyroid- and adrenal-friendly exercise: walk, yoga, cardio, light weights, Pilates, dancing, playing actively with your kids.

Before dinner

- Use lamps with amber lightbulbs exclusively or put on amber eyeglasses.
- Make sure your phone and computer are set to "f.lux app" or nighttime settings.

Dinner

- *Curried Coconut Soup with Shrimp and Veggies (pages 332–334)*
- Take your dinnertime supplements (page 269).

After dinner

- Spend at least thirty minutes doing something that brings you joy: socializing, reading, crafting, yoga, writing/journaling, taking a walk.

Before bed

- Relax with HeartMath, Muse, binaural beats, brain-wave entrainment, meditation, prayer, breath work for ten to thirty minutes.
- Enjoy a warm bath with epsom salt and your favorite essential oils.
- Drink your bedtime herbal tea.
- If you are following the SIBO, yeast overgrowth, or parasite protocol, take your bedtime supplements.

Bedtime

- Turn off all electronics.
- Make sure your room is dark or use an eye mask.
- Lower your thermostat to a cool and relaxing temperature.
- Enjoy seven and a half to nine hours of deep, restful sleep.

DAY 12

Morning

- Take your supplemental thyroid hormone, if applicable.
- If you are following the SIBO, yeast overgrowth, or parasite protocol, take your upon-waking supplements.
- Drink one to two cups filtered water with juice from ½ lemon.
- Go outside for at least five minutes within twenty minutes of waking to let the natural daylight hit your eyes and skin.
- Relax with HeartMath, Muse, binaural beats, brain-wave entrainment, meditation, prayer, breath work for ten to thirty minutes.
- Morning: caffeine-free herbal tea or herbal coffee

Breakfast

- Leftover *Sweet Potato and Greens Breakfast Hash* with *Cinnamon Apple Breakfast Sausage*
- Take your breakfast supplements (page 268).

One daily snack (enjoyed either before lunch or before dinner)

- Avocado with mixed raw veggies: cucumbers, carrots, celery, zucchini

Lunch

- Leftover *Kelp Noodle Stir-Fry with Chicken and Veggies*
- Take your lunchtime supplements (pages 268–269).

After your workday is done

- Choose your thyroid- and adrenal-friendly exercise: walk, yoga, cardio, light weights, Pilates, dancing, playing actively with your kids.

Before dinner

- Use lamps with amber lightbulbs exclusively or put on amber eyeglasses.
- Make sure your phone and computer are set to "f.lux app" or nighttime settings.

Dinner

- *Sautéed Cranberry Kale with Bacon over Sweet Potatoes (pages 345– 346)* with *Spinach Salad with Outstanding Dressing (page 330)*
- Take your dinnertime supplements (page 269).

After dinner

- Spend at least thirty minutes doing something that brings you joy: socializing, reading, crafting, yoga, writing/journaling, taking a walk.

Before bed

- Relax with HeartMath, Muse, binaural beats, brain-wave entrainment, meditation, prayer, breath work for ten to thirty minutes.
- Enjoy a warm bath with epsom salt and your favorite essential oils.
- Drink your bedtime herbal tea.
- If you are following the SIBO, yeast overgrowth, or parasite protocol, take your bedtime supplements.

Bedtime

- Turn off all electronics.
- Make sure your room is dark or use an eye mask.
- Lower your thermostat to a cool and relaxing temperature.
- Enjoy seven and a half to nine hours of deep, restful sleep.

DAY 13

Morning

- Take your supplemental thyroid hormone, if applicable.
- If you are following the SIBO, yeast overgrowth, or parasite protocol, take your upon-waking supplements.
- Drink one to two cups filtered water with juice from ½ lemon.
- Go outside for at least five minutes within twenty minutes of waking to let the natural daylight hit your eyes and skin.
- Relax with HeartMath, Muse, binaural beats, brain-wave entrainment, meditation, prayer, breath work for ten to thirty minutes.
- Enjoy one cup of leftover *Gut-Healing Bone Broth* or *The Myers Way Gut-Healing Collagen Tea (page 322)*.

Breakfast

- *Blueberries and Cream Smoothie (pages 318–319)*
- Take your breakfast supplements (page 268).

One daily snack (enjoyed either before lunch or before dinner)

- *Classic Green Juice (page 321)*

Lunch

- Leftover *Curried Coconut Soup with Shrimp and Veggies*
- Take your lunchtime supplements (pages 268–269).

After your workday is done

- Choose your thyroid- and adrenal-friendly exercise: walk, yoga, cardio, light weights, Pilates, dancing, playing actively with your kids.

Before dinner

- Use lamps with amber lightbulbs exclusively or put on amber eyeglasses.
- Make sure your phone and computer are set to "f.lux app" or nighttime settings.

Dinner

- *Hawaiian Fish "Tacos" with Mango Salsa (pages 341–342)*
- Take your dinnertime supplements (page 269).

After dinner

- Spend at least thirty minutes doing something that brings you joy: socializing, reading, crafting, yoga, writing/journaling, taking a walk.

Before bed

- Relax with HeartMath, Muse, binaural beats, brain-wave entrainment, meditation, prayer, breath work for ten to thirty minutes.
- Enjoy a warm bath with epsom salt and your favorite essential oils.
- Drink your bedtime herbal tea.
- If you are following the SIBO, yeast overgrowth, or parasite protocol, take your bedtime supplements.

Bedtime

- Turn off all electronics.
- Make sure your room is dark or use an eye mask.
- Lower your thermostat to a cool and relaxing temperature.
- Enjoy seven and a half to nine hours of deep, restful sleep.

DAY 14

Morning

- Take your supplemental thyroid hormone, if applicable.
- If you are following the SIBO, yeast overgrowth, or parasite protocol, take your upon-waking supplements.
- Drink one to two cups filtered water with juice from ½ lemon.
- Go outside for at least five minutes within twenty minutes of waking to let the natural daylight hit your eyes and skin.
- Relax with HeartMath, Muse, binaural beats, brain-wave entrainment, meditation, prayer, breath work for ten to thirty minutes.
- Enjoy 1 cup of caffeine-free herbal tea or herbal coffee

Breakfast

- *Cinnamon Cocoa Smoothie (page 319)*
- Take your breakfast supplements (page 268).

One daily snack (enjoyed either before lunch or before dinner)

- *Beet Fennel Juice (pages 320–321)*

Lunch

- Leftover *Sautéed Cranberry Kale with Bacon over Sweet Potatoes* with *Spinach Salad with Outstanding Dressing*
- Take your lunchtime supplements (pages 268–269).

After your workday is done

- Choose your thyroid- and adrenal-friendly exercise: walk, yoga, cardio, light weights, Pilates, dancing, playing actively with your kids.

Before dinner

- Use lamps with amber lightbulbs exclusively or put on amber eyeglasses.
- Make sure your phone and computer are set to "f.lux app" or nighttime settings.

Dinner

- *Grass-Fed Steak with Thyme-Roasted Root Veggies (pages 344–345)* with *Spinach Salad with Outstanding Dressing (page 330)*
- Dessert: *Decadent Cocoa Pudding (pages 350–351)*
- Take your dinnertime supplements (page 269).

After dinner

- Spend at least thirty minutes doing something that brings you joy: socializing, reading, crafting, yoga, writing/journaling, taking a walk.

Before bed

- Relax with HeartMath, Muse, binaural beats, brain-wave entrainment, meditation, prayer, breath work for ten to thirty minutes.
- Enjoy a warm bath with epsom salt and your favorite essential oils.
- Drink your bedtime herbal tea.
- If you are following the SIBO, yeast overgrowth, or parasite protocol, take your bedtime supplements.

Bedtime

- Turn off all electronics.
- Make sure your room is dark or use an eye mask.
- Lower your thermostat to a cool and relaxing temperature.
- Enjoy seven and a half to nine hours of deep, restful sleep.

DAY 15

Morning

- Take your supplemental thyroid hormone, if applicable.
- If you are following the SIBO, yeast overgrowth, or parasite protocol, take your upon-waking supplements.
- Drink one to two cups filtered water with juice from ½ lemon.
- Go outside for at least five minutes within twenty minutes of waking to let the natural daylight hit your eyes and skin.
- Relax with HeartMath, Muse, binaural beats, brain-wave entrainment, meditation, prayer, breath work for ten to thirty minutes.
- Enjoy one cup of *The Myers Way "Spa" Water (pages 321–322)*

Breakfast

- *Pear and Parsley Smoothie (page 319)*
- Take your breakfast supplements (page 268).

One daily snack (enjoyed either before lunch or before dinner)

- *Simple Sardine Snack (page 349)*

Lunch

- Leftover *Hawaiian Fish "Tacos" with Mango Salsa*
- Take your lunchtime supplements (pages 268–269).

After your workday is done

- Choose your thyroid- and adrenal-friendly exercise: walk, yoga, cardio, light weights, Pilates, dancing, playing actively with your kids.

Before dinner

- Use lamps with amber lightbulbs exclusively or put on amber eyeglasses.
- Make sure your phone and computer are set to "f.lux app" or nighttime settings.

Dinner

- *Oven-Roasted Chicken (pages 336–337)* with *Texas Grapefruit and Avocado Spinach Salad with Shredded Chicken (pages 326–327)*
- Put *Gut-Healing Bone Broth (page 331)* in crockpot overnight.
- Take your dinnertime supplements (page 269).

After dinner

- Spend at least thirty minutes doing something that brings you joy: socializing, reading, crafting, yoga, writing/journaling, taking a walk.

Before bed

- Relax with HeartMath, Muse, binaural beats, brain-wave entrainment, meditation, prayer, breath work for ten to thirty minutes.
- Enjoy a warm bath with epsom salt and your favorite essential oils.
- Drink your bedtime herbal tea.
- If you are following the SIBO, yeast overgrowth, or parasite protocol, take your bedtime supplements.

Bedtime

- Turn off all electronics.
- Make sure your room is dark or use an eye mask.
- Lower your thermostat to a cool and relaxing temperature.
- Enjoy seven and a half to nine hours of deep, restful sleep.

Once a week I would love you to try a new relaxation technique, for example acupuncture, float tank, massage, or neurofeedback (see pages 226–228). Once you find one or more techniques that work for you, enjoy them as often as your schedule and budget permit.

DAY 16

Morning

- Take your supplemental thyroid hormone, if applicable.
- If you are following the SIBO, yeast overgrowth, or parasite protocol, take your upon-waking supplements.
- Drink one to two cups filtered water with juice from ½ lemon.
- Go outside for at least five minutes within twenty minutes of waking to let the natural daylight hit your eyes and skin.
- Relax with HeartMath, Muse, binaural beats, brain-wave entrainment, meditation, prayer, breath work for ten to thirty minutes.
- Enjoy one cup of leftover *Gut-Healing Bone Broth,* made the night before

Breakfast
- *Grass-Fed Beef and Veggie Breakfast Scramble (page 323)*
- Take your breakfast supplements (page 268).

One daily snack (enjoyed either before lunch or before dinner)
- ½ cup mixed berries

Lunch
- Leftover *Grass-Fed Steak with Thyme-Roasted Root Veggies* with *Spinach Salad with Outstanding Dressing*
- Take your lunchtime supplements (pages 268–269).

After your workday is done
- Choose your thyroid- and adrenal-friendly exercise: walk, yoga, cardio, light weights, Pilates, dancing, playing actively with your kids.

Before dinner
- Use lamps with amber lightbulbs exclusively or put on amber eyeglasses.
- Make sure your phone and computer are set to "f.lux app" or nighttime settings.

Dinner
- *Wild-Caught Shrimp Sushi Rolls with Spinach, Carrots, and Cucumber (pages 339–340)* with *Cucumber Seaweed Salad (page 350)*
- Take your dinnertime supplements (page 269).

After dinner
- Spend at least thirty minutes doing something that brings you joy: socializing, reading, crafting, yoga, writing/journaling, taking a walk.

Before bed
- Relax with HeartMath, Muse, binaural beats, brain-wave entrainment, meditation, prayer, breath work for ten to thirty minutes.
- Enjoy a warm bath with epsom salt and your favorite essential oils.
- Drink your bedtime herbal tea.
- If you are following the SIBO, yeast overgrowth, or parasite protocol, take your bedtime supplements.

Bedtime
- Turn off all electronics.
- Make sure your room is dark or use an eye mask.

- Lower your thermostat to a cool and relaxing temperature.
- Enjoy seven and a half to nine hours of deep, restful sleep.

DAY 17

Morning

- Take your supplemental thyroid hormone, if applicable.
- If you are following the SIBO, yeast overgrowth, or parasite protocol, take your upon-waking supplements.
- Drink one to two cups filtered water with juice from ½ lemon.
- Go outside for at least five minutes within twenty minutes of waking to let the natural daylight hit your eyes and skin.
- Relax with HeartMath, Muse, binaural beats, brain-wave entrainment, meditation, prayer, breath work for ten to thirty minutes.
- Enjoy one cup of *The Myers Way "Spa" Water (pages 321–322)*

Breakfast

- *Ginger Avocado Green Smoothie* (page 320)
- Take your breakfast supplements (page 268).

One daily snack (enjoyed either before lunch or before dinner)

- Leftover *Cucumber Seaweed Salad*

Lunch

- Leftover *Texas Grapefruit and Avocado Spinach Salad with Shredded Chicken*
- Take your lunchtime supplements (pages 268–269).

After your workday is done

- Choose your thyroid- and adrenal-friendly exercise: walk, yoga, cardio, light weights, Pilates, dancing, playing actively with your kids.

Before dinner

- Use lamps with amber lightbulbs exclusively or put on amber eyeglasses.
- Make sure your phone and computer are set to "f.lux app" or nighttime settings.

Dinner

- *White Sweet Potato and Parsnip Clam Chowder (page 332)* with *Spinach Salad with Outstanding Dressing (page 330)*

- Take your dinnertime supplements (page 269).

After dinner

- Spend at least thirty minutes doing something that brings you joy: socializing, reading, crafting, yoga, writing/journaling, taking a walk.

Before bed

- Relax with HeartMath, Muse, binaural beats, brain-wave entrainment, meditation, prayer, breath work for ten to thirty minutes.
- Enjoy a warm bath with epsom salt and your favorite essential oils.
- Drink your bedtime herbal tea.
- If you are following the SIBO, yeast overgrowth, or parasite protocol, take your bedtime supplements.

Bedtime

- Turn off all electronics.
- Make sure your room is dark or use an eye mask.
- Lower your thermostat to a cool and relaxing temperature.
- Enjoy seven and a half to nine hours of deep, restful sleep.

DAY 18

Morning

- Take your supplemental thyroid hormone, if applicable.
- If you are following the SIBO, yeast overgrowth, or parasite protocol, take your upon-waking supplements.
- Drink one to two cups filtered water with juice from ½ lemon.
- Go outside for at least five minutes within twenty minutes of waking to let the natural daylight hit your eyes and skin.
- Relax with HeartMath, Muse, binaural beats, brain-wave entrainment, meditation, prayer, breath work for ten to thirty minutes.
- Enjoy one cup of leftover *Gut-Healing Bone Broth*

Breakfast

- *Berry Coconut Breakfast Parfait with Cocoa Dust and Orange Zest (page 324)*
- Take your breakfast supplements (page 268).

One daily snack (enjoyed either before lunch or before dinner)

- *Cranberry Ginger Juice (page 321)*

Lunch

- Leftover *Grass-Fed Beef and Veggie Breakfast Scramble*
- Take your lunchtime supplements (pages 268–269).

After your workday is done

- Choose your thyroid- and adrenal-friendly exercise: walk, yoga, cardio, light weights, Pilates, dancing, playing actively with your kids.

Before dinner

- Use lamps with amber lightbulbs exclusively or put on amber eyeglasses.
- Make sure your phone and computer are set to "f.lux app" or nighttime settings.

Dinner

- *Beef Liver with Bacon and Rosemary (page 344)* with *Spinach Salad with Outstanding Dressing (page 330)*
- Take your dinnertime supplements (page 269).

After dinner

- Spend at least thirty minutes doing something that brings you joy: socializing, reading, crafting, yoga, writing/journaling, taking a walk.

Before bed

- Relax with HeartMath, Muse, binaural beats, brain-wave entrainment, meditation, prayer, breath work for ten to thirty minutes.
- Enjoy a warm bath with epsom salt and your favorite essential oils.
- Drink your bedtime herbal tea.
- If you are following the SIBO, yeast overgrowth, or parasite protocol, take your bedtime supplements.

Bedtime

- Turn off all electronics.
- Make sure your room is dark or use an eye mask.
- Lower your thermostat to a cool and relaxing temperature.
- Enjoy seven and a half to nine hours of deep, restful sleep.

DAY 19

Morning

- Take your supplemental thyroid hormone, if applicable.
- If you are following the SIBO, yeast overgrowth, or parasite protocol, take your upon-waking supplements.
- Drink one to two cups filtered water with juice from ½ lemon.
- Go outside for at least five minutes within twenty minutes of waking to let the natural daylight hit your eyes and skin.
- Relax with HeartMath, Muse, binaural beats, brain-wave entrainment, meditation, prayer, breath work for ten to thirty minutes.
- Enjoy one cup of leftover *Gut-Healing Bone Broth* or *The Myers Way Gut-Healing Collagen Tea (page 322)*.

Breakfast

- *Blueberries and Cream Smoothie (pages 318–319)*
- Take your breakfast supplements (page 268).

One daily snack (enjoyed either before lunch or before dinner)

- *Classic Green Juice (page 321)*

Lunch

- Leftover *White Sweet Potato and Parsnip Clam Chowder* with *Spinach Salad with Outstanding Dressing*
- Take your lunchtime supplements (pages 268–269).

After your workday is done

- Choose your thyroid- and adrenal-friendly exercise: walk, yoga, cardio, light weights, Pilates, dancing, playing actively with your kids.

Before dinner

- Use lamps with amber lightbulbs exclusively or put on amber eyeglasses.
- Make sure your phone and computer are set to "f.lux app" or nighttime settings.

Dinner

- *Wild-Caught Salmon with Zucchini Noodle Pesto and Garlic Butternut Squash (pages 340–341)*

- Put *Gut-Healing Bone Broth (page 331)* in crockpot overnight.
- Take your dinnertime supplements (page 269).

After dinner

- Spend at least thirty minutes doing something that brings you joy: socializing, reading, crafting, yoga, writing/journaling, taking a walk.

Before bed

- Relax with HeartMath, Muse, binaural beats, brain-wave entrainment, meditation, prayer, breath work for ten to thirty minutes.
- Enjoy a warm bath with epsom salt and your favorite essential oils.
- Drink your bedtime herbal tea.
- If you are following the SIBO, yeast overgrowth, or parasite protocol, take your bedtime supplements.

Bedtime

- Turn off all electronics.
- Make sure your room is dark or use an eye mask.
- Lower your thermostat to a cool and relaxing temperature.
- Enjoy seven and a half to nine hours of deep, restful sleep.

DAY 20

Morning

- Take your supplemental thyroid hormone, if applicable.
- If you are following the SIBO, yeast overgrowth, or parasite protocol, take your upon-waking supplements.
- Drink one to two cups filtered water with juice from ½ lemon.
- Go outside for at least five minutes within twenty minutes of waking to let the natural daylight hit your eyes and skin.
- Relax with HeartMath, Muse, binaural beats, brain-wave entrainment, meditation, prayer, breath work for ten to thirty minutes.
- Enjoy one cup of leftover *Gut-Healing Bone Broth.*

Breakfast

- *Cinnamon Cocoa Smoothie (page 319)*
- Take your breakfast supplements (page 268).

One daily snack (enjoyed either before lunch or before dinner)
- *Beet Fennel Juice (pages 320–321)*

Lunch
- Leftover *White Sweet Potato and Parsnip Clam Chowder* with *Spinach Salad with Outstanding Dressing*
- Take your lunchtime supplements (pages 268–269).

After your workday is done
- Choose your thyroid- and adrenal-friendly exercise: walk, yoga, cardio, light weights, Pilates, dancing, playing actively with your kids.

Before dinner
- Use lamps with amber lightbulbs exclusively or put on amber eyeglasses.
- Make sure your phone and computer are set to "f.lux app" or nighttime settings.

Dinner
- *Turkey Meatballs over Spaghetti Squash with Tuscan Kale Pesto (pages 337–338)* with *Spinach Salad with Outstanding Dressing (page 330)*
- Take your dinnertime supplements (page 269).

After dinner
- Spend at least thirty minutes doing something that brings you joy: socializing, reading, crafting, yoga, writing/journaling, taking a walk.

Before bed
- Relax with HeartMath, Muse, binaural beats, brain-wave entrainment, meditation, prayer, breath work for ten to thirty minutes.
- Enjoy a warm bath with epsom salt and your favorite essential oils.
- Drink your bedtime herbal tea.
- If you are following the SIBO, yeast overgrowth, or parasite protocol, take your bedtime supplements.

Bedtime
- Turn off all electronics.
- Make sure your room is dark or use an eye mask.
- Lower your thermostat to a cool and relaxing temperature.
- Enjoy seven and a half to nine hours of deep, restful sleep.

DAY 21

Morning

- Take your supplemental thyroid hormone, if applicable.
- If you are following the SIBO, yeast overgrowth, or parasite protocol, take your upon-waking supplements.
- Drink one to two cups filtered water with juice from ½ lemon.
- Go outside for at least five minutes within twenty minutes of waking to let the natural daylight hit your eyes and skin.
- Relax with HeartMath, Muse, binaural beats, brain-wave entrainment, meditation, prayer, breath work for ten to thirty minutes.
- Enjoy one cup of leftover *Gut-Healing Bone Broth* or *The Myers Way Gut-Healing Collagen Tea (page 322).*

Breakfast

- *Sweet Potato and Greens Breakfast Hash (pages 322–323)* with *Cinnamon Apple Breakfast Sausages (page 324)*
- Take your breakfast supplements (page 268).

One daily snack (enjoyed either before lunch or before dinner)

- ½ cup mixed berries

Lunch

- Leftover *Wild-Caught Salmon with Zucchini Noodle Pesto and Garlic Butternut Squash*
- Take your lunchtime supplements (pages 268–269).

After your workday is done

- Choose your thyroid- and adrenal-friendly exercise: walk, yoga, cardio, light weights, Pilates, dancing, playing actively with your kids.

Before dinner

- Use lamps with amber lightbulbs exclusively or put on amber eyeglasses.
- Make sure your phone and computer are set to "f.lux app" or nighttime settings.

Dinner

- *Baked Chicken Breasts with Sautéed Brussels Sprouts, Spinach, and Bacon (pages 338–339)*

- Dessert: *Creamy Fruit Smoothie Pops (page 351)*
- Take your dinnertime supplements (page 269).

After dinner

- Spend at least thirty minutes doing something that brings you joy: socializing, reading, crafting, yoga, writing/journaling, taking a walk.

Before bed

- Relax with HeartMath, Muse, binaural beats, brain-wave entrainment, meditation, prayer, breath work for ten to thirty minutes.
- Enjoy a warm bath with epsom salt and your favorite essential oils.
- Drink your bedtime herbal tea.
- If you are following the SIBO, yeast overgrowth, or parasite protocol, take your bedtime supplements.

Bedtime

- Turn off all electronics.
- Make sure your room is dark or use an eye mask.
- Lower your thermostat to a cool and relaxing temperature.
- Enjoy seven and a half to nine hours of deep, restful sleep.

DAY 22

Morning

- Take your supplemental thyroid hormone, if applicable.
- If you are following the SIBO, yeast overgrowth, or parasite protocol, take your upon-waking supplements.
- Drink one to two cups filtered water with juice from ½ lemon.
- Go outside for at least five minutes within twenty minutes of waking to let the natural daylight hit your eyes and skin.
- Relax with HeartMath, Muse, binaural beats, brain-wave entrainment, meditation, prayer, breath work for ten to thirty minutes.
- Enjoy one cup of caffeine-free herbal tea or herbal coffee.

Breakfast

- *Ginger Avocado Green Smoothie (page 320)*
- Take your breakfast supplements (page 268).

One daily snack (enjoyed either before lunch or before dinner)

- Avocado with mixed raw veggies: cucumbers, carrots, celery, zucchini

Lunch

- Leftover *Turkey Meatballs over Spaghetti Squash with Tuscan Kale Pesto* with *Spinach Salad with Outstanding Dressing*
- Take your lunchtime supplements (pages 268–269).

After your workday is done

- Choose your thyroid- and adrenal-friendly exercise: walk, yoga, cardio, light weights, Pilates, dancing, playing actively with your kids.

Before dinner

- Use lamps with amber lightbulbs exclusively or put on amber eyeglasses.
- Make sure your phone and computer are set to "f.lux app" or nighttime settings.

Dinner

- *Wild-Caught Cod with Sage Parsnip Mash and Asparagus (pages 342–343)*
- Take your dinnertime supplements (page 269).

After dinner

- Spend at least thirty minutes doing something that brings you joy: socializing, reading, crafting, yoga, writing/journaling, taking a walk.

Before bed

- Relax with HeartMath, Muse, binaural beats, brain-wave entrainment, meditation, prayer, breath work for ten to thirty minutes.
- Enjoy a warm bath with epsom salt and your favorite essential oils.
- Drink your bedtime herbal tea.
- If you are following the SIBO, yeast overgrowth, or parasite protocol, take your bedtime supplements.

Bedtime

- Turn off all electronics.
- Make sure your room is dark or use an eye mask.
- Lower your thermostat to a cool and relaxing temperature.
- Enjoy seven and a half to nine hours of deep, restful sleep.

Once a week I would love you to try a new relaxation technique, for example acupuncture, float tank, massage, or neuro-feedback (see pages 226–228). Once you find one or more techniques that work for you, enjoy them as often as your schedule and budget permit.

DAY 23

Morning
- Take your supplemental thyroid hormone, if applicable.
- If you are following the SIBO, yeast overgrowth, or parasite protocol, take your upon-waking supplements.
- Drink one to two cups filtered water with juice from ½ lemon.
- Go outside for at least five minutes within twenty minutes of waking to let the natural daylight hit your eyes and skin.
- Relax with HeartMath, Muse, binaural beats, brain-wave entrainment, meditation, prayer, breath work for ten to thirty minutes.
- Enjoy one cup of leftover *Gut-Healing Bone Broth* or *The Myers Way Gut-Healing Collagen Tea (page 322)*.

Breakfast
- *Berry Coconut Breakfast Parfait with Cocoa Dust and Orange Zest (pages 324–325)*
- Take your breakfast supplements (page 268).

One daily snack (enjoyed either before lunch or before dinner)
- *Cranberry Ginger Juice (page 321)*

Lunch
- Leftover *Baked Chicken Breasts with Sautéed Brussels Sprouts, Spinach, and Bacon*
- Take your lunchtime supplements (pages 268–269).

After your workday is done
- Choose your thyroid- and adrenal-friendly exercise: walk, yoga, cardio, light weights, Pilates, dancing, playing actively with your kids.

Before dinner

- Use lamps with amber lightbulbs exclusively or put on amber eyeglasses.
- Make sure your phone and computer are set to "f.lux app" or nighttime settings.

Dinner

- *Chimichurri Grass-Fed Skirt Steak Salad with Garlic Lime Asparagus (pages 328–329)*
- Take your dinnertime supplements (page 269).

After dinner

- Spend at least thirty minutes doing something that brings you joy: socializing, reading, crafting, yoga, writing/journaling, taking a walk.

Before bed

- Relax with HeartMath, Muse, binaural beats, brain-wave entrainment, meditation, prayer, breath work for ten to thirty minutes.
- Enjoy a warm bath with epsom salt and your favorite essential oils.
- Drink your bedtime herbal tea.
- If you are following the SIBO, yeast overgrowth, or parasite protocol, take your bedtime supplements.

Bedtime

- Turn off all electronics.
- Make sure your room is dark or use an eye mask.
- Lower your thermostat to a cool and relaxing temperature.
- Enjoy seven and a half to nine hours of deep, restful sleep.

DAY 24

Morning

- Take your supplemental thyroid hormone, if applicable.
- If you are following the SIBO, yeast overgrowth, or parasite protocol, take your upon-waking supplements.
- Drink one to two cups filtered water with juice from ½ lemon.
- Go outside for at least five minutes within twenty minutes of waking to let the natural daylight hit your eyes and skin.

- Relax with HeartMath, Muse, binaural beats, brain-wave entrainment, meditation, prayer, breath work for ten to thirty minutes.
- Enjoy one cup of: caffeine-free herbal tea or herbal coffee

Breakfast

- *Blueberries and Cream Smoothie (pages 318–319)*
- Take your breakfast supplements (page 268).

One daily snack (enjoyed either before lunch or before dinner)

- *Simple Sardine Snack (page 349)* or leftover *Sweet Potato and Greens Breakfast Hash* with *Cinnamon Apple Breakfast Sausages*

Lunch

- Leftover *Wild-Caught Cod with Sage Parsnip Mash and Asparagus*
- Take your lunchtime supplements (pages 268–269).

After your workday is done

- Choose your thyroid- and adrenal-friendly exercise: walk, yoga, cardio, light weights, Pilates, dancing, playing actively with your kids.

Before dinner

- Use lamps with amber lightbulbs exclusively or put on amber eyeglasses.
- Make sure your phone and computer are set to "f.lux app" or nighttime settings.

Dinner

- *Coconut Chicken Curry (pages 335–336)*
- Take your dinnertime supplements (page 269).

After dinner

- Spend at least thirty minutes doing something that brings you joy: socializing, reading, crafting, yoga, writing/journaling, taking a walk.

Before bed

- Relax with HeartMath, Muse, binaural beats, brain-wave entrainment, meditation, prayer, breath work for ten to thirty minutes.
- Enjoy a warm bath with epsom salt and your favorite essential oils.
- Drink your bedtime herbal tea.
- If you are following the SIBO, yeast overgrowth, or parasite protocol, take your bedtime supplements.

Bedtime
- Turn off all electronics.
- Make sure your room is dark or use an eye mask.
- Lower your thermostat to a cool and relaxing temperature.
- Enjoy seven and a half to nine hours of deep, restful sleep.

DAY 25

Morning
- Take your supplemental thyroid hormone, if applicable.
- If you are following the SIBO, yeast overgrowth, or parasite protocol, take your upon-waking supplements.
- Drink one to two cups filtered water with juice from ½ lemon.
- Go outside for at least five minutes within twenty minutes of waking to let the natural daylight hit your eyes and skin.
- Relax with HeartMath, Muse, binaural beats, brain-wave entrainment, meditation, prayer, breath work for ten to thirty minutes.
- Enjoy one cup of *The Myers Way "Spa" Water (pages 321–322)*

Breakfast
- *Pear and Parsley Smoothie (page 319)*
- Take your breakfast supplements (page 268).

One daily snack (enjoyed either before lunch or before dinner)
- *Classic Green Juice (page 321)*

Lunch
- Leftover *Chimichurri Grass-Fed Skirt Steak Salad with Garlic Lime Asparagus*
- Take your lunchtime supplements (pages 268–269).

After your workday is done
- Choose your thyroid- and adrenal-friendly exercise: walk, yoga, cardio, light weights, Pilates, dancing, playing actively with your kids.

Before dinner
- Use lamps with amber lightbulbs exclusively or put on amber eyeglasses.
- Make sure your phone and computer are set to "f.lux app" or nighttime settings.

Dinner

- *Hawaiian Fish "Tacos" with Mango Salsa (pages 341–342)*
- Take your dinnertime supplements (page 269).

After dinner

- Spend at least thirty minutes doing something that brings you joy: socializing, reading, crafting, yoga, writing/journaling, taking a walk.

Before bed

- Relax with HeartMath, Muse, binaural beats, brain-wave entrainment, meditation, prayer, breath work for ten to thirty minutes.
- Enjoy a warm bath with epsom salt and your favorite essential oils.
- Drink your bedtime herbal tea.
- If you are following the SIBO, yeast overgrowth, or parasite protocol, take your bedtime supplements.

Bedtime

- Turn off all electronics.
- Make sure your room is dark or use an eye mask.
- Lower your thermostat to a cool and relaxing temperature.
- Enjoy seven and a half to nine hours of deep, restful sleep.

DAY 26

Morning

- Take your supplemental thyroid hormone, if applicable.
- If you are following the SIBO, yeast overgrowth, or parasite protocol, take your upon-waking supplements.
- Drink one to two cups filtered water with juice from ½ lemon.
- Go outside for at least five minutes within twenty minutes of waking to let the natural daylight hit your eyes and skin.
- Relax with HeartMath, Muse, binaural beats, brain-wave entrainment, meditation, prayer, breath work for ten to thirty minutes.
- Enjoy one cup of caffeine-free herbal tea or herbal coffee

Breakfast

- *Grass-Fed Beef and Veggie Breakfast Scramble (page 323)*
- Take your breakfast supplements (page 268).

One daily snack (enjoyed either before lunch or before dinner)

- ½ cup mixed berries

Lunch

- Leftover *Coconut Chicken Curry*
- Take your lunchtime supplements (pages 268–269).

After your workday is done

- Choose your thyroid- and adrenal-friendly exercise: walk, yoga, cardio, light weights, Pilates, dancing, playing actively with your kids.

Before dinner

- Use lamps with amber lightbulbs exclusively or put on amber eyeglasses.
- Make sure your phone and computer are set to "f.lux app" or nighttime settings.

Dinner

- *Citrus Shrimp over Red Leaf Lettuce Salad (pages 329–330)*
- Take your dinnertime supplements (page 269).

After dinner

- Spend at least thirty minutes doing something that brings you joy: socializing, reading, crafting, yoga, writing/journaling, taking a walk.

Before bed

- Relax with HeartMath, Muse, binaural beats, brain-wave entrainment, meditation, prayer, breath work for ten to thirty minutes.
- Enjoy a warm bath with epsom salt and your favorite essential oils.
- Drink your bedtime herbal tea.
- If you are following the SIBO, yeast overgrowth, or parasite protocol, take your bedtime supplements.

Bedtime

- Turn off all electronics.
- Make sure your room is dark or use an eye mask.
- Lower your thermostat to a cool and relaxing temperature.
- Enjoy seven and a half to nine hours of deep, restful sleep.

DAY 27

Morning

- Take your supplemental thyroid hormone, if applicable.
- If you are following the SIBO, yeast overgrowth, or parasite protocol, take your upon-waking supplements.
- Drink one to two cups filtered water with juice from ½ lemon.
- Go outside for at least five minutes within twenty minutes of waking to let the natural daylight hit your eyes and skin.
- Relax with HeartMath, Muse, binaural beats, brain-wave entrainment, meditation, prayer, breath work for ten to thirty minutes.
- Enjoy one cup of leftover *The Myers Way "Spa" Water*

Breakfast

- *Cinnamon Cocoa Smoothie (page 319)*
- Take your breakfast supplements (page 268).

One daily snack (enjoyed either before lunch or before dinner)

- ½ cup mixed berries

Lunch

- Leftover *Hawaiian Fish "Tacos" with Mango Salsa*
- Take your lunchtime supplements (pages 268–269).

After your workday is done

- Choose your thyroid- and adrenal-friendly exercise: walk, yoga, cardio, light weights, Pilates, dancing, playing actively with your kids.

Before dinner

- Use lamps with amber lightbulbs exclusively or put on amber eyeglasses.
- Make sure your phone and computer are set to "f.lux app" or nighttime settings.

Dinner

- *Baked Chicken Breasts with Sautéed Brussels Sprouts, Spinach, and Bacon (pages 338–339)*
- Take your dinnertime supplements (page 269).

After dinner

- Spend at least thirty minutes doing something that brings you joy: socializing, reading, crafting, yoga, writing/journaling, taking a walk.

Before bed

- Relax with HeartMath, Muse, binaural beats, brain-wave entrainment, meditation, prayer, breath work for ten to thirty minutes.
- Enjoy a warm bath with epsom salt and your favorite essential oils.
- Drink your bedtime herbal tea.
- If you are following the SIBO, yeast overgrowth, or parasite protocol, take your bedtime supplements.

Bedtime

- Turn off all electronics.
- Make sure your room is dark or use an eye mask.
- Lower your thermostat to a cool and relaxing temperature.
- Enjoy seven and a half to nine hours of deep, restful sleep.

DAY 28

Morning

- Take your supplemental thyroid hormone, if applicable.
- If you are following the SIBO, yeast overgrowth, or parasite protocol, take your upon-waking supplements.
- Drink one to two cups filtered water with juice from ½ lemon.
- Go outside for at least five minutes within twenty minutes of waking to let the natural daylight hit your eyes and skin.
- Relax with HeartMath, Muse, binaural beats, brain-wave entrainment, meditation, prayer, breath work for ten to thirty minutes.
- Enjoy one cup of caffeine-free herbal tea or herbal coffee

Breakfast

- Leftover *Grass-Fed Beef and Veggie Breakfast Scramble*
- Take your breakfast supplements (page 268).

One daily snack (enjoyed either before lunch or before dinner)

- Avocado with mixed raw veggies: cucumbers, carrots, celery, zucchini

Lunch

- Leftover *Citrus Shrimp over Red Leaf Lettuce Salad*
- Take your lunchtime supplements (pages 268–269).

After your workday is done

- Choose your thyroid- and adrenal-friendly exercise: walk, yoga, cardio, light weights, Pilates, dancing, playing actively with your kids.

Before dinner

- Use lamps with amber lightbulbs exclusively or put on amber eyeglasses.
- Make sure your phone and computer are set to "f.lux app" or nighttime settings.

Dinner

- *Kelp Noodle Stir-Fry with Chicken and Veggies (page 335)*
- Dessert: *Zesty Fruit Salad with Whipped Coconut Cream (pages 351–352)*
- Take your dinnertime supplements (page 269).

After dinner

- Spend at least thirty minutes doing something that brings you joy: socializing, reading, crafting, yoga, writing/journaling, taking a walk.

Before bed

- Relax with HeartMath, Muse, binaural beats, brain-wave entrainment, meditation, prayer, breath work for ten to thirty minutes.
- Enjoy a warm bath with epsom salt and your favorite essential oils.
- Drink your bedtime herbal tea.
- If you are following the SIBO, yeast overgrowth, or parasite protocol, take your bedtime supplements.

Bedtime

- Turn off all electronics.
- Make sure your room is dark or use an eye mask.
- Lower your thermostat to a cool and relaxing temperature.
- Enjoy seven and a half to nine hours of deep, restful sleep.

CHAPTER 13

The Myers Way Thyroid Connection Plan...for Life

Congratulations on completing The Myers Way Thyroid Connection twenty-eight-day plan! Now you're probably wondering, "What's next?"

What's next is a lifetime of excellent thyroid and immune health. If you are doing well and don't want to add any foods back in, no problem! Enjoy the abundant nutritious foods that are available for you on The Myers Way Thyroid Connection Plan. You are not missing any nutrients if you choose to stay on the program indefinitely.

However, if you'd like to get some more variety in your diet, now is the time. One by one, you are going to add some foods back into your diet and see whether your body can tolerate them. Let me talk you through it.

SOME GENERAL GUIDELINES

- If you have autoimmune thyroid, either Hashimoto's or Graves', and your condition has not improved or your thyroid antibodies have not lowered, then I encourage you to stay on the plan for another few months. It will be best for you to avoid gluten/grains, legumes, and dairy indefinitely to reverse the autoimmune process your body has suffered. When your symptoms have disappeared and your antibodies are within optimal range, you can begin adding foods back in.

- If you are hypothyroid and do not have autoimmune thyroid dysfunction, and if things are not improving for you, I encourage you to work with your doctor to find the supplemental thyroid hormone form and dose that works best for you. Even if your diet is spot on, you might not feel better until your supplemental thyroid hormone is optimal for you. You can also stay on the twenty-eight-day plan longer to see if your body needs more time for healing. If you have thyroid dysfunction, autoimmune or not, I do not recommend that you ever add back in gluten or cow's milk dairy. Some of you may be able to tolerate sheep's and/or goat's milk dairy.
- Once you are at a place to add foods back in, remember to enjoy the following only in small amounts: caffeine, sugar, alcohol, grains, and legumes.
- Always avoid such toxic foods as artificial sweeteners, genetically modified foods, artificial colors, artificial preservatives, dyes, high-fructose corn syrup, trans fats, and hydrogenated fats.
- Here's what I'd like you to do as far as supplements:
  - Continue the multivitamin, Omega-3, and probiotic indefinitely.
  - Continue to work with your doctor to monitor your vitamin D levels and continue to supplement as needed.
  - If you have the MTHFR SNP, continue to take the recommended additional B vitamins indefinitely.
  - If you have the GSTM1 SNP, continue to take the recommended additional glutathione indefinitely.
  - For all other supplements, continue to take them until your condition has resolved and your symptoms are gone — then stop.
- If you are not satisfied with your results after two or three months, you might want to consult a functional medicine practitioner (see Resources) to assess other possible root causes (see appendices for more information).
- Remember, your health is a spectrum. During different times in your life, you might be able to tolerate different foods.

POTENTIAL CHALLENGES

- You might not always feel a difference in your symptoms even if your body is becoming inflamed or reactive.
  - Suggestion: Work with your doctor to get a complete thyroid blood panel, checking all markers, especially your thyroid antibodies, before and after food reintroductions.
- If you are on medications to suppress your immune system, you might not notice a reaction even if you have one.
  - Suggestion: Work with your doctor to reduce any unnecessary medications; this should be possible now that you have healed your gut, reduced inflammation, tamed toxins, healed your infections, and relieved your stress. When you've been able to get off your immunosuppressive drugs, you can begin reintroducing foods to see how your body is really responding.

FOODS TO TEST

- Eggs
- Tomatoes
- Potatoes
- Eggplant
- Peppers
- Goat dairy
- Sheep dairy

Test the following items by having them only in small amounts as part of a single meal or snack. Going forward, you should enjoy them only occasionally:

- Alcoholic drinks
- Caffeinated drinks
- Sugar
- Nuts and seeds

- Gluten-free grains
- Legumes
- Gluten-free and dairy-free baked goods for special occasions

HOW TO TEST FOODS

For the first seven foods listed above (eggs, tomatoes, potatoes, egg-plant, peppers, goat dairy, sheep dairy), I recommend a specific proto-col of bombarding your system with each of the foods by eating **one food at a time three times a day for three days.** If a food is a trig-ger of inflammation for you, I want you to have the best chance to determine that right away, rather than allowing silent inflammation to sneak in, causing you unwanted health problems.

- Reintroduce only *one* food at a time.
- Reintroduce by consuming it three times a day for three days.
- Return to The Myers Way for three days before trying the next food.
- If you have a reaction, stop eating that food and wait until you are symptom-free before you try the next food.
- If you don't have a reaction, leave that food out of your diet, spend three days on The Myers Way, and then continue on to other foods one at a time. Test only one food at a time—if you test two foods on the same day, you won't know which one you had an adverse reaction to!
- Add each food that you have tested and found safe back into your diet at the end of the food-reintroduction phase.

For the remaining seven types of foods listed above (alcohol, caf-feine, sugar, etc.), add them back in slowly, one at a time, to determine if you can tolerate them in small amounts without any of your symp-toms returning. If you do not notice any unwanted symptoms, then you may enjoy these on occasion and in small amounts as you toler-ate them.

WHAT SHOULD I WATCH FOR?

Here's where you'll have to develop your own body awareness, because an inflammatory response or food-sensitivity reaction can take just about any form, including, but not limited to

- Increasing autoimmune blood markers
- Brain fog
- Depression/anxiety
- Diarrhea/constipation
- Disruptions in sleep
- Fatigue
- Gas/bloating
- Headache
- Heightened emotions
- Increasing inflammatory blood markers
- Joint pain
- Mood swings
- Rash
- Sleepiness after meals
- Swelling or puffiness in hands, face, feet, legs
- Water retention
- Weight gain

If you notice one or any combination of these symptoms, then stop eating the new food immediately. You can keep track of how your body responds to these foods using The Myers Way Symptom Tracker on my website (www.amymyersmd.com). Tracking your symptoms on the chart will allow you to gauge which foods you should permanently avoid due to sensitivities or intolerances.

CHAPTER 14

The Myers Way Thyroid Connection Plan Recipes

Note: Organic food is so much healthier—and pesticides, additives, and other toxins can make it that much harder to heal. Please use only organic ingredients wherever possible, especially for the next twenty-eight days (see pages 184–186 for more on eating organic). Your thyroid will thank you!

SMOOTHIES

The following smoothies provide large servings of flavor-filled and energy-packed nutrition. They contain The Myers Way Paleo Protein powder so you can start your day with those crucial amino acids. Blend it in with the other ingredients, or if the powder is clumping, mix it with ¼ cup of room-temperature or warm water to help dissolve it before blending.

Each smoothie recipe serves two. If you are making it just for yourself, either cut the recipe in half or enjoy a bigger breakfast.

Blueberries and Cream Smoothie   SERVES 2

For this smoothie, you can use unsweetened coconut cream or any coconut cream left over from the Berry Coconut Breakfast Parfait with Cocoa Dust and Orange Zest recipe on pages 324–325. You can also simply use full-fat coconut milk. If you top the smoothie with a dollop of coconut cream, you'll feel like you're eating dessert for breakfast!

  2 cups frozen or fresh blueberries
  ½ cup coconut cream (or full-fat coconut milk, well mixed)

2 scoops The Myers Way Paleo Protein powder
2 heaping tablespoons grass-fed beef collagen
3 handfuls ice
Dollops of coconut cream for topping (optional)

Place all ingredients except extra coconut cream in high-speed blender and blend until desired consistency is reached. Top each smoothie with a dollop of coconut cream if desired.

Pear and Parsley Smoothie   SERVES 2

Parsley is a great source of vitamin K, vitamin C, and vitamin A. Combining it with pear makes it sweet and delicious. The spinach has lots of thyroid-supportive iron. And the avocado makes it all smooth and creamy. Mmm!

4 cups spinach
2 pears, peeled and cored
2 handfuls fresh parsley, stemmed
2 cups water (or less for thicker consistency)
1 avocado
2 scoops The Myers Way Paleo Protein powder
1 heaping tablespoon grass-fed beef collagen
1 handful ice

Place all ingredients in high-speed blender and blend until desired consistency is reached.

Cinnamon Cocoa Smoothie   SERVES 2

Cinnamon helps support healthy blood-sugar levels. You'll feel full and satisfied, and you won't get hungry again until it's time for your next meal.

2 ripe bananas
2 scoops The Myers Way Paleo Protein powder
2 tablespoons unsweetened cocoa
1 avocado
2 cups water or coconut milk (reduce to 1 cup if full-fat coconut milk)
1 tablespoon cinnamon, or more to taste
3 handfuls ice

Place all ingredients in high-speed blender and blend until desired consistency is reached.

Ginger Avocado Green Smoothie   SERVES 2

This smoothie has great greens and healthy fats plus The Myers Way Paleo Protein powder for more thyroid support. If you need more sweetness, feel free to add a banana.

    4 cups spinach
    2 stalks celery
    1 cucumber, peeled, halved lengthwise, and seeds scooped out
    2 handfuls fresh parsley, stemmed
    1 avocado
    1-inch piece fresh ginger, peeled and minced
    Juice of 1 lemon
    ⅔ cup water (or more to desired consistency)
    2 handfuls ice
    2 scoops The Myers Way Paleo Protein powder or 2 tablespoons
        grass-fed beef collagen
    1 ripe banana (optional)

Place all ingredients in high-speed blender and blend until desired consistency is reached.

BEVERAGES

Any of the following juices can be made with either a juicer or a blender. If you use a blender, after blending well, you can strain the pulp and fiber out with a cheesecloth or nut milk bag to get the quick nutrition from pure juice. Don't worry—you are getting plenty of fiber from all the great veggies you'll be eating throughout the rest of the day. These juices are great for shots of nutrition to start your day or for an energy treat in the afternoon.

Beet Fennel Juice   SERVES 2

If you haven't tried fennel before, it has a wonderful sweet licorice taste. Plus it's rich in potassium. One of my favorites to juice with! The beet juice is also sweet, and the lemon provides zing.

1 large red beet, peeled and quartered

1 fennel bulb, stalks and fronds included, trimmed and roughly chopped

1 lemon, peeled

1 cucumber, peeled and roughly chopped

Juice all ingredients in a juicer or a blender. Enjoy as is or over ice.

Cranberry Ginger Juice   SERVES 2

Cranberry is a great antioxidant and a good source of iodine for your thyroid. Ginger is excellent for your digestion—and I love its spicy taste.

1 cup fresh or frozen cranberries

1-inch piece fresh ginger, peeled

2 stalks celery, roughly chopped

½ cucumber, peeled and roughly chopped

4 cups spinach

1 handful cilantro, stemmed

Juice all ingredients in a juicer or a blender. Enjoy as is or over ice.

Classic Green Juice   SERVES 2

Gotta love green juice! Feel free to make this drink your own by using different greens and herbs.

4 cups spinach

2 cucumbers, peeled and roughly chopped

1-inch piece fresh ginger, peeled

1 lemon, peeled

1 handful mint, stemmed

1 green apple, cored, peeled, and roughly chopped (optional)

Juice all ingredients in a juicer or a blender. Enjoy as is or over ice.

The Myers Way "Spa" Water   SERVES 2

This recipe brings the luxury of the spa to you! There are so many ways to enjoy water with a little flavor. Here's one of my favorites.

2 cups water
½ cucumber, sliced, with or without the peel
½ cup packed mint leaves
1 cup strawberries, sliced

Combine ingredients in a glass jar or pitcher and let sit in the fridge to collect flavor. You can refill the water as much as you want to enjoy this spa water for 2 to 3 days.

The Myers Way Gut-Healing Collagen Tea   SERVES 2

Collagen is especially healing for your gut and great for your skin and joints. It mixes well with your favorite tea for a warm morning treat.

2–4 tablespoons grass-fed beef collagen
12 ounces boiling water
2 tea bags or servings of loose-leaf tea

Divide 1 to 2 tablespoons of the collagen into each teacup. Add 6 ounces of boiling water to each cup and mix well. Add tea and steep as directed.

BREAKFAST

Sweet Potato and Greens Breakfast Hash   SERVES 4

This recipe takes off from the popular sweet potato hash in my first book. The spinach gives you lots of iron, which your thyroid depends on. The kale is rich in calcium, potassium, antioxidants, and magnesium. Feel free to slice in some avocado for another serving of healthy fats!

1 tablespoon coconut oil
2 sweet potatoes, peeled and diced ¼ inch
1 sweet onion, diced
½ teaspoon cinnamon
¼ teaspoon nutmeg
¼ teaspoon sea salt
Pinch of ground black pepper

3 cups baby kale

3 cups baby spinach

1 large avocado, sliced (optional)

Heat a large skillet over medium heat. Add coconut oil, sweet potatoes, and onions. Cover and cook for about 8 minutes, stirring frequently. Uncover and add cinnamon, nutmeg, salt, and pepper. Mix well and add kale and spinach. Cook uncovered for 2 to 3 minutes until potatoes are soft and slightly browned and greens are wilted. Serve with avocado slices if desired.

Grass-Fed Beef and Veggie Breakfast Scramble   SERVES 4

After you've been fasting all night, you need a healthy dose of protein to start your morning. With this scramble, you can enjoy the comfort of sweet potatoes combined with nutrient-packed veggies and grass-fed beef. You can easily make this ahead and heat it up in the morning, or you can prep the ingredients the night before for quicker cooking in the morning. You can also substitute a different starchy veggie, such as cubed butternut squash, for the sweet potato if you wish.

1 pound ground grass-fed beef

¼ teaspoon sea salt

2 tablespoons coconut oil

1 large sweet onion, roughly chopped

1 large sweet potato, peeled and diced

1 zucchini, sliced into half-moons

6 asparagus spears, woody ends removed and spears cut into bite-size
  pieces

½ teaspoon cinnamon

¼ teaspoon nutmeg

2 large avocados, sliced

In a large skillet, brown beef over medium-low heat and season with sea salt. Set aside. In another large skillet, heat coconut oil over medium heat. Add onions and cook for 3 minutes. Add sweet potatoes or squash and cook for 3 to 5 minutes. Add zucchini and asparagus and cook for another 5 minutes until veggies are soft. Season with cinnamon and nutmeg, and stir well. Combine browned beef with veggies and serve topped with sliced avocado.

Cinnamon Apple Breakfast Sausages   SERVES 4

Another variation on a favorite staple from my first book, *The Autoimmune Solution*. These sausages are so easy to make ahead of time and heat up in the morning as part of a quick and nutritious breakfast. If you don't have any broth on hand, feel free to use water.

> 1 pound ground grass-fed beef or lamb, free-range turkey or chicken, or pork
> 1 small green apple, peeled and grated
> 1 teaspoon cinnamon
> ¼ teaspoon nutmeg
> ¼ teaspoon salt
> 2 tablespoons coconut oil
> ¼ cup Gut-Healing Bone Broth (see page 33) or water

Let meat come to room temperature in a large mixing bowl. Combine with grated apple, cinnamon, nutmeg, and salt. Mix ingredients together to incorporate spices well into meat. Form mixture into 8 sausage patties.

Heat coconut oil in large sauté pan over medium-high heat. Add sausages to hot oil and cook for about 5 minutes total, flipping throughout to brown both sides — cooking time will depend on your choice of meat. Add broth or water to pan, lower the heat to medium, cover, and cook for another 3 to 5 minutes, until cooked through.

Berry Coconut Breakfast Parfait with Cocoa Dust and Orange Zest   SERVES 2

This is easy to make the night before for a quick breakfast in the morning. To save even more time, you can purchase unsweetened coconut cream instead of making it yourself. The parfait is equally delicious with berries or dark cherries, so switch it up depending on your preference.

For the coconut cream

> One 13.5-ounce can full-fat coconut milk, chilled in fridge for at least 3 hours
> ¾ teaspoon cinnamon
> ¼ teaspoon sea salt
> Stevia to taste (optional)

For the parfait toppings
½ cup mixed berries or dark cherries
Sprinkle of unsweetened cocoa
2 teaspoons orange zest

Skim off the top layer of coconut cream from the chilled can of coconut milk and place into a medium bowl, reserving the rest for other recipes. Add cinnamon, salt, and stevia, if desired. Beat the coconut cream and spices with a whisk or an electric mixer until thickened. Divide into serving bowls and top with berries or cherries. Sprinkle with unsweetened cocoa and orange zest.

SALADS

Pineapple Taco Salad with Grass-Fed Beef   SERVES 4

This recipe has lots of protein from the beef—and tons of flavor! Don't be intimidated by the long list of ingredients; most are just seasonings that give great depth of flavor to the beef. Coconut aminos is a seasoning similar to soy sauce. However, it is made from coconut and is free of all soy, wheat, and gluten. You can find coconut aminos at Whole Foods or online at Thrive Market.

For the beef
1 pound ground grass-fed beef
2 tablespoons apple cider vinegar
2 tablespoons olive oil
1 tablespoon coconut aminos (avoid on the yeast overgrowth/SIBO protocol)
2 cloves garlic, minced
¼ teaspoon cinnamon
½ teaspoon turmeric
½ teaspoon cumin
½ teaspoon sea salt
¼ teaspoon ground black pepper
¼ green cabbage, sliced

For the salad

8 cups salad greens

1 carrot, peeled and julienned

½ small pineapple, chopped into bite-size pieces

Begin to brown beef in a large skillet over medium heat. After a few minutes, pour off any excess fat and add apple cider vinegar, olive oil, coconut aminos, garlic, cinnamon, turmeric, cumin, salt, and ground black pepper. Mix well. Add cabbage to beef as it is browning. Cover and simmer for 5 to 10 minutes. Meanwhile, divide salad greens among serving plates. Top with cooked beef, carrots, and pineapple. If you are planning leftovers, keep beef and cold ingredients separate until you enjoy them. When you are in the food-reintroduction phase, this recipe can be enjoyed with tomatoes or peppers or organic corn chips.

Texas Grapefruit and Avocado Spinach Salad with Shredded Chicken   SERVES 4

Texas grapefruit is delicious in season! If you can get your hands on it, I definitely recommend it, but this recipe is delicious with any grapefruit. Using leftover chicken makes this recipe quick and nutritious! If you are following the meal plan as directed for two people, you will have two servings to enjoy for leftovers. I like to prep my leftovers as much as possible to simply grab and go in the morning.

8 ounces baby spinach

2 Texas grapefruits

1 large avocado, thinly sliced

2 cups shredded cooked Oven-Roasted Chicken

4 teaspoons mustard

2 teaspoons apple cider vinegar

¼ cup olive oil

Dash of sea salt

Dash of ground black pepper

½ red onion, minced

Divide spinach among serving plates. If you are planning leftovers, reserve remaining spinach servings in glass storage dishes in the refrigerator for later.

I like to get as much fruit as possible from the grapefruit. Cut the peel off each end, then scoop your knife carefully around the sides of the grapefruit between the peel and fruit to remove the peel. When peel is gone, cut each grapefruit segment from its white membrane. Divide grapefruit, avocado slices, and shredded chicken among the serving plates. Whisk together mustard, apple cider vinegar, olive oil, salt, and ground black pepper for creamy mustard dressing. When whisked well, add minced red onions to dressing before drizzling over salad. For your leftover salad, wait to add dressing until right before eating.

Wild-Caught Scallop Spinach Salad with Pomegranate Vinaigrette   SERVES 4

Scallops are a great source of selenium and zinc, which are crucial for thyroid function. Bragg has a great organic pomegranate vinaigrette dressing that you can find at your local health-food store or online (see Resources). If you prefer, in place of the Organic Pomegranate Vinaigrette dressing, you can use the Outstanding Dressing from the Spinach Side Salad with Outstanding Dressing recipe, page 330.

   16 wild-caught scallops
   Pinch of sea salt
   Pinch of ground black pepper
   2 tablespoons coconut oil
   2 cloves garlic, minced
   Juice from ½ lemon
   10 ounces baby spinach
   Bragg Organic Pomegranate Vinaigrette, as desired

Season scallops with salt and pepper and set aside. Heat coconut oil in large skillet over medium heat. Add garlic and stir until fragrant. Add scallops to the skillet in batches so each scallop fully touches the surface of the pan. Cook for about 2 minutes, then flip. Cook for another 2 to 3 minutes until cooked through. Sprinkle with lemon juice and remove from heat. Divide baby spinach among serving plates. Top spinach with cooked scallops and drizzle with pomegranate vinaigrette. Keep cooked scallops, spinach, and dressing separate for leftovers.

Chimichurri Grass-Fed Skirt Steak
Salad with Garlic Lime Asparagus   SERVES 4

This chimichurri sauce has such a fresh flavor profile against the rich steak. You may want to make some extra to enjoy later in the week with grilled vegetables or on a salad. There are a lot of ingredients for the chimichurri sauce but it only takes a minute to whip it up!

For the steak

1¼ pounds grass-fed skirt steak
Large pinch of sea salt
Large pinch of ground black pepper
1 tablespoon coconut oil

For the chimichurri sauce

¾ cup olive oil
3 tablespoons apple cider vinegar
Juice from 2 lemons
1 bunch parsley
½ bunch cilantro
1 teaspoon sea salt
½ teaspoon ground black pepper
¼ small yellow onion
4 cloves garlic

For the asparagus and salad

1 tablespoon coconut oil
2 cloves garlic, minced
12 stalks asparagus, woody ends removed
Juice from 1 lime
8 cups salad greens

Season steak with salt and pepper, then set aside at room temperature. Heat large skillet with oil over medium-high heat. When pan is hot, add steak and sear for about 4 to 5 minutes, until browned. Flip steak and sear on other side for 4 to 5 minutes. Remove from heat and set aside to rest for 5 to 7 minutes.

While steak is resting, combine olive oil, apple cider vinegar, lemon juice, parsley, cilantro, sea salt, ground black pepper, yellow onion, and garlic in a food processor with s-blade and mix until herbs, onion, and garlic are finely chopped.

Heat coconut oil in medium skillet over medium heat. Add garlic and stir until fragrant. Add asparagus and cook for 4 minutes, until beginning to soften. Add lime juice and stir to coat asparagus.

Then slice the steak thinly, against the grain. Divide salad greens among serving plates, top with sliced steak and drizzle with chimichurri sauce. Serve asparagus on the side. For leftovers, keep greens, steak, asparagus, and dressing separate. Reheat steak and asparagus. Combine greens, steak, and chimichurri sauce before serving with asparagus.

Citrus Shrimp over Red Leaf Lettuce Salad   SERVES 4

The shrimp is best if it has about two hours to marinate, so plan ahead. If you have a grill you can thread the shrimp onto skewers and grill instead of cooking them on the stovetop. Radish is a cruciferous vegetable, which makes it a mild goitrogen, so try not to eat too much of it raw. However, the one radish per serving in this recipe is just fine—and you'll get lots of other nutritional benefits, including fiber that nourishes your friendly gut bacteria.

For the shrimp
½ cup olive oil
¼ bunch parsley, chopped
2 tablespoons minced garlic
2 tablespoons coconut aminos (avoid on the yeast overgrowth/SIBO protocol)
2 tablespoons orange or lemon juice
½ teaspoon sea salt
½ teaspoon ground black pepper
1 to 2 pounds wild-caught shrimp, peeled and deveined

For the salad
2 heads red leaf lettuce, roughly torn
1 cucumber, sliced into thin disks, with or without peel
4 radishes, thinly sliced
¼ red onion, minced
2 stalks celery, finely chopped
2 tablespoons olive oil
2 tablespoons orange juice
2 teaspoons apple cider vinegar

Whisk together olive oil, parsley, garlic, coconut aminos, orange or lemon juice, salt, and pepper in a large bowl. Add shrimp and toss to coat. Cover and let marinate for 1 to 2 hours in the refrigerator.

Divide lettuce among serving bowls. Top with cucumber, radishes, red onion, and celery.

Heat a large sauté pan over medium heat and cook shrimp for a couple of minutes until they are an opaque, whitish color. Top salad with cooked shrimp. Drizzle with olive oil, orange juice, and apple cider vinegar. For leftovers, reserve undressed salad and store ingredients separately to compose salad for a later meal.

Spinach Salad with Outstanding Dressing
SERVES 2; DRESSING MAKES ABOUT 1 CUP

When I bring this dressing to work, everyone in my clinic marvels at how good it looks. Well, it tastes even better, so I want to share it with you! It's best if you can use all organic spices and ingredients, as I do. This is a great way to incorporate more vegetables throughout your day. You can substitute other spring greens or lettuce for the spinach if you prefer.

For the dressing
1 cup olive oil
4 cloves garlic, minced
½ teaspoon turmeric
½ teaspoon ginger powder or freshly grated ginger
¼ red onion, minced
1 tablespoon yellow mustard or Dijon mustard
½ cup apple cider vinegar
½ teaspoon sea salt

For the salad
4 packed cups spinach
1 cup chopped vegetables, such as cucumbers, celery, carrots, asparagus, zucchini (optional)

Put all the dressing ingredients in a medium bowl and whisk together. Drizzle desired amount of dressing over spinach and vegetables. Store dressing in a sealed glass jar in the refrigerator for up to 14 days.

Gut-Healing Bone Broth   MAKES ABOUT 8 CUPS

Gut-Healing Bone Broth is a terrific foundation for any meal plan! The nutrients in bone broth work to heal the mucosal lining of the digestive tract, reduce inflammation, and help to promote sleep and a calm mind—all great benefits for your thyroid. I recommend savoring this in the morning in your favorite mug. You can also use it when you cook vegetables, meat, and soups. If you find yourself with some extra after three or four days, freeze the leftovers in small glass containers to enjoy later on. If you have a great local place that serves bone broth or want to buy it online (see Resources, page 359), you don't have to make it yourself from scratch. But don't do this unless you trust the quality and that every ingredient is approved.

1 organic pasture-raised chicken carcass or 1 pound bones (marrow
    bones, chicken bones, knucklebones)
2 tablespoons apple cider vinegar
1 teaspoon salt
2 cloves garlic, peeled and smashed with blade of knife
8 cups water
1–2 cups chopped carrots, celery, white or yellow onions (optional)

Put chicken carcass or bones in a slow cooker. If you prefer, you can use a large soup pot instead. Add vinegar, salt, garlic, water, and vegetables, if desired. Depending on the bones you use and the size of your slow cooker or pot, you can add more water to cover bones.

Cook in the slow cooker on low for at least 24 hours or simmer over the stove for 8 to 10 hours. You can start using broth any time after 8 hours, but I recommend waiting till at least 24 hours.

When broth is done, use a slotted spoon to discard bones and veggies. Then pour through a fine-mesh strainer to separate and discard any solid pieces. Once cooled, store in the fridge in glass jars or containers. The excess fat will rise to the top; skim off fat and heat individual portions for drinking or using in recipes.

White Sweet Potato and Parsnip Clam Chowder   SERVES 6

I don't typically cook with clams, but since they are such a good source of iron, I thought I would try them in this chowder. It's easiest to use canned wild-caught calms and clam juice, but you can also use fresh clams if you prefer. In the Resources on page 359, you can find places to order these ingredients online if you can't locate them locally. If you are using fresh shelled clams, start with about 4 pounds and bring to a boil in 2 cups water in a large pot over high heat. Cook for 6 to 8 minutes until clams open, then strain through a fine mesh strainer. After they have slightly cooled, remove from shell and set aside.

- 1 8-ounce package of bacon (e.g., Pederson's or find at your local farmers' market)
- 1 large sweet onion, finely chopped
- 4 white sweet potatoes, peeled and cubed
- 4 parsnips, peeled and chopped
- 1 small head cauliflower, chopped
- 1 cup clam juice
- Water, as needed
- One 13-ounce can full-fat coconut milk
- 10 ounces canned wild-caught clams
- Sea salt to taste
- Ground black pepper to taste

Heat large skillet over medium-high heat. Add bacon slices and cook a few minutes on each side until crispy. Set bacon on paper-towel-lined plate to remove excess grease. Pour bacon grease from the pan into a large soup pot. Heat pot over medium heat and stir in chopped onion. After 3 minutes add sweet potatoes, parsnips, and cauliflower. Add clam juice and enough water to cover the vegetables. Bring to a boil, then simmer, covered, for 30 minutes. Add coconut milk, then, using an immersion blender, blend until smooth. Be careful—hot soup! If you do not have an immersion blender you can transfer soup in batches to your blender and blend carefully. Add clams. Stir well and season to taste with salt and pepper. Serve hot.

Curried Coconut Soup with Shrimp and Veggies   SERVES 4

One of the most popular recipes from my first book is the Thai Green Curry with Shrimp. This is a very similar dish with a slightly different spin. If you love the curry paste as much as I do, you can double or triple the recipe and freeze in small glass containers to have quick curry cubes for another night.

For the green curry paste
1 shallot

4 cloves garlic

1-inch piece of fresh ginger, peeled

½ bunch cilantro

½ bunch basil leaves picked

½ teaspoon cumin

½ teaspoon ground black pepper

3 tablespoons gluten-free fish sauce (avoid on the yeast overgrowth/ SIBO protocol)

2 tablespoons lime juice

2 tablespoons full-fat coconut milk

For the shrimp curry
2 tablespoons coconut oil, divided

1 red onion, sliced

2 heads broccoli, cut into bite-size pieces

1 head cauliflower, cut into bite-size pieces

3 carrots, peeled and julienned

2½ cups Gut-Healing Bone Broth (see page 331) or store-bought bone broth

2 cups mushrooms, sliced

Two 13.5-ounce cans full-fat coconut milk

3 pounds shrimp, peeled and deveined

1 small bunch kale, thinly sliced

½ teaspoon sea salt

1 large avocado, sliced

Blend curry paste ingredients in a food processer or blender until smooth. Heat 1 tablespoon coconut oil in large soup pot over medium heat. Add blended curry paste and let cook for about 1 minute. Add red onion. Let cook for about 3 minutes until onions are soft. Add broccoli, cauliflower, carrots, and remaining coconut oil. Let cook for 3 minutes. Add Gut-Healing Bone Broth. Bring to a boil and turn down heat to simmer for 10 minutes. Add mushrooms and cook for 3 minutes. Add coconut milk and stir well. Add shrimp and kale and cook for a few minutes to let shrimp cook through. Season with salt and serve with avocado.

MAIN DISHES

POULTRY

Apricot Chicken Salad   SERVES 6

This recipe is super-easy to mix up and has a freshness that you don't generally find in traditional chicken salads. Enjoy this on a Sunday picnic. You can use homemade Coconut Milk Yogurt or store-bought yogurt. If you are really busy, use a cooked rotisserie chicken from your local grocery store.

- 1 Oven-Roasted Chicken (page 336–337), shredded
- ¼ bunch basil leaves
- ¼ bunch parsley
- ¼ bunch cilantro
- ½ teaspoon sea salt
- ¼ teaspoon ground black pepper
- 1½ cups dried unsweetened apricots
- 2 packed cups spinach
- ½ small red onion, peeled and halved
- Juice from 1 lemon
- 2 cups Coconut Milk Yogurt (see page 348) or store-bought unsweetened coconut milk yogurt
- 1 head romaine or 1 large cucumber, sliced

Put shredded chicken in a food processor in batches with basil, parsley, cilantro, salt, and pepper. Process on low to mix chicken and herbs. Transfer to large mixing bowl. Next put apricots, spinach, red onion, and lemon juice in food processer. Process until onions are chopped to desired texture. Stir into chicken and herb mix. Toss with coconut milk yogurt. Refrigerate and serve chilled over romaine lettuce leaves or with cucumber slices.

Kelp Noodle Stir-Fry with Chicken and Veggies SERVES 4

This recipe is packed with thyroid-supporting nutrition! Kelp noodles are a great source of iodine, while chicken contains selenium and iron to help your thyroid function properly.

2 to 3 tablespoons olive or coconut oil

3 chicken breasts, butterflied

2 sweet onions, diced

4 cloves garlic, minced

2-inch piece fresh ginger, peeled and minced

4 carrots, peeled and thinly sliced

8 ounces spinach

4 scallions, thinly sliced

½ teaspoon sea salt

2 tablespoons coconut aminos (avoid on the yeast overgrowth/SIBO protocol)

16 ounces kelp noodles, rinsed

2 avocados, sliced

Heat oil in large skillet over medium heat. Add chicken and cook for about 10 minutes, flipping halfway through, until fully cooked. Transfer cooked chicken to a covered plate.

Add onions to the skillet once the chicken is set aside and let cook for 2 to 3 minutes. Add garlic and ginger. After a minute, add carrots and cook for about 5 minutes, until they begin to soften. Add spinach, scallions, salt, and coconut aminos. Mix well and let spinach wilt. Finally, add the kelp noodles, mixing well until noodles are hot. Divide among serving plates, top with avocado slices, and serve with sliced chicken breast.

Coconut Chicken Curry SERVES 4

This recipe has been a favorite of mine and my patients for years! It was in my first book, and we just had to include it here for you to enjoy on your thyroid-healing journey.

For the curry
1 tablespoon olive oil

2 cloves garlic, chopped

1 onion, diced

½ tablespoon turmeric

½ tablespoon cumin

1 tablespoon coriander

1 sweet potato, peeled and cut into ½-inch cubes

2 stalks celery, chopped

4 scallions, thinly sliced

1 cup water

1 teaspoon sea salt

1 13.5-ounce can full-fat coconut milk

1 avocado, sliced

For the chicken

1 tablespoon coconut oil

Pinch of sea salt

2 chicken breasts, cut into bite-size pieces

Heat large skillet on medium heat. Coat the pan with olive oil. When hot, add garlic and cook until slightly browned. Add onions and more oil, if needed. Cover and cook until onions are translucent, about 3 minutes. Stir in turmeric, cumin, and coriander. Add sweet potatoes, celery, scallions, water, and salt. Cover and cook until sweet potatoes are soft (5 to 7 minutes).

While veggies are cooking, heat coconut oil in a sauté pan over medium heat. Add chicken and sauté until cooked through, 5 to 10 minutes, stirring occasionally.

Add cooked chicken and coconut milk to veggies. Let simmer for a few minutes to mix flavors. Serve topped with sliced avocado.

Oven-Roasted Chicken   SERVES 6

This recipe is so easy to make, so full of flavor, and great to have on hand for delicious salads, like the Apricot Chicken Salad on page 334. And of course, you can use the carcass for Gut-Healing Bone Broth (page 331). Store the cooked chicken whole, or remove the meat and store the bones separately.

1 whole chicken (about 5 pounds), giblets removed

1 tablespoon olive oil

¾ teaspoon sea salt

½ teaspoon ground black pepper

3 cloves garlic, peeled and smashed

1 lemon, sliced

2 tablespoons Gut-Healing Bone Broth (see page 331) or store-bought broth (optional)

1 tablespoon apple cider vinegar (optional)

Preheat oven to 375 degrees F. Rub chicken with olive oil, then salt and pepper. Put garlic cloves and lemon slices inside chicken cavity. Place chicken in baking dish and add broth and vinegar in bottom of dish. Bake for about 1½ hours or until the chicken is cooked through and has reached an internal temperature of 165 degrees.

Turkey Meatballs over Spaghetti Squash with Tuscan Kale Pesto   SERVES 4

Turkey is a good source of selenium, which helps support your thyroid. In the meal plan, I put this recipe after the Wild-Caught Salmon with Zucchini Noodle Pesto and Garlic Butternut Squash so that you will already have made the pesto. If you are not following the meal plan, just make the pesto fresh for this meal.

For spaghetti squash

1 large spaghetti squash, cut in half lengthwise and seeds discarded

2 teaspoons coconut oil

For meatballs

1½ pounds ground turkey (or 1 pound ground turkey and ½ pound ground pork)

2 cloves garlic, minced

¼ onion, finely chopped

1½ teaspoons turmeric

1½ teaspoons ground ginger

1 teaspoon rosemary

¼ teaspoon sea salt

¼ teaspoon ground black pepper

2 tablespoons coconut oil

¼ cup Gut-Healing Bone Broth (see page 331) or water

¾ cup Tuscan Kale Pesto (see page 349)

Preheat oven to 375 degrees F. Rub the edge of the squash that will be touching the baking sheet, with coconut oil. Place squash cut-side down on baking sheet or oven-safe glass dish and bake for about 35 minutes, until soft.

While squash is baking, put meat, garlic, onions, turmeric, ginger, rosemary, salt, and pepper in a large mixing bowl. Using your hands, mash ingredients together to incorporate spices into meat. Form into 12 medium meatballs or 24 small meatballs.

Heat coconut oil in large sauté pan over medium-high heat. Add meatballs and cook for about 5 minutes, flipping to brown all sides. Add broth or water and cook covered over medium heat for another 3 to 5 minutes, until cooked through.

When squash is soft to touch with an oven mitt, remove from the oven and let cool, turning cut-side up with tongs or oven mitt. When cooled enough, scoop out squash with a spoon and divide among serving plates. If you are not using all right away, store in a covered glass container (see Resources on page 359) in the refrigerator. Top squash with meatballs and dollops of pesto.

Baked Chicken Breasts with Sautéed
Brussels Sprouts, Spinach, and Bacon   SERVES 4

Bone-in chicken does a great job of retaining its juiciness. If you prefer, you can use boneless breasts, but the bones definitely enhance the flavor. Cooking times may vary depending on your oven and the type of chicken you use. Use a meat thermometer or regularly check for doneness.

    4 bone-in chicken breasts
    ¼ cup olive oil
    ½ teaspoon sea salt
    ¼ teaspoon ground black pepper
    1 clove garlic, minced
    1 teaspoon dried thyme
    4 slices bacon (e.g., Pederson's or find at your local farmers' market)
    16 ounces Brussels sprouts, stemmed and halved
    8 cups spinach

Drizzle chicken with olive oil and flip to coat both sides. Season with salt, pepper, garlic, and thyme. Let it reach room temperature as oven preheats to 350 degrees F. Bake in an oven-safe dish for 30 to 40 minutes until internal temperature reaches 165 degrees F. While chicken is baking, heat large skillet over medium-high heat and cook bacon until crispy. Set bacon aside on a paper-towel-lined plate to remove excess grease. Pour bacon grease into a heat-safe glass dish. Add ¼ cup bacon grease back to pan. Add Brussels sprouts and toss to coat with grease. Cook for about 5 minutes, until sprouts are softening. Add spinach and cook a couple minutes, until spinach is wilted. Crumble cooked bacon into sautéed sprouts and spinach. When chicken is done, serve with sautéed sprouts and spinach.

MAIN DISHES

SEAFOOD

Wild-Caught Shrimp Sushi Rolls with
Spinach, Carrots, and Cucumber   SERVES 2

When I wrote my thyroid blog series, this was one of my most popular recipes. Nori is a great sea-veggie treat full of the iodine, zinc, and iron that your thyroid needs. Be patient with making the rolls—it might take you a little while to get the hang of it. No matter what they look like, though, they will taste delicious.

- 4 sheets nori
- 1 large avocado, mashed
- 1 inch fresh ginger, peeled and grated
- 1 cup packed baby spinach leaves
- 10 wild-caught shrimp, cooked
- 2 small carrots, peeled and julienned
- 1 small cucumber, thinly sliced into sticks the length of the nori sheet
- 2 lemon wedges
- ¼ cup coconut aminos (avoid on the yeast overgrowth/SIBO protocol)

Place 1 nori sheet on a sushi mat or cutting board. With a flat spoon, spread the avocado very thinly over the entire surface of the nori sheet. Sprinkle some grated ginger on top of the avocado, then top with spinach. Place a row of shrimp along the nearest edge of the avocado-covered nori sheet.

Create a second row of carrots just above the shrimp. Then create a third row of cucumber slices above the carrots. Starting from the bottom, fold the nori over all the ingredients, then roll tightly until you have a compact sushi roll. With a very sharp knife, cut the roll into about 8 pieces. Set them aside and repeat the steps with the remaining ingredients to create more rolls. Squeeze lemon on individual rolls and dip in coconut aminos as desired.

Wild-Caught Salmon with Zucchini Noodle Pesto and Garlic Butternut Squash   SERVES 4

If you are following the meal plan, make the full Tuscan Kale Pesto recipe (page 349) so you can enjoy the extra ¾ cup of pesto with the Turkey Meatballs over Spaghetti Squash with Tuscan Kale Pesto (pages 337–338) this week. This recipe has a lot of components and steps, but it's all quite simple and methodical—and much easier than it looks!

For the butternut squash
1 small butternut squash
Pinch of sea salt

For the salmon
4 wild-caught salmon fillets
2 tablespoons olive oil
Pinch of sea salt
Pinch of ground black pepper

For the zucchini noodles
3 zucchini
Pinch of sea salt
1 tablespoon coconut oil
3 cloves garlic, minced
¾ cup Tuscan Kale Pesto (see page 349)

Preheat oven to 400 degrees F. There are a couple ways to prepare the butternut squash. You can cut the squash in half lengthwise before cooking—be careful since the rind is hard and can be difficult to cut! Then scoop out the seeds and put the squash in a large baking dish cut-side down. Add a little water to slightly cover the bottom. The other option is to make a few slits in the whole squash with a sharp knife. Add the whole squash to a glass baking dish with a little water covering the bottom. Either way, let the squash cook for 30 to 45 minutes, until soft to touch through your oven mitt. If you are cooking it whole, it will take longer than if you cut it prior to cooking.

While the squash is cooking, place salmon in a glass baking dish, skin-side down. Drizzle with olive oil and sprinkle with salt and pepper. Set aside to reach room temperature.

Using a julienne peeler or spiral slicer, cut zucchini into noodles. Put noodles in a bowl and sprinkle with salt. Heat coconut oil in large skillet over medium heat and add minced garlic. When garlic is beginning to brown, carefully remove two-thirds of it and set aside in small dish for butternut squash. Add zucchini noodles to hot pan and toss in oil. Let cook on low heat for about 5 minutes.

When squash is soft, remove from oven. Put salmon in oven and cook for about 15 to 20 minutes, while you are finishing the squash and making the pesto, until salmon is flaky.

After the squash has cooled for about 5 minutes, scoop out flesh into a mixing bowl, reserving ½ cup for pesto. Season with reserved browned garlic and a pinch of salt and mix well. Use reserved squash to make Tuscan Kale Pesto. Set aside.

When salmon is done, serve with garlic butternut squash and sautéed zucchini noodles topped with pesto.

Hawaiian Fish "Tacos" with Mango Salsa   SERVES 4

This mango salsa is a favorite! Enjoy it with these delicious fish tacos. As you saw from the approved-food list, radish is a cruciferous vegetable, so don't each too much of it raw. If you prefer, you can eliminate the radish, but it's full of so many nutrients—including vitamin C and fiber to nourish your friendly gut bacteria—that I'd rather you ate the one radish per serving that is allowed for this recipe.

For the fish
4 wild-caught red snapper fillets
2 tablespoons olive oil

2 lemons, cut into slices

4 sprigs rosemary

For the salsa

1 mango, chopped

1 avocado, chopped

½ red onion, chopped

¼ bunch cilantro, chopped

Juice of 1 small lemon

2 to 3 teaspoons lemon zest

1 tablespoon olive oil

Pinch of sea salt, or more to taste

Pinch of ground black pepper, or more to taste

For "tacos"

8 iceberg lettuce or red leaf lettuce leaves

4 watermelon radishes, sliced

Preheat oven to 425 degrees F. Place snapper fillets in large baking dish. Drizzle with olive oil and top with lemon slices and rosemary sprigs. Set aside to bring to room temperature while oven preheats.

In a mixing bowl, combine mango, avocado, red onion, cilantro, lemon juice, lemon zest, olive oil, salt, and pepper. Toss to mix well.

Cook snapper for about 15 minutes, until it flakes easily. Flake snapper into lettuce leaves and top with mango salsa and watermelon radish slices.

Wild-Caught Cod with Sage Parsnip Mash and Asparagus   SERVES 4

Cod is a great source of iodine and selenium, which your thyroid needs for optimal function. The fish pairs well with the creamy parsnip mash and roasted asparagus. If you have an immersion blender, you can use it to blend the parsnip mash in the pot instead of transferring into a blender or food processor.

For the fish

4 wild-caught cod fillets

2 tablespoons olive oil

Juice from 1 lemon

Pinch of sea salt

For the asparagus

2 bunches asparagus, washed and woody ends removed

2 tablespoons olive oil

For the parsnip mash

3 to 4 parsnips, peeled and chopped

6 carrots, peeled and chopped

1 clove garlic, peeled and smashed

2 stalks celery, chopped

2 scallions, thinly sliced

½ small yellow onion, chopped

3 cups Gut-Healing Bone Broth (see page 331) or water

½ cup full-fat unsweetened coconut milk

5 sage leaves

½ teaspoon sea salt

¼ teaspoon ground black pepper

Preheat oven to 400 degrees F.

Place cod fillets in baking dish. Drizzle with olive oil and lemon juice and season with salt. Set aside to reach room temperature.

In a separate dish or baking sheet, scatter asparagus and drizzle with olive oil. Set aside while oven preheats.

Combine chopped parsnips, carrots, garlic, celery, scallions, and onion in a large pot with bone broth. Bring to a boil, then simmer for 25 minutes.

While vegetables are cooking, put cod fillets and asparagus in oven and bake for about 20 minutes, until fish flakes easily and asparagus is soft.

Drain liquid from cooked vegetables (you can reserve liquid for cooking veggies later if you like), then add vegetables to blender or food processor with coconut milk, sage leaves, salt, and pepper. Blend until creamy, like mashed potatoes. Serve with cod and asparagus.

MAIN DISHES

BEEF

Beef Liver with
Bacon and Rosemary   SERVES 2 TO 4

Liver is commonly known as a superfood but it may not be a staple in your kitchen yet. Let's change that right now, because this recipe is delicious! Liver is very high in fat-soluble vitamins, iron, and B vitamins, so you can see why it's become a superfood. And don't worry about toxins, because the liver doesn't store them; it actually works hard to help process them. A cast-iron skillet gives it the best flavor, but you can use a regular skillet as well.

    6 slices bacon (Pederson's or find at your local farmers' market)
    8 ounces grass-fed beef liver
    2 teaspoons rosemary, divided

Heat cast-iron skillet over medium heat. Add 3 pieces of bacon, top with liver, then cover liver with remaining 3 pieces of bacon. Sprinkle 1 teaspoon rosemary on top. Let cook for about 5 minutes, then flip. Add remaining rosemary and let cook for another 5 minutes. Flip again and let cook for another 1 to 3 minutes, until liver is cooked through and bacon is crispy.

Grass-Fed Steak with
Thyme-Roasted Root Veggies   SERVES 2

You can cook the steak in a skillet or on the grill. This is a simple recipe that showcases how elegant and delicious The Myers Way Thyroid Connection Plan can be!

    8 to 10 ounces grass-fed steak
    1 teaspoon sea salt
    ¼ teaspoon ground black pepper
    1 to 2 teaspoons olive oil
    1 sweet potato, peeled and cubed
    2 carrots, peeled and sliced
    2 parsnips, peeled and sliced

3 teaspoons olive oil

½ teaspoon sea salt

2 teaspoons dried thyme

Preheat oven to 375 degrees F.

Sprinkle steak with salt and pepper. Let sit at room temperature for about 30 minutes.

Place sweet potatoes, carrots, and parsnips on a baking sheet and coat with 3 teaspoons olive oil. Sprinkle with salt and thyme. Bake in oven for about 45 minutes, until veggies are soft.

About 20 to 30 minutes into the vegetables' roasting, heat a large skillet over high heat. Drizzle steak with olive oil. Carefully place steak in hot pan and cook. Wait until steak is not sticking before flipping, about 3 to 4 minutes. Cook the other side until steak is cooked through to desired doneness. Remove steak from pan and let it rest for 10 minutes before serving. Enjoy with root veggies and Spinach Salad with Outstanding Dressing (see page 330).

MAIN DISHES

PORK

Sautéed Cranberry Kale with Bacon over Sweet Potatoes   SERVES 4

Cranberries are a good source of iodine to help support your thyroid. Even friends and family who think they don't like kale will love this recipe!

For the sweet potatoes

4 sweet potatoes, cut in half lengthwise

4 teaspoons coconut oil

For the cranberry kale with bacon

8 slices bacon (e.g., Pederson's or find at your local farmers' market)

1 bunch kale (about 12 stalks), stems removed and leaves sliced into thin strips

⅓ cup unsweetened dried cranberries

    1 tablespoon apple cider vinegar

    ¼ teaspoon sea salt

Preheat oven to 400 degrees F. Spread about ½ teaspoon of coconut oil on the inside flesh of each sweet potato half. Place each half cut-side down on a baking sheet and bake for about 45 minutes, until they are soft to touch with an oven mitt and slightly caramelized.

    While sweet potatoes are baking, heat large sauté pan over medium-high heat and cook bacon in batches, until crisp. Let bacon sit on paper-towel-lined plate to get rid of excess grease. Add kale to bacon grease in the pan and cook on low heat. After kale begins to soften, remove excess fat as desired, and add dried cranberries, apple cider vinegar, and sea salt. Crumble bacon into pan. Toss to mix well and serve over cooked sweet potatoes.

MAIN DISHES

LAMB

Greek Lamb Burger with Coconut Tzatziki and Zucchini Half-Moons   SERVES 4

Lamb is a great source of zinc to help support your thyroid. The rich pork in this recipe helps to balance out the leanness of the lamb, but you can choose to use all lamb instead. The many components of this dish combine to make wonderfully nutritious and complex flavors. I want you to enjoy them all—but if you prefer, you can simplify as desired. As you saw from the approved-food list, arugula is a cruciferous vegetable, so don't eat too much of it raw. You may substitute mixed greens, but the 1 cup per serving is definitely fine.

For the tzatziki sauce

    1 cup Coconut Milk Yogurt (see page 348)

    1 tablespoon lemon juice

    1 tablespoon olive oil

    1 tablespoon chopped fresh dill

½ teaspoon sea salt

1 large cucumber

For the burgers

3 tablespoons coconut oil, divided

1 sweet onion, minced

3 cloves garlic, minced

1-inch piece fresh ginger, peeled and minced

1 pound grass-fed ground lamb

½ pound ground pork

1 cup olives, pitted and chopped

1½ tablespoons fresh chopped dill

1 tablespoon fresh chopped mint

½ teaspoon cumin

½ teaspoon dried thyme

1 teaspoon sea salt

1 teaspoon ground black pepper

4 cups arugula

For the zucchini

1 tablespoon coconut oil

2 zucchini, cut into half-moons

To make the tzatziki sauce, combine yogurt, lemon juice, olive oil, dill, and salt in a medium bowl. Cut cucumber in half crosswise. Slice one-half into thin disk and reserve. Dice the other into small cubes, and add to the tzatziki sauce. Mix well and store in the fridge with cucumber disks while making the burgers.

Heat 2 tablespoons of the coconut oil in a large sauté pan over medium heat. Add onions and cook until beginning to brown. Add garlic and ginger and cook for 1 more minute. Turn off heat and transfer onion mixture to a large bowl. Set pan aside to cook burgers later. Add lamb, pork, chopped olives, dill, mint, cumin, thyme, salt, and ground black pepper to the cooked onions and combine. Form into 4 patties.

Add remaining coconut oil to the sauté pan and heat over medium-high heat. Cook the burgers for about 5 minutes on each side, until cooked through. If you are using lamb only, you may not need as much time. When the burgers are done, transfer to plate. If needed, add additional coconut oil to the pan and sauté zucchini half-moons for about 5 minutes until beginning to brown.

Serve the burgers over arugula and top with tzatziki. Serve with reserved cucumber disks and zucchini half-moons.

SIDES AND SNACKS

Coconut Milk Yogurt   MAKES ABOUT 1 CUP

It can be difficult to find a coconut milk yogurt that doesn't have a lot of sugar or ingredients that are not approved on The Myers Way, but you can make this at home anytime. Please note that you will need to ferment the yogurt overnight or all day, so plan ahead to have the yogurt ready when you want it. See Resources to find places to buy a store-bought alternative. This recipe uses tapioca starch as a thickener, but you can also use grass-fed beef gelatin. This is very similar to the collagen we use in tea and smoothies, but it thickens to a different consistency. See Resources to find places online to buy this gelatin. If you use gelatin instead of tapioca, you will only need about ¾ teaspoon gelatin.

- 1 13.5-ounce can full-fat coconut milk
- 1 capsule dairy-free probiotic
- 1 tablespoon tapioca starch
- ½ scoop The Myers Way Paleo Protein powder (optional)

Spoon the coconut milk into a medium-size bowl. Empty the contents of the probiotic capsule into the coconut milk and whisk together. Add tapioca starch to coconut milk mixture and whisk. Pour contents into a clean glass mason jar and seal the lid.

Place the sealed jar in a warm environment such as an unheated oven with the light on or a stable environment slightly above 100 degrees F. Allow the coconut milk to ferment for about 15 to 24 hours, and then place in refrigerator to halt the fermentation process. The flavor of the yogurt is directly related to the time it spends fermenting, so if you want a tangier, tarter flavor, let your yogurt ferment longer. Allow yogurt to cool in refrigerator for about 5 hours. If you would like to add The Myers Way Paleo Protein powder for increased protein, dissolve it in ¼ cup warm water, then stir into the yogurt.

Tuscan Kale Pesto   MAKES ABOUT 1½ CUPS

This recipe is great to make when you are already cooking a butternut squash. I like to do that on the weekends to have some starch ready for the week. This pesto is a terrific source of vitamin A and vitamin K and is wonderful with any protein or salad or used as a veggie dip.

    2 tablespoons coconut oil
    1 bunch Tuscan kale, roughly chopped
    2 cups loosely packed spinach
    8 cloves garlic, peeled and smashed
    1 bunch basil
    ½ cup olive oil
    ¼ cup lemon juice
    ½ teaspoon sea salt
    ½ cup cooked butternut squash (optional but ideal)

Heat coconut oil in large skillet over medium heat. Add kale, spinach, and garlic. Cook to soften, about 5 minutes. Transfer to blender and add basil, olive oil, lemon juice, salt, and squash. Blend until smooth. Store in a sealed glass container in the fridge for up to 5 days. If you have leftovers after 5 days, you can freeze individual portions in an ice-cube tray and store for 3 to 6 months.

Simple Sardine Snack   SERVES 2

This may not be your typical snack but it's a great way to get iodine and selenium into your diet. You could wrap the sardines in nori for some added iodine.

    1 tablespoon coconut oil
    ¾ red onion, thinly sliced
    2 cloves garlic, minced
    2 3.75-ounce cans sardines, in oil or water
    Juice from 1 lemon
    Pinch of sea salt

Heat coconut oil in medium skillet over medium heat. Add onions and let cook for 1 to 2 minutes. Add garlic and cook for 1 minute. Add sardines and lemon juice. Mix well and cook until sardines are heated through, about 4 to 5 minutes, flipping halfway through. Season with sea salt.

Cucumber Seaweed Salad   SERVES 4

Enjoy this seaweed salad as a snack or pair it with your favorite fish dish. Either way, you'll get lots of iodine from the seaweed.

¾ ounce wakame seaweed, cut into 1-inch pieces
2 cucumbers, peeled, seeded, and diced

For the dressing

1½ tablespoons coconut aminos (avoid on the yeast overgrowth/SIBO
    protocol)
2 tablespoons apple cider vinegar
1 tablespoon olive oil
Juice from ½ small lemon
½-inch piece fresh ginger, peeled and minced
Pinch of sea salt, to taste

Soak seaweed 5 to 10 minutes in warm water, then drain liquid. Mix the seaweed and cucumber in a large bowl.

Whisk together coconut aminos, apple cider vinegar, olive oil, lemon juice, ginger, and salt. Drizzle desired amount of dressing over seaweed and cucumbers.

DESSERTS

Decadent Cocoa Pudding   SERVES 4–6

I know what you're thinking: *Can I really have chocolate pudding?* Yes, you can! However, since it does have honey, enjoy it in small amounts, perhaps as a weekend treat.

2 large avocados
3 tablespoons cocoa
2 dates
1 ripe banana
2 tablespoons coconut butter (or coconut manna)
3 tablespoons raw honey
1 teaspoon cinnamon
1 teaspoon vanilla

¼ teaspoon sea salt

⅛ teaspoon stevia (more or less, to taste)

1 teaspoon orange zest (optional)

Soak the dates in filtered water for 30 minutes or until soft. Drain the dates. Put all ingredients except orange zest in a food processer or high-speed blender and blend until smooth. Chill for 60 minutes before serving. Garnish with orange zest if desired.

Creamy Fruit Smoothie Pops   MAKES 10 4-INCH POPS

These homemade Popsicles are sure to be a hit at home with kids and adults, and they are packed full of nutrition for every age. Paired with the spinach, mango and pineapple yield a fresh bright green pop. Using a darker fruit, like raspberries or cherries, will give you a darker green color.

1 avocado

2 bananas

4 cups baby spinach

1 cup full-fat coconut milk

1½ cups frozen fruit (e.g., mango and pineapple)

Blend all ingredients together until smooth. Pour into Popsicle molds. Lightly drop filled molds onto counter a few times to get any air bubbles out. Insert Popsicle sticks. Freeze until solid, about 3 or more hours. You may need to dip the Popsicle mold in warm water to remove pops.

Zesty Fruit Salad with Whipped Coconut Cream   SERVES 4

In this delicious dessert, fresh fruit is topped off with the satisfying creaminess of whipped coconut cream.

For the whipped coconut cream

1 13.5-ounce can full-fat coconut milk, chilled in refrigerator for at least 3 hours

¼ teaspoon cinnamon

¼ teaspoon sea salt

Stevia to taste (optional)

For the fruit salad

1 cup blackberries

1 cup strawberries, trimmed and halved

1 cup blueberries

½ small pineapple, cut into bite-size pieces

1 small lemon

Skim off the top layer of coconut cream from the chilled can of coconut milk and place into a medium bowl, reserving the rest for other recipes. Add cinnamon, salt, and stevia (if desired). Beat the coconut cream and spices with a whisk or an electric mixer until thickened.

Wash blackberries, strawberries, blueberries, and pineapple and lightly toss in large glass dish. Zest lemon, then slice lemon into thin slices for garnish. Sprinkle lemon zest over fruit and garnish with lemon-scattered slices on top of the fruit. Serve with coconut cream.

Lemon Coconut Macaroons with Dark Chocolate Drizzle   MAKES 20 MACAROONS

These are delicious! They are the perfect solution when you feel the need for a "carby" treat. I used a round squeeze-handle cookie scoop (size 50, which is about a tablespoon) to portion these macaroons. Pack them in the scoop for density, then use the squeezing feature to push the macaroons out. You can also just use a rounded tablespoon and scoop each one out with your finger.

For the macaroons

2 cups unsweetened coconut flakes

5 dates, pitted and roughly chopped

1 teaspoon vanilla

¼ teaspoon sea salt

¼ cup lemon juice

1 teaspoon lemon zest

2 tablespoons full-fat coconut milk

For the chocolate drizzle

2 tablespoons cocoa

2 tablespoons coconut oil

Pinch of sea salt

Put coconut flakes, dates, vanilla, salt, lemon juice, lemon zest, and coconut milk into a food processor and blend for a few minutes. Transfer to a medium mixing bowl. Pack macaroon mixture well into a cookie scoop and turn out each macaroon onto a cookie sheet.

For the chocolate drizzle, heat the cocoa, coconut oil, and salt in a small saucepan over low heat, stirring frequently. When combined, drizzle over macaroons. Refrigerate for at least 20 minutes before serving. Store in an airtight container in the refrigerator.

Resources

Amy Myers, MD, Online

Connect with me online for empowering information and helpful tips.
Website: www.amymyersmd.com
The Myers Way Community: www.amymyersmd.com/community
The Myers Way Podcast: http://www.amymyersmd.com/category/podcast
Facebook: www.facebook.com/amymyersmd
Twitter: @amymyersmd
Instagram: @amymyersmd
Pinterest: www.pinterest.com/amymyersmd

Dr. Myers's Books, Summits, and Programs

You can find these resources on my website, www.amymyersmd.com:
The Autoimmune Solution (book)
The Autoimmune Solution Summit
The Thyroid Connection Summit
The Myers Way Autoimmune Solution Program
The Myers Way Comprehensive Elimination Diet Program
The Myers Way Guide to the Gut Program
The Myers Way Candida Control Program
The Myers Way Meal Planning Tool

The Thyroid Connection Downloadable Guides and Resources

I've put together tons of handy guides, eBooks, and other resources to support you during and after the Thyroid Connection Plan. You can find all of them at www.thethyroidconnection.com.

The Thyroid Connection Guide to Working with Your Doctor

A downloadable and printable version of the letter for your doctor, questions to ask, and labs to request.

The Power of Food Guide

Sources and links for purchasing organic, non-GMO foods online plus tips for shopping at your grocery store.

The Tame Your Toxins Guide

A room-by-room guide to removing toxic chemicals and materials from your home, with recommended brands for toxin-free home goods, makeup, and body-care products.

The Stress Solution Guide

De-stressing exercises, a stress diary, tips for rejuvenating relaxation, and resources to learn more about stress management, including where to find HeartMath, Binaural Beats, and other recommended products.

The Thyroid Connection Shopping List

Weekly shopping lists, broken down by type of food, for all of the meals in the twenty-eight-day plan.

The Myers Way Meal-Planning Tool

Access the twenty-eight-day Thyroid Connection Plan meal plan in an interactive tool that allows you to adjust serving sizes, add and remove dishes and snacks, and then auto-generate an updated shopping list.

The Thyroid Connection Symptom Tracker

A tool to track your symptoms and inflammation during the twenty-eight-day plan and the weeks after when you are reintroducing foods.

The Thyroid Connection Supplements

A list of all of the supplements recommended in the plan accompanied by trusted, high-quality sources and links to purchase.

Food Reintroduction Recipe eBook

Recipes for reintroducing foods after you have completed the twenty-eight-day plan.

The Thyroid Connection Summit

I personally interviewed thirty-five leaders about the causes of thyroid dysfunction for the Thyroid Connection Summit online event (release date October 24, 2016); www.thyroidconnectionsummit.com.

Working with a Functional Medicine Doctor

Functional medicine practitioners are a great resource for identifying and addressing the root cause of your thyroid dysfunction.

Austin UltraHealth

The physicians, nurse practitioners, and registered dietitians at my functional medicine clinic treat patients from all over the world who are overcoming thyroid disease, autoimmune disease, gut infections, and other chronic health conditions.

5656 Bee Caves Rd., Suite D-203
Austin, Texas 78746
(512) 383-5343
info@amymyersmd.com
www.amymyersmd.com/become-a-patient

The Institute for Functional Medicine (IFM)

I did my functional medicine training through IFM. If you are not able to make an appointment with us at Austin UltraHealth, I would suggest you check the IFM's website to locate a practitioner in your area. Functional medicine addresses the underlying causes of disease using a systems-oriented approach and engaging both patient and practitioner in a therapeutic partnership. It is an evolution in the practice of medicine that better addresses the health-care needs of the twenty-first century; see www.functionalmedicine.org.

American Academy of Environmental Medicine

The mission of the American Academy of Environmental Medicine is "to promote optimal health through prevention, and safe and effective treatment of the causes of illness by supporting physicians and other professionals in serving the public through education about the interaction between humans and their environment." The AAEM is an international organization representing physicians who specialize in environmental medicine, a type of medicine that focuses on the environmental causes of poor health; see www.aaemon line.org.

Lab Resources

The Thyroid Connection Guide to Working with Your Doctor

A downloadable and printable version of the letter for your doctor, questions to ask, and labs to request. www.thethyroidconnection.com. If your doctor is unwilling to order any of the recommended labs for you, I have partnered with a lab that allows you to order your own labs online at a discounted price; see http://www.mylabsforlife.com.

Thyroid Resources and Support

The Myers Way Community: www.amymyersmd.com/community

Hashimoto's Awareness: www.hashimotosawareness.org

Thyroid Change: www.thyroidchange.org

National Academy of Hypothyroidism: www.nahypothyroid ism.org

American Thyroid Association: www.thyroid.org

Graves' Disease and Thyroid Foundation: www.gdatf.org

Hashimoto's Disease: www.hashimotosawareness.org

Gluten Intolerance Group: www.gluten.net

Healthy Eating

The Power of Food Guide

Find a list of my favorite online sources for organic, non-GMO foods, as well as tips for purchasing healthy, whole foods at your grocery store; see www.thethyroidconnection.com.

The Myers Way Meal-Planning Tool

An interactive tool that allows you to browse hundreds of The Myers Way Thyroid Connection–approved recipes to build a customized weekly meal plan and personalized shopping list; see http://store.amy myersmd.com/shop/the-myers-way-meal-planning/.

Thrive Market

Thrive Market offers the best in organic, non-GMO, paleo, gluten-free/dairy-free foods and toxin-free household goods for 25 to 50 percent less than you'll find in the grocery store; see http://thrv.me/ amymyersgift.

US Wellness Meats

Depending on where you live, it can be difficult to find 100 percent grass-fed meat, free of hormones and antibiotics. US Wellness Meats has a huge selection of beef, bison, poultry, pork, seafood, and other meats. I like to order in bulk a few times a year; see www.grass landbeef.com.

Vital Choice

I recommend enjoying wild-caught seafood during the twenty-eight-day plan and beyond. Vital Choice has excellent options for low-mercury seafood, including wild-caught salmon; see www.vitalchoice.com.

Genetically Modified Organisms (GMOs)

Institute for Responsible Technology

The IRT is a comprehensive resource for GMO research that also offers practical tips for making informed decisions about GMOs; see www .responsibletechnology.org.

The Environmental Working Group

EWG offers a huge range of reports, resources, and tools to help you minimize your exposure to toxins. On their website you can find their Dirty Dozen and Clean Fifteen lists, guides to avoiding GMO foods, lists of low-mercury fish, their Skin Deep app to rate the safety of your beauty products, and much more; see www.ewg.org.

Food Democracy Now!

Food Democracy Now! is a grassroots community dedicated to building a sustainable food system for the planet. They help members organize at the local and national level to protect our food systems; see www.fooddemocracynow.org.

Just Label It

Studies show that more than 90 percent of Americans support mandatory labeling of genetically modified foods. Ever since GMOs entered the market twenty years ago, we've been kept in the dark about whether foods we feed our families contain GMOs. This organization works for complete mandatory labeling of all GMOs; see www.just labelit.org.

Toxins

The Tame Your Toxins Guide

This guide includes all of the tools, guides, and lists mentioned in this book, plus a room-by-room guide to removing toxic chemicals and materials from your home, with recommended brands for toxin-free home goods, makeup, and body-care products; see www.thethyroid connection.com.

Natural Resources Defense Council

The NRDC offers guides and tips for avoiding mercury in your air, water, food, and home; see www.nrdc.org/health/effects/mercury/ guide.asp.

Center for Media and Democracy's Interactive Coal-Burning Power Plants Map

Coal-burning plants expose you to mercury; use this map to find out whether any such plants are located near you: www.sourcewatch.org/index.php/Existing_U.S._Coal_Plants.

Biological Dentistry

To find a biological dentist in your area, you can check out either of these two great organizations:

> International Academy of Biological Dentistry and Medicine; see www.iabdm.org.
> International Academy of Oral Medicine and Toxicology; see www.iaomt.org.

Surviving Mold

This is one of my go-to resources for everything related to chronic inflammatory response syndrome, which is caused by mold and mycotoxins. You can order labs, do online sensitivity testing, and find a practitioner who can help you cope with mold; see www.survivingmold.com.

CitriSafe

Find safe shampoos, laundry detergent, household cleaners, and pet shampoos for removing mold from your home, your pets, and your clothing; see www.citrisafecertified.com.

Stress Management

The Stress-Solution Guide

You can find all of the stress-relieving products I recommend in this book in a free downloadable guide on my website. This guide includes de-stressing exercises as well as a de-stressing diary, tips for rejuvenating relaxation, and resources to learn more about stress management, including where to find HeartMath, Binaural Beats, and other recommended products; see www.thethyroidconnection.com.

National Certification Commission for Acupuncture and Oriental Medicine

Find a certified acupuncturist in your area; see www.nccaom.org.

International Society for Neurofeedback and Research

Learn more about neurofeedback and find a practitioner in your area who offers this amazing therapy see www.isnr.org.

Float Locations

Find a facility in your area that offers sensory deprivation float tank sessions; see www.floatationlocations.com/category/united-states/.

Acknowledgments

While writing this book I had a significant mold exposure. If you have followed me and my story, you know that I am genetically susceptible to molds wreaking havoc on my health, and this was not my first exposure. There is a saying in the mold community—you get "sicker quicker" upon repeated exposures. I can attest to the truth of this statement. Midway through this book, my world and my health turned upside down. Writing a book and regaining your health are no small feats, and conquering them simultaneously seemed insurmountable. It truly took a village for me to finish this book, put the pieces of my life back together, and regain my health. It is through the love, dedication, strength, and support of the following people that I was able to do just that. I honestly could not have done this without you all. Thank you from the bottom of my heart for being part of my village.

My Book Village

Rachel Kranz: With you at my side, we are the dynamic duo. I appreciate your lightning-fast pace, incredible organization, and creative mind. Thank you for keeping everything going on the days I needed to put my health first.

Brianne Williams, RD, LD, you are a godsend. Our patients and I have been so blessed to have you in our lives. I am excited for your next adventure—motherhood! You will be an incredible mother, and Rowan will be one well-fed baby.

Tracy Behar, thank you for believing in me and helping to bring my message to the world. Your editing is amazing and so spot on!

Stephanie Tade, you are so much more than an agent — you are a confidante, cheerleader, and adviser, and above all, you are my friend. Thank you for all your pep talks and for reminding me to just breathe.

Thank you to the entire team at Little, Brown for all your support and for getting this book out so quickly!

My Austin UltraHealth Village

My incredible team at my clinic, Austin UltraHealth. It is because of you that the patients are so well taken care of, that the clinic runs so smoothly, and that I am able to do all the other things I do outside of the clinic. Thank you, Kathryn Arenz, Seth Osgood, Christine Maren, Taylor Morgan, Taylor Hohmann, Caroline Balter, and the rest of the team.

My patients. A deep, heartfelt thank-you to you for placing your faith and trust in me. I appreciate each of you for your dedication to The Myers Way program and to reclaiming your health. You are what gets me up in the morning, and I am so blessed to be able to work with each of you. I am so thankful for your flexibility and your understanding over the last several months while I was focused on my health and this book.

My AMMD, LLC Village

My absolutely amazing online store and marketing team at AMMD, LLC. It is because of you that we are able to help support people from around the word on their health journey, whether through our free online community, summits, blogs, newsletters, online programs, social media posts, high-quality supplements, phone calls, or personal e-mails. Thank you Jordyn Davenport, Susan Scambray, Ali Fine (who also created the illustrations in this book), and the rest of the team for all that you do for me and for our community. You ladies *rock!*

And to all of you whom I have not met but who have followed The Myers Way and shared it with your family, friends, and anyone who will listen — you are the grassroots movement that will help change the face of medicine. I applaud you and send a huge thank-you to each of you.

My Health Village

I would be nowhere without the village of functional medicine physicians, alternative practitioners, and consultants who helped restore my health during this most difficult time in my life. I am forever grateful to Drs. Darin Ingles, David Haase, John Bandy, Richie Shoemaker, and Robert Thoreson, as well as to Kimberly Patterson, Cassandra Bradford, Tony Hoffman, Eric Althouse, Walter and Sandy Hayhurst, and Connie Zack at Sunlighten Sauna.

Very few people can truly comprehend what it's like to be so affected by mold that you must get rid of everything you own. To my village of mold warriors who genuinely understood what I was going through, thank you for your generosity, for the endless phone calls, support, and advice, and for bringing me back to my breath one step at a time: Suzanne, Ann, Sophia, Ryen, Margaret, Carla, and Adam.

My IFM Village

I appreciate those who blazed the trail before me, shared their wisdom with me, and mentored me. Thank you for your continued support and generosity, Drs. Mark Hyman, David Perlmutter, Jeff Bland, Sidney Baker, and Frank Lipman.

Each of you in journal club inspire me with your brilliance and dedication to the field. I am so lucky to call you my colleagues and friends! Thank you to Drs. Kara Fitzgerald, Todd Lepine, David Brady, Patrick Hanaway, Bethany Hays, Michael Stone, Tom Shultz.

My Home Village

Cresta, Kaylee, Kenzie, and Eric Foster, thank you for loving Mocha with all your heart and for always helping out in times of need. I so appreciate all that you do for us.

Thank you for your unconditional love and support, Dad, Chris, Janie, big Xave, and all our extended family. Christian, thank you for helping me with the Selected Bibliography.

My sweet guardian angel, my mother. She taught me never to accept the status quo, to be curious and to question, to take the road less traveled, to be authentic, and never to be afraid to be different or stand up for what I believe. I am the woman and the doctor I am today because of my mother.

Most important, I want to thank my dear, sweet husband and soul mate, Xavier. This first year of our marriage has been a complete whirlwind. We experienced more highs and more lows in one year than many marriages do in a lifetime. This man literally gave up everything he owned and helped to nurse me back to health. Xavier, you are my everything and you are all I need. I love you more!

Letter to Your Doctor

You can share this letter with your doctor as part of your strategy to get more complete medical care.

Dear Colleague:

I'm the author of *The Thyroid Connection* (Little, Brown, 2017), and a physician who has treated several thousand patients with a wide variety of thyroid conditions, including non-autoimmune hypo- and hyperthyroidism, Hashimoto's thyroiditis, and Graves' disease. In the spirit of collegiality and commitment to patient care, I wanted to share with you some of the information that I have found helpful in the hopes that you will find it helpful too.

As you know, a number of factors can intersect to produce thyroid dysfunction—factors that are often neglected in our medical school training but that are well documented in the literature. For example, thyroid function is profoundly affected by chronic inflammation, and both thyroid function and inflammation are made worse by poor gut function. When an autoimmune disorder is involved, we have the makings of a vicious cycle. Add in adrenal dysfunction—which, as part of the endocrine system, is intimately linked to thyroid function—and problems can become even worse. In addition, the xenoestrogens that result from industrial chemicals and toxins further contribute to thyroid dysfunction and put an additional strain on the immune system.

Another key aspect of thyroid function involves nutrition, particularly having sufficient levels of iodine and tyrosine for thyroid hormone formation as well as enough selenium, iron, and zinc to facilitate the conversion of T4 to T3. Vitamins D and A are also crucial for the immune system and to enable T3 to enter the cells.

Moreover, the literature as well as my own clinical experience suggests that a great many people with hypothyroidism are underdiagnosed and undertreated. If a complete panel of thyroid blood work is not performed—for instance, if physicians test only TSH, or only TSH and free T4—many people who could benefit from medical care will not get it. Likewise, if standard reference ranges are used, many people who fall within those ranges will continue to suffer from suboptimal thyroid function. As you are undoubtedly aware, in 2002, the American Association of Clinical Endocrinologists recommended the use of more stringent reference ranges, given that the initial ranges were developed based on the inclusion of many people with hypothyroidism. I have found that even narrower optimal ranges enable me to treat the full spectrum of patients who need medical help.

Finally, I have found that testing thyroid antibodies is of primary importance because they often predict the onset of autoimmune disease by up to five years. If a patient knows that he or she has antibodies, he or she can support an autoimmune condition with the diet and lifestyle changes that I recommend in *The Thyroid Connection* and in my previous book, *The Autoimmune Solution* (HarperOne, 2015).

To these ends, I have recommended in my book a complete panel of thyroid and nutritional blood work, as well as a more stringent set of reference ranges, both of which are attached to this letter. I urge you to run these tests and analyze them based on these reference ranges so that this patient can get the very best that medical care has to offer. You can find further information on my website, www.amymyersmd.com.

With gratitude for your time and attention,

Amy Myers, MD

Recommended Blood Work and Reference Ranges

Blood Work and Reference Ranges for Thyroid Hormones

- TSH: 1–2 μIU/mL or lower (desiccated T4/T3 or compounded T3, as T3 can artificially suppress TSH)
- Free T4: >1.1 ng/dL
- Free T3: > 3.2 pg/mL
- Reverse T3: less than a 10:1 ratio of RT3 to FT3
- Thyroid peroxidase antibody (TPO): < 9 IU/mL or negative
- Thyroglobulin antibody (TgAb): <4 IU/mL or negative
- TSH receptor antibodies (TRAb or TSHRAb): 1.75 IU/L or negative
- Thyroids-stimulating immunoglobin (TSI or TSAb): <1.3 TSI index

Blood Work and Reference Ranges for the Nutrients Needed for Optimal Thyroid Function

- Iron/ferritin (serum): normal 12–150 ng/mL; optimal 75–100 ng/mL
- Vitamin D (serum): normal 30–100 ng/mL; optimal 50–70 ng/mL
- Vitamin A (serum): normal 0.30–1.20 mg/L; optimal 0.8–1 mg/L
- Homocysteine (serum): normal 4–15 mmol/L; optimal 7–8 mmol/L
- Selenium (RBC): 120-300 mcg/L, optimal 200–250 mcg/L
- Zinc (RBC): normal 790–1,500 mcg/dL; optimal 1,000–1,200 mcg/dL
- Magnesium (RBC): normal 1.5–3.1 mmol/L; optimal 2.5–3.0 mmol/L

Home Detox

In chapter 8, you read my first line of defense against the toxins that surround us in our homes. If you'd like to go further, here's what I recommend, listed in order of importance. For where to purchase related products, see Resources.

Choose Clean Cleaning Products
Home-cleaning products contain brominated flame retardants, which disrupt thyroid function, and perfluorinated chemicals, which do the same. Your immune system isn't happy about them either.

Get a Clean Mattress
And if you think those conventional mattresses are clean, think again. Considering that you detox when you sleep and that you spend hours each day on your mattress, having a clean mattress is absolutely crucial to protect thyroid function and immune health. Do you want continual, nightly exposure to industrial chemicals and fire retardants? I didn't think so! A better choice would be a 100 percent natural latex mattress and an organic wool mattress topper.

Clean Up Your Bedding
Those fire retardants are in your commercial bedding too, along with pesticides, bleaches, and dyes. Look for organic, untreated sheets, blankets, and pillows.

Pick a Clean Sofa

You probably spend hours on your sofa too. The flame retardants and industrial chemicals used to protect it don't really make it less flammable, but they do make it more toxic. Upholstered furniture can also contain petroleum-based polyurethane foams, which likewise contain fire retardants and industrial toxins. Particleboard ups the ante by emitting formaldehyde. Instead, look for a sofa with a label that says, *Contains no added flame retardant chemicals,* and go for furniture made with solid wood, natural latex foam, wool cushions, and organic fabrics.

Choose Area Rugs or Safe Carpeting

You can be exposed to up to 120 hazardous chemicals from the synthetic, petroleum-based material used to carpet your floors. And older stain-resistant carpets contain PFOA, which, as we saw, disrupts your thyroid while putting you at risk for cancer. The newer carpets are treated with another type of chemical, PFAS, which has been linked to birth defects and cancer as well. Finally, the rubber padding and adhesive glues can further contribute to asthma, allergies, neurological problems, and cancer. You will do better with recycled carpet tiles (no adhesives) or with area rugs of organic wool, cotton, sisal, or no rug at all.

Choose Safe Paints

Many paints contain VOCs, but you can find non-VOC paints. Just verify that they really *are* nontoxic through and through. Sometimes a paint advertised as non-VOC is good only for the base white paint. The added color can make them toxic again, so do a bit of research to be sure.

Choose Safe Window Treatments

By now you will not be surprised to find that fire retardants, pesticides, bleaches, and dyes are routinely used to treat curtains. Go with organic, untreated cotton or linen curtains and valences, or with bamboo shades—and problem solved!

...And One Last Thing

Hand sanitizer isn't a great idea to begin with, because it kills off the friendly bacteria you need for a healthy microbiome. Adding insult to injury, the ingredient triclosan has been linked to liver cancer in mice. A substitute that many manufacturers are using, *benzalkonium chloride,* might exacerbate asthma. If you like hand sanitizers for those times when you travel and can't wash your hands, find one that relies on ethyl alcohol.

Biological Dentistry

It's not just mercury fillings that can cause problems in our mouths. Root canals, extracted wisdom teeth, braces, retainers, fillings, crowns, and posts can all trigger inflammation, which will burden your immune system and disrupt thyroid function. I cannot recommend highly enough a trip to a biological dentist—a dentist who understands the hazards of conventional dentistry and can help make sure that only biocompatible materials are used in your mouth.

Remember, your mouth is part of your body, so anything that stays there is exposed to your immune system. You don't want a permanent trigger to remain within your body.

Your biological dentist can do a blood test to find out which dental materials will work for you and which might cause reactions. You can also request products made by VOCO, a German company, which are almost always biocompatible.

Your top priority is to get any amalgam out of your mouth. The amalgam fillings contain a mixture of mercury, silver, tin, and copper. The video prepared by the International Academy of Oral Medicine and Toxicology (IAOMT) shows plumes of mercury vapors actually rising off a tooth with a mercury filling (www.youtube.com/watch?v= 9ylnQ-T7oiA). I know it's hard to believe that the standard practice in conventional dentistry is so deadly to your health. Believe me, it is.

In addition to the mercury being toxic, tin is also. And when they added the copper, they found that the level of mercury exposure increased by a factor of fifty. If you've had a crown put in on top of a filling, it will exacerbate the effect of mercury, partly by potentially creating a galvanic current—an electric current at odds with the natural currents running through your body.

So, please, work with a biological dentist, and do *not* let a conventional dentist switch out your fillings. They simply don't know how to do it safely, and you—and they—might be exposed to mercury vapors in the process.

Root canals can also create inflammation. A root canal kills the nerve of a tooth but leaves the tooth in your mouth, where toxic bacteria can breed freely. In a living part of your body, blood flows, bringing with it immune factors and killer chemicals to neutralize these bacteria. But a root canal produces a dead tooth, whose bacteria cannot be removed even with antibiotics. If you have autoimmune thyroid dysfunction in particular, I advise you to either give the dead tooth an ozone treatment or have it extracted.

A third concern is *cavitations:* holes or spaces inside a bone, most commonly the jaw. Say you've had a wisdom tooth extracted. Your gum tissue grows over the open area, and bone grows over that—but toxic bacteria remain within the cavitation. Your immune system is confronted with these bacteria daily, and if you're struggling with other immune challenges, this can make them worse.

A biological dentist will make a small surgical incision, irrigate the area, and attack the bacteria with ozone. Your immune system will be super-grateful.

Finally, braces and retainers frequently contain nickel and titanium—yes, they are part of the stainless steel that you were told was safe. The titanium might be, but the nickel is something you don't want to be exposed to. Work with a biological dentist to clean up the problem.

You can find a biological dentist on the IOAMT website (www .iaomt.org), through your functional medicine physician, or by doing an online search. You can double-check that your dentist is safe by asking if he or she uses a rubber dam to protect patients whose fillings are being removed. You can also find out how dentists protect themselves and their staffs; that's a good clue of whether they're aware of how dangerous mercury can be. Finally, you can ask dentists if they have *an amalgam separator,* which prevents mercury from ending up in the local wastewater.

If you want to read more about the hazards of dentistry, I can recommend two excellent books: *It's All in Your Head: The Link Between Mercury Amalgams and Illness* (Avery Publishing, 1993), by Hal A. Huggins, and *Uninformed Consent: The Hidden Dangers in Dental Care* (Hampton Roads Publishing, 1999), by Hal A. Huggins and Thomas E. Levy.

Do I Need Chelation?

As you saw in chapter 8, heavy metals can be hazardous to your thyroid, your immune system, and your overall health. If you haven't seen the improvement you'd like to see after three months of following The Myers Way Thyroid Connection Plan, heavy metals might be part of the problem, especially if you have one or more of the following risk factors:

- You regularly drink or shower in unfiltered water.
- You have amalgam fillings, either currently or in the past.
- You eat tuna more than once a week (tuna is heavily laden with mercury).
- You have recurrent yeast overgrowth (sometimes you develop yeast to protect you from the mercury).
- You live near a coal-burning plant, which emits mercury (find out more from this link: www.epa.gov/mats/where.html).
- You've spent time in China, where they burn a lot of coal—which emits mercury.
- You have one or more SNPs in the MTHFR gene (see page 191).

If you think heavy metals are a factor in your condition, get a functional medicine physician to test you. You will likely be given one or both of these tests:

○ A red blood cell (RBC) test, which measures your exposure to heavy metals over the previous three months (the life of a red blood cell).

○ A challenge test, which measures accumulated metals in your body. This involves you giving a baseline urine sample, then swallowing a solution of 2,3-dimercapto-1-propanesulfonic acid (DMPS), which will help your body chelate, or filter out, the heavy metals from where they have been stored, primarily in your bones. The urine is collected for the next six hours so the lab can measure how much heavy metal is stored there.

If your functional medicine doctor thinks you need it, you might undergo *chelation*—a process of filtering heavy metals from your system. Cilantro and other natural substances might be all you need. High concentrations of heavy metals require dimercaptosuccinic acid (DMSA), which the FDA has approved for chelating lead, although it's used to chelate other heavy metals too. You will likely take DMSA a few times a day for a number of days, then take some time off. The whole process can take three to seven months, usually with a follow-up test three months later. You want to support your detox pathways throughout, with lots of glutathione and minerals.

Make *sure* you have fully healed your gut and supported your detox pathways before you even begin to think about chelation! Chelation pulls toxins out of your bones and into your system so you can then excrete them through your urine. If your gut is leaky and your detox pathways are not working properly, you might reabsorb huge quantities of toxins into your system. Make sure you and your doctor are working together to prevent this.

Coping with Toxic Mold

Toxic mold is a health hazard for the 25 percent of the population that is vulnerable to it. That's why I ask all of my patients about the possibility of a toxic mold exposure. Of course, I always begin by addressing diet, gut, toxins, infections, and stress. But if you've tried those key approaches and you're still struggling with thyroid symptoms, recurrent Candida or yeast overgrowth, or an autoimmune condition that developed suddenly and seemingly out of nowhere, then mold is the next place I'd look.

Don't forget: three-fourths of the population is *not* vulnerable to mold, and that might well include your family or roommates or coworkers. Just because you're the only one at home or work who's getting sick does *not* mean that mold is not a problem.

These are the most common types of mold that give off mycotoxins—that is, gases known as volatile organic compounds (VOCs):

- *Aspergillus*
- *Fusarium*
- *Paecilomyces*
- *Penicillium*
- *Stachybotrys*
- *Trichoderma*

Symptoms of mold exposure include the following:

- ADD/ADHD
- anxiety
- autoimmunity
- chronic fatigue syndrome
- depression
- fatigue
- fibromyalgia
- headaches
- insomnia
- skin rashes of all types, including eczema
- neurologic dysfunction

I start thinking mold might be a problem when I hear about the following risk factors:

- older homes
- homes with known leaks
- homes with crawl spaces
- homes with basements
- homes built into hillsides
- homes with flat roofs
- humid climates

Likewise, if you live in a large apartment complex, work in a large office building, or spend time in a hotel or school, you have a higher risk of being exposed to mold. Be especially aware of homes or workplaces with a shared HVAC (heating, ventilating, and air-conditioning) system, because it can transmit the toxins from a moldy space to a seemingly dry one.

Testing for Toxic Mold

You're not interested in air quality and mold spores, which are what most typical tests look for. You're interested only in the specific types of mold that release mycotoxins or VOCs. You can either cut off a piece of your air filter and send it to RealTime Laboratories (see Resources) or look for a company that does an ERMI (environmental relative moldiness index) test. If you're testing your own home, you will be legally obligated to disclose the results of an ERMI test to the next buyer, which could lead to some real headaches if you can't easily identify the source of the mold.

You don't have to test your home, though. You can try to test yourself. A urine test can detect four specific mycotoxins, but it won't tell you anything about the others. A more effective solution — if you can manage it — is to stay somewhere else for two weeks: a friend's home, a motel, anywhere you think might be mold-free. Take as little with you as possible — no pillows, stuffed animals, or anything else that might have picked up microscopic amounts of mold. If you feel better when you leave home and worse when you return, mold might be your culprit.

Now, how do you know if you're reacting to mold at home or at work? You can always get others in your home tested. If they test positive for mycotoxins, they've been exposed to mold — even if they don't have any symptoms. If they test negative, the mold is probably somewhere else where you spend a lot of time, either work or school.

Solving the Problem

First, you have to permanently remove yourself from the environment (i.e., find another place to live or work) or fix the environment (i.e., remove all traces of the mold from the environment). Then you need to detoxify yourself, binding the mycotoxins so you can excrete them from your body. Here's the protocol I recommend:

- Hire a certified mold remediator. You'll need to stay away from your home until the work is complete.
- Take 300 mg of glutathione up to three times a day, which helps your body detoxify. See Resources for the brand I recommend. Most of the others are very hard for your body to absorb and are frankly a waste of money.

- Take 1.5 to 3 grams of glucomannan twice a day, which will bind the toxins so you can safely excrete them. Alternatively, you can take 4 grams of cholestyramine three times a day, but for that, you will need a prescription.

Look for a functional medicine physician who can prescribe anti-fungal medications and order blood tests to help identify the source and to help restore you to health.

One of my favorite go-to resources for mold toxicity is www.survivingmold.com.

Selected Bibliography

Chapter 1. The Thyroid Crisis

About Your Thyroid. *AACE Thyroid Awareness*. http://www.thyroidawareness.com/about-your-thyroid.

Bahn, R, Burch, H, Cooper, D, et al. Hyperthyroidism and Other Causes of Thyrotoxicosis: Management Guidelines of the American Thyroid Association and American Association of Clinical Endocrinologists. *Endocrine Practice*. 2011;17(3):456–520. doi:10.4158/ep.17.3.456.

Blackwell, J. Evaluation and Treatment of Hyperthyroidism and Hypothyroidism. *Journal of the American Academy of Nurse Practitioners*. 2004;16(10):422–425.

Blum, MR, Wijsman, LW, Virgini, VS, et al. Subclinical Thyroid Dysfunction and Depressive Symptoms among Elderly: A Prospective Cohort Study. *Neuroendocrinology*. 2015.

Cappola, AR, Cooper, DS. Screening and Treating Subclinical Thyroid Disease: Getting Past the Impasse. *Annals of Internal Medicine*. 2015;162(9):664. doi:10.7326/m15-0640.

Garber, JR, Cobin, RH, Gharib, H, et al. Clinical Practice Guidelines for Hypothyroidism in Adults: Cosponsored by the American Association of Clinical Endocrinologists and the American Thyroid Association. *Thyroid*. 2012;22(12):1200–1235.

General Information/Press Room. American Thyroid Association. 2016. http://www.thyroid.org/media-main/about-hypothyroidism/.

Hashimoto's Disease. National Institute of Diabetes and Digestive and Kidney Diseases. 2014. http://www.niddk.nih.gov/health-information/health-topics/endocrine/hashimotos-disease/Pages/fact-sheet.aspx.

Hypothyroidism. National Institute of Diabetes and Digestive and Kidney Diseases. 2013. http://www.niddk.nih.gov/health-information/health-topics/endocrine/hypothyroidism/Pages/fact-sheet.aspx.

Ittermann, T, Völzke, H, Baumeister, SE, Appel, K, Grabe, HJ. Diagnosed thyroid disorders are associated with depression and anxiety. *Social Psychiatry and Psychiatric Epidemiology*. 2015;50(9):1417–1425.

Krysiak, R, Drosdzol-Cop, A, Skrzypulec-Plinta, V, Okopien, B. Sexual function and depressive symptoms in young women with thyroid autoimmunity and subclinical hypothyroidism. *Clinical Endocrinology*. 2015;84(6):925–931.

Lefevre, ML. Screening for Thyroid Dysfunction: U.S. Preventive Services Task Force Recommendation Statement. *Annals of Internal Medicine.* 2015;162(9):641. doi:10.7326/m15-0483.

Marinò, M, Latrofa, F, Menconi, F, Chiovato, L, Vitti, P. Role of genetic and non-genetic factors in the etiology of Graves' disease. *Journal of Endocrinological Investigation.* 2014;38(3):283–294.

Massoudi, MS, et al. Prevalence of thyroid antibodies among healthy middle-aged women. Findings from the thyroid study in healthy women. *Annals of Epidemiology.* 1995;5(3):229–233.

Mayo Clinic Staff. Hyperthyroidism Symptoms. Mayo Clinic. 2015. http://www.mayoclinic.org/diseases-conditions/hyperthyroidism/basics/symptoms/con-20020986.

———. Hypothyroidism (underactive thyroid): Symptoms and Causes. Mayo Clinic. 2015. http://www.mayoclinic.org/diseases-conditions/hypothyroidism/symptoms-causes/dxc-20155382.

Najafi, L, Malek, M, Hadian, A, Valojerdi, AE, Khamseh, ME, Aghili, R. Depressive symptoms in patients with subclinical hypothyroidism—the effect of treatment with levothyroxine: a double-blind randomized clinical trial. *Endocrine Research.* 2015;40(3):121–126.

Orth, DN, Shelton, RC, Nicholson, WE, et al. Serum Thyrotropin Concentrations and Bioactivity During Sleep Deprivation in Depression. *Archives of General Psychiatry.* 2001;58(1):77.

Patil, A. Link between hypothyroidism and small intestinal bacterial overgrowth. *Indian Journal of Endocrinology and Metabolism.* 2014;18(3):307.

Saran, S, Gupta, B, Philip, R, et al. Effect of hypothyroidism on female reproductive hormones. *Indian Journal of Endocrinology and Metabolism.* 2016;20(1):108.

Schindler, AE. Thyroid function and postmenopause. *Gynecological Endocrinology.* 2003;17(1):79–85.

Stagnaro-Green, A, Abalovich, M, Alexander, E, et al. Guidelines of the American Thyroid Association for the Diagnosis and Management of Thyroid Disease During Pregnancy and Postpartum. *Thyroid.* 2011;21(10):1081–1125.

Stockigt, JR, and Braverman, LE. Update on the Sick Euthyroid Syndrome. *Diseases of the Thyroid.* Totowa, NJ: Humana Press, 1997, 49–68.

Thyroid Disease: Know the Facts. Thyroid Foundation of Canada. 2016. http://www.thyroid.ca/know_the_facts.php.

Thyroid Disease and Menopause: Symptoms, Causes, Treatments. *WebMD.* 2015. http://www.webmd.com/menopause/guide/symptoms-thyroid-vs-menopause.

The Thyroid and You: Coping with a Common Condition. *NIH Medline Plus,* 2012:22–23.

Treatment Options. Graves' Disease and Thyroid Foundation. http://www.gdatf.org/about/about-graves-disease/treatment-options/.

Yeung, S. Graves' Disease. *Medscape.* May 2014. http://emedicine.medscape.com/article/120619-overview.

Chapter 2. *You* Can *Be Helped*

Arem, R. The Thyroid Solution: A Mind–Body Program for Beating Depression and Regaining Your Emotional and Physical Health. New York: Ballantine Books, 1999.

Davis, W. Wheat belly: lose the wheat, lose the weight, and find your path back to health. Emmaus, PA: Rodale, 2011.

Kimura, H, Caturegli, P. Chemokine Orchestration of Autoimmune Thyroiditis. *Thyroid*. 2007;17(10):1005–1011.

Ruggeri, RM, Vicchio, TM, Cristani, M, et al. Oxidative Stress and Advanced Glycation End Products in Hashimoto's Thyroiditis. *Thyroid*. 2016;26(4):504–511.

Shomon, MJ. *Living Well with Hypothyroidism: What Your Doctor Doesn't Tell You . . . That You Need to Know*. New York: Harper Collins, 2002.

Wu, H, Gu, G, Zhou, W, Wu, Y, Jiang, K, Yu, S. Relationship between occupational stressors and serum levels of thyroid hormones in policemen. *Zhonghua Lao Dong Wei Sheng Zhi Ye Bing Za Zhi*. 2015;33(10):727–730.

Chapter 3. *What Is the Thyroid?*

Abdullatif, HD, Ashraf, AP. Reversible Subclinical Hypothyroidism in the Presence of Adrenal Insufficiency. *Endocrine Practice*. 2006;12(5):572–575.

Andersson, M, Takkouche, B, Egli, I, et al. Current global iodine status and progress over the last decade towards the elimination of iodine deficiency. *Bulletin of the World Health Organization*. 2005;83:518–525.

Canaris, GJ, Tape, TG, Wigton, RS. Thyroid disease awareness is associated with high rates of identifying subjects with previously undiagnosed thyroid dysfunction. *BMC Public Health*. 2013;13(1):351.

Chen, K, Yan, B, Wang, F, et al. Type 1 5'-deiodinase activity is inhibited by oxidative stress and restored by alpha-lipoic acid in HepG2 cells. *Biochemical and Biophysical Research Communications*. 2016;472(3):496–501.

Devdhar, M, Ousman, YH, Burman, KD. Hypothyroidism. *Endocrinology and Metabolism Clinics of North America*. 2007;36:595–615.

Flores-Rebollar, A, Moreno-Castañeda, L, Vega-Servín, NS, López-Carrasco, G, Ruiz-Juvera, A. Prevalence of autoimmune thyroiditis and thyroid dysfunction in healthy adult Mexicans with a slightly excessive iodine intake. *Nutrición Hospitalaria*. 2015;32(2):918–924.

Fukao, A, Takamatsu, J, Miyauchi, A, Hanafusa, T. Stress and Thyroid Disease. Endocrine Diseases. iConcept Press, 2015.

Hanaway, P. Thyroid Dysfunction: The Role of Nutrients, Toxins and Stress. 2012. https://www.gdx.net/presentations/webinars/thyroid-dysfunction-the-role-of-nutrients-toxins-stress.pdf.

Hernandez, A, Quignodon, L, Martinez, ME, Flamant, F, Germain, DLS. Type 3 Deiodinase Deficiency Causes Spatial and Temporal Alterations in Brain T3 Signaling that Are Dissociated from Serum Thyroid Hormone Levels. *Endocrinology*. 2010;151(11):5550–5558.

How does the thyroid work? *PubMed Health*. 2015. http://www.ncbi.nlm.nih.gov/pubmedhealth/pmh0072572/.

Kawicka, A, Regulska-Ilow, B, Regulska-Ilow, B. Metabolic disorders and nutritional status in autoimmune thyroid diseases. *Postepy Hig Med Dosw Postępy Higieny i Medycyny Doświadczalnej.*

Kellman, R. Low Thyroid in Men: Not Just a Woman's Issue. *US News and World Report Health.* 2015.http://health.usnews.com/health-news/patient-advice/articles/2015/07/21/low-thyroid-in-men-not-just-a-womans-issue.

Kimura, H, Caturegli, P. Chemokine Orchestration of Autoimmune Thyroiditis. *Thyroid.* 2007;17(10):1005–1011.

Lazarus, JH. The importance of iodine in public health. *Environmental Geochemistry and Health.* 2015;37(4):605–618.

Liu, L, Wang, D, Liu, P, et al. The relationship between iodine nutrition and thyroid disease in lactating women with different iodine intakes. *British Journal of Nutrition.* 2015;114(09):1487–1495.

Mizokami, T, Li, AW, El-Kaissi, S, Wall, JR. Stress and Thyroid Autoimmunity. *Thyroid.* 2004;14(12):1047–1055.

Patrick, L. Thyroid disruption: mechanism and clinical implications in human health. *Alternative Medicine Review.* 2009 Dec;14(4):326–46. Erratum in *Alternative Medicine Review.* 2010 Apr;15(1):58.

Shivaraj, G, Prakash, BD, Sonal, V, et al. Thyroid function tests: a review. *European Review for Medical and Pharmacological Sciences.* 2009;13:341–349.

Sikic, D, Lüdecke, G, Lieb, V, Keck, B. Side effect management of tyrosine kinase inhibitors in urology: Fatigue and hypothyroidism. *Urolege A.* 2016.

Stone, MB, Wallace, RB. Pathophysiology and Diagnosis of Thyroid Disease. In *Medicare coverage of routine screening for thyroid dysfunction.* Washington, DC: National Academies Press, 2003, 14–20.

Thyroid Function Tests. American Thyroid Association. http://www.thyroid.org/thyroid-function-tests/.

Vanderpump, MP. The epidemiology of thyroid diseases. In Braverman, LE, Utiger, RD, ed. *The Thyroid: A Fundamental and Clinical Text.* 9th edition. Philadelphia: Lippincott, Williams and Wilkins, 2004, 398–406.

Warrell, DA, Cox, TM, Firth, JD, Weetman, AP. The thyroid gland and disorders of thyroid function. In *Oxford Textbook of Medicine.* Oxford: Oxford University Press, 2012. http://oxfordindex.oup.com/view/10.1093/med/9780199204854.003.1304_update_002#fulltextlinks.

Wu, Q, Rayman, MP, Lv, H, et al. Low Population Selenium Status Is Associated with Increased Prevalence of Thyroid Disease. *Journal of Clinical Endocrinology and Metabolism.* 2015;100(11):4037–4047.

Chapter 4. *The Autoimmune Connection*

Abu-Shakra, et al. The Mosaic of Autoimmunity: Hormonal and Environmental Factors Involved in Autoimmune Diseases—2008. *Israel Medical Association Journal.* 2008;10(1): 8–12.

Ashraf, R, Shah, NP. Immune System Stimulation by Probiotic Microorganisms. *Critical Reviews in Food Science and Nutrition.* 2014;54(7):938–956.

Bahn, R. Immunogenetics, Epigenetics and Environmental Triggers of Autoimmune Thyroid Disorders. Paper presented at Spring Meeting of the American

Thyroid Association Thyroid Disorders in the Era of Personalized Medicine; 2010; Minneapolis, Minnesota.

Bonds, RS, Midoro-Horiuti, T, Goldblum, R. A structural basis for food allergy: the role of cross-reactivity. *Current Opinion in Allergy and Clinical Immunology.* 2008;8(1):82–86.

Brandtzaeg, P. "Gatekeeper Function of the Intestinal Epithelium." *Beneficial Microbes.* 2013;4(1):67–82.

Brown, K, DeCoffe, D, Molcan, E, Gibson, DL. Corrections to Article: Diet-Induced Dysbiosis of the Intestinal Microbiota and the Effects on Immunity and Disease. *Nutrients.* 2012;4(11):1552–1553.

———. Diet-Induced Dysbiosis of the Intestinal Microbiota and the Effects on Immunity and Disease. *Nutrients.* 2012;4(8):1095–119.

Catassi, C, Bai, J, Bonaz, B, et al. Non-Celiac Gluten Sensitivity: The New Frontier of Gluten Related Disorders. *Nutrients.* 2013;5(10):3839–3853.

Chen, J, He, X, Huang, J. Diet Effects in Gut Microbiome and Obesity. *Journal of Food Science.* 2014;79(4):R442–451.

Cordain, L, Toohey, L, Smith, MJ, Hickey, MS. Modulation of immune function by dietary lectins in rheumatoid arthritis. *British Journal of Nutrition.* 2000; 83(3):207–217.

Crook, WG. *The Yeast Connection: A Medical Breakthrough.* New York: Vintage, 1986.

Decker, E, Engelmann, G, Findeisen, A, et al. Cesarean Delivery Is Associated with Celiac Disease but Not Inflammatory Bowel Disease in Children. *Pediatrics.* 2010;125(6).

Dieterich, W. Cross linking to tissue transglutaminase and collagen favours gliadin toxicity in coeliac disease. *Gut.* 2006;55(4):478–484.

Doe, WF. The Intestinal Immune System. *Gut.* 1989;30:1679–1685.

Drago, S, Asmar, RE, Pierro, MD, et al. Gliadin, zonulin and gut permeability: Effects on celiac and non-celiac intestinal mucosa and intestinal cell lines. *Scandinavian Journal of Gastroenterology.* 2006;41(4):408–419.

Eberl, G. A New Vision of Immunity: Homeostasis of the Superorganism. *Mucosal Immunology.* 2010;3(5):450–460.

Eswaran, S, Tack, J, Chey, WD. Food: The Forgotten Factor in the Irritable Bowel Syndrome. *Gastroenterological Clinics of North America.* 2011;40(1):141–162.

Farrell, RJ, Kelly, CP. Celiac Sprue. *New England Journal of Medicine.* 2002;346(3): 180–188.

Fasano, A. Celiac Disease Insights: Clues to Solving Autoimmunity. *Scientific American.* 2009.

———. Leaky Gut and Autoimmune Diseases. *Clinical Reviews in Allergy and Immunology.* 2012;42(1):71–78.

Fasano, A. Physiological, Pathological, and Therapeutic Implications of Zonulin-Mediated Intestinal Barrier Modulation: Living Life on the Edge of the Wall. *American Journal of Pathology.* 2008;173(5):1243–1252.

———. Zonulin and Its Regulation of Intestinal Barrier Function: The Biological Door to Inflammation, Autoimmunity, and Cancer. *Physiological Reviews.* 2011;91(1):151–175.

————. Zonulin, Regulation of Tight Junctions, and Autoimmune Diseases. *Annals of the New York Academy of Sciences.* 2012;1258(1):25–33.

Fasano, A, Shea-Donohue, T. Mechanisms of Disease: The Role of Intestinal Barrier Function in the Pathogenesis of Gastrointestinal Autoimmune Diseases. *Nature Clinical Practice: Gastroenterology and Hepatology.* 2005;2(9):416–422.

Fleiner, HF, Bjøro, T, Midthjell, K, Grill, V, Åsvold, BO. Prevalence of Thyroid Dysfunction in Autoimmune and Type 2 Diabetes: The Population-Based HUNT Study in Norway. *Journal of Clinical Endocrinology and Metabolism.* 2016;101(2):669–677.

Hardy, H, Harris, J, Lyon, E, Beal, J, Foey, A. Probiotics, Prebiotics and Immunomodulation of Gut Mucosal Defences: Homeostasis and Immunopathology. *Nutrients.* 2013;5(6):1869–1912.

Hausch, F, Shan, L, Santiago, NA, Gray, GM, Khosla, C. Intestinal digestive resistance of immunodominant gliadin peptides. *American Journal of Physiology—Gastrointestinal and Liver Physiology.* 2002;283(4).

Hawrelak, JA, Myers, SP. The Causes of Intestinal Dysbiosis: A Review. *Alternative Medicine Review.* 2004;9(2):180–197.

Hering, NA, Schulzke, JD. Therapeutic Options to Modulate Barrier Defects in Inflammatory Bowel Disease. *Digestive Diseases.* 2009;27(4):450–454.

Hybenova, M, Hrda, P, Procházková, J, Stejskal, V, Sterzl, I. The role of environmental factors in autoimmune thyroiditis. *Neuro Endocrinology Letters.* 2010; 31(3):283–289.

Institute for Functional Medicine. Advanced Practice GI Module.

————. *Textbook of Functional Medicine.* 2010.

Institute for Responsible Technology. Health Risks. www.responsibletecnology .org/health-risks.

Ji, S. *The Dark Side of Wheat: A Critical Appraisal of the Role of Wheat in Human Disease.* http://curezone.com/upload/PDF/Articles/jurplesman/DarkSideWheat _GreenMedInfo.pdf.

Junker, Y, Zeissig, S, Kim, S-J, et al. Wheat amylase trypsin inhibitors drive intestinal inflammation via activation of toll-like receptor 4. *Journal of Experimental Medicine.* 2012;209(13):2395–2408.

Kagnoff, MF. Celiac Disease: Pathogenesis of a Model Immunogenetic Disease. *Journal of Clinical Investigation.* 2007;117(1):41–49.

Kharrazian, D. The Gluten, Leaky Gut, Autoimmune Connection Seminar. Apex Semina. 2013.

Kitano, H, Oda, K. Robustness Trade-Offs and Host–Microbial Symbiosis in the Immune System. *Molecular Systems Biology.* 2006;2:2006.0022.

Kumar, V, Jarzabek-Chorzelska, M, Sulej, J, Karnewska, K, Farrell, T, Jablonska, S. Celiac Disease and Immunoglobulin A Deficiency: How Effective Are the Serological Methods of Diagnosis? *Clinical and Vaccine Immunology.* 2002;9(6): 1295–1300.

Lammers, KM, Lu, R, Brownley, J, et al. Gliadin Induces an Increase in Intestinal Permeability and Zonulin Release by Binding to the Chemokine Receptor CXCR3. *Gastroenterology.* 2008;135(1).

Lankelma, JM, Nieuwdorp, M, de Vos, WM, Wiersinga, WJ. The Gut Microbiota in Sickness and Health. [In Dutch.] *Nederlands Tijdschrift voor Geneeskunde.* 2014;157:A5901.

McDermott, AJ, Huffnagle, GB. The Microbiome and Regulation of Mucosal Immunity. *Immunology.* 2014;142(1):24–31.

Myers, A. *The Autoimmune Solution: Prevent and Reverse the Full Spectrum of Inflammatory Symptoms and Diseases.* New York: HarperOne, 2015.

Pellegrina, CD, Perbellini, O, Scupoli, MT, et al. Effects of wheat germ agglutinin on human gastrointestinal epithelium: Insights from an experimental model of immune/epithelial cell interaction. *Toxicology and Applied Pharmacology.* 2009;237(2):146–153.

Pizzorno, JE, Murray, MT. *Textbook of Natural Medicine.* 4th ed. London: Churchill Livingstone, 2012.

Proal, AD, Albert, PJ, Marshall, TG. The Human Microbiome and Autoimmunity. *Current Opinion in Rheumatology.* 2013;25(2):234–240.

Rescigno, M. Intestinal Microbiota and Its Effects on the Immune System. *Cellular Microbiology.* 2014.

Rogier, EW, Frantz, AL, Bruno, MEC, et al. Secretory antibodies in breast milk promote long-term intestinal homeostasis by regulating the gut microbiota and host gene expression. *Proceedings of the National Academy of Sciences.* 2014;111(8):3074–3079.

Sapone, A, Lammers, KM, Casolaro, V, et al. Divergence of gut permeability and mucosal immune gene expression in two gluten-associated conditions: celiac disease and gluten sensitivity. *BMC Medicine.* 2011;9(1):23.

Sapone, A, Lammers, KM, Mazzarella, G, et al. Differential Mucosal IL-17 Expression in Two Gliadin-Induced Disorders: Gluten Sensitivity and the Autoimmune Enteropathy Celiac Disease. *International Archives of Allergy and Immunology.* 2010;152(1):75–80.

Sapone, A, Magistris, LD, Pietzak, M, et al. Zonulin Upregulation Is Associated with Increased Gut Permeability in Subjects with Type 1 Diabetes and Their Relatives. *Diabetes.* 2006;55(5):1443–1449.

Sathyabama, S, Khan, N, Agrewala, JN. Friendly pathogens: prevent or provoke autoimmunity. *Critical Reviews in Microbiology.* 2013;40(3):273–280.

Shaoul, R, Lerner, A. Associated Autoantibodies in Celiac Disease. *Autoimmunity Reviews.* 2007;6(8):559–565.

Shoaie, S, Nielsen, J. Elucidating the interactions between the human gut microbiota and its host through metabolic modeling. *Front Genet Frontiers in Genetics.* 2014;5.

Shor, DB-A, Barzilai, O, Ram, M, et al. Gluten Sensitivity in Multiple Sclerosis. *Annals of the New York Academy of Sciences.* 2009;1173(1):343–349.

Sollid, LM, Jabri, B. Triggers and Drivers of Autoimmunity: Lessons from Coeliac Disease. *Nature Reviews: Immunology.* 2013;13(4):294–302.

Thompson, T, Lee, AR, Grace, T. Gluten Contamination of Grains, Seeds, and Flours in the United States: A Pilot Study. *Journal of the American Dietetic Association.* 2010;110(6):937–940.

Togami, K, Hayashi, Y, Chono, S, Morimoto, K. Involvement of intestinal permeability in the oral absorption of clarithromycin and telithromycin. *Biopharmaceutics and Drug Disposition*. 2014;35(6):321–329.

Tripathi, A, Lammers, KM, Goldblum, S, et al. Identification of human zonulin, a physiological modulator of tight junctions, as prehaptoglobin-2. *Proceedings of the National Academy of Sciences*. 2009;106(39):16799–16804.

Vieira, S, Pagovich, O, Kriegel, M. Diet, microbiota and autoimmune diseases. *Lupus*. 2014;23(6):518–526.

Vojdani, A, Tarash, I. Cross-Reaction Between Gliadin and Different Food and Tissue Antigens. *Food and Nutrition Sciences*. 2013;4(1):20–32.

West, CE, Jenmalm, MC, Prescott, SL. The gut microbiota and its role in the development of allergic disease: a wider perspective. *Clinical and Experimental Allergy*. 2014;45(1):43–53.

Yu, LC-H. Host-microbial interactions and regulation of intestinal epithelial barrier function: From physiology to pathology. *World Journal of Gastrointestinal Pathophysiology*. 2012;3(1):27.

Chapter 5. Why Your Doctor Gets It Wrong

AACE Medical Guidelines for Clinical Practice for the Evaluation and Treatment of Hyperthyroidism and Hypothyroidism. *Endocrine Practice*. 2002;8(6).

Anjana, Y, Tandon, OP, Vaney, N, Madhu, SV. Cognitive status in hypothyroid female patients: event-related evoked potential study. *Neuroendocrinology*. 2008;88(1):59–66.

Bahn, RS, Burch, HB, Cooper, DS, et al. Hyperthyroidism and Other Causes of Thyrotoxicosis: Management Guidelines of the American Thyroid Association and American Association of Clinical Endocrinologists. *Thyroid*. 2011; 21(6):593–646.

Christenson, RH, Duh, S-H, Clarisse, DE, Zorn, N. Thyroid function testing evaluated on three immunoassay systems. *Journal of Clinical Laboratory Analysis*. 1995;9(3):178–183.

Cordova, RA, Vignola, G. The utility of FT4 serum in newborns at risk for congenital hypothyroidism (CH). *Southeastern Asian Journal of Tropical Medicine Public Health*. 2003;34(3):152–153.

Duntas, LH, Biondi, B. New insights into subclinical hypothyroidism and cardiovascular risk. *Semin Thromb Hemost*. 2011;37(1):27–34.

Ehrenkranz, J, Bach, PR, Snow, GL, et al. Circadian and Circannual Rhythms in Thyroid Hormones: Determining the TSH and Free T4 Reference Intervals Based Upon Time of Day, Age, and Sex. *Thyroid*. 2015;25(8):954–961.

Faix, JD. Principles and pitfalls of free hormone measurements. *Best Practice and Research Clinical Endocrinology and Metabolism*. 2013;27(5):631–645.

Fatourechi, V, Klee, GG, Grebe, SK, et al. Effects of reducing the upper limit of normal TSH values. *Journal of the American Medical Association*. 2003;290:3195–3196.

Friedberg, RC, Souers, R, Wagar, EA, Stankovic, AK, Valenstein, PN, College of American Pathologists. The origin of reference intervals. *Archives of Pathology and Laboratory Medicine*. 2007;131(3):348–357.

Fröhlich, E, Wahl, R. Mechanisms in Endocrinology: Impact of isolated TSH levels in and out of normal range on different tissues. *European Journal of Endocrinology*. 2015;174(2).

Garber, JR, Cobin, RH, Gharib, H, et al. Clinical Practice Guidelines for Hypothyroidism in Adults: Cosponsored by the American Association of Clinical Endocrinologists and the American Thyroid Association. *Thyroid*. 2012; 22(12):1200–1235.

Garber, J. New Campaign Urges People to "Think Thyroid" at Critical Life Stages and Get Tested. Hypothyroidism—Talking Points 2006. *U.S. Endocrine Disease 2006*. 2006.

Gharib, H, Cobin, R, Baskin, J. Subclinical Thyroid Disease. American Association of Clinical Endocrinologists. https://www.aace.com/files/position-statements/subclinical.pdf.

Hennessey, JV, Espaillat, R. Diagnosis and Management of Subclinical Hypothyroidism in Elderly Adults: A Review of the Literature. *Journal of the American Geriatrics Society*. 2015;63(8):1663–1673.

Hogervorst, E, Huppert, F, Matthews, FE, Brayne, C. Thyroid function and cognitive decline in the MRC Cognitive Function and Ageing Study. *Psychoneuroendocrinology*. 2008;33(7):1013–1022.

Kritz-Silverstein, D, Schultz, ST, Palinska, LA, Wingard, DL, Barrett-Connor, E. The association of thyroid stimulating hormone levels with cognitive function and depressed mood: the Rancho Bernardo study. *Journal of Nutrition, Health, and Aging*. 2009;13(4):317–321.

Kvetny, J, Heldgaard, PE, Bladbjerg, EM, Gram, J. Subclinical hypothyroidism is associated with a low-grade inflammation, increased triglyceride levels and predicts cardiovascular disease in males below 50 years. *Clinical Endocrinology (Oxford)*. 2004;61(2):232–238.

Pasqualetti, G, Pagano, G, Rengo, G, Ferrara, N, Monzani, F. Subclinical Hypothyroidism and Cognitive Impairment: Systematic Review and Meta-Analysis. *Journal of Clinical Endocrinology and Metabolism*. 2015;100(11):4240–4248.

Ray, RA, Howanitz, PJ, Howanitz, JH. Controversies in thyroid function testing. *Clinics in Laboratory Medicine*. 1984;4(4):671–682.

Samuels, MH, Schuff, KG, Carlson, NE, et al. Health status, mood, and cognition in experimentally induced subclinical hypothyroidism. *Journal of Clinical Endocrinology and Metabolism*. 2007;92(7):2545–2551.

Surks, MI, Ortiz, E, Daniels, GH, et al. Subclinical Thyroid Disease. *Journal of the American Medical Association*. 2004;291(2):228.

Temizkan, S, Balaforlou, B, Ozderya, A, et al. Effects of Thyrotropin, Thyroid Hormones, and Thyroid Antibodies on Metabolic Parameters in a Euthyroid Population with Obesity. *Clinical Endocrinology*. 2016.

Thienpont, LM, Uytfanghe, KV, Houcke, SV. Standardization activities in the field of thyroid function tests: a status report. *Clinical Chemistry and Laboratory Medicine*. 2010;48(11).

Volpé, R, Ginsberg, J. Rational Use of Thyroid Function Tests. *Critical Reviews in Clinical Laboratory Sciences*. 1997;34(5):405–438.

Wang, ZG, Hu, LT. Internal Quality Control Practice of Thyroid Disease Related

Tests and Imprecision Analysis in China. *Clinical Laboratory.* 2014;60(2):301–308.

Witte, T, Ittermann, T, Thamm, M, Riblet, NBV, Völzke, H. Association Between Serum Thyroid-Stimulating Hormone Levels and Serum Lipids in Children and Adolescents: A Population-Based Study of German Youth. *Journal of Clinical Endocrinology and Metabolism.* 2015;100(5):2090–2097.

Chapter 6. How to Ask Your Doctor for More

Armour Thyroid. *Armour Thyroid.* 2016. http://www.armourthyroid.com/.

Azezli, AD, Bayraktaroglu, T, Orhan, Y. The Use of Konjac Glucomannan to Lower Serum Thyroid Hormones in Hyperthyroidism. *Journal of the American College of Nutrition.* 2007;26(6):663–668.

Bastemir, M, Emral, R, Erdogan, G, Gullu, S. High Prevalence of Thyroid Dysfunction and Autoimmune Thyroiditis in Adolescents after Elimination of Iodine Deficiency in the Eastern Black Sea Region of Turkey. *Thyroid.* 2006;16(12):1265–1271.

Benvenga, S, Lakshmanan, M, Trimarchi, F. Carnitine Is a Naturally Occurring Inhibitor of Thyroid Hormone Nuclear Uptake. *Thyroid.* 2000;10(12):1043–1050.

Benvenga, S, Ruggeri, RM, Russo, A, Lapa, D, Campenni, A, Trimarchi, F. Usefulness of l-Carnitine, a Naturally Occurring Peripheral Antagonist of Thyroid Hormone Action, in Iatrogenic Hyperthyroidism: A Randomized, Double-Blind, Placebo-Controlled Clinical Trial. *Journal of Clinical Endocrinology and Metabolism.* 2001;86(8):3579–3594.

Bernatoniene, J, Kopustinskiene, D, Jakstas, V, et al. The Effect of Leonurus cardiaca Herb Extract and Some of Its Flavonoids on Mitochondrial Oxidative Phosphorylation in the Heart. *Planta Medica.* 2014;80(7):525–532.

Bischoff-Ferrari, HA. Optimal Serum 25-Hydroxyvitamin D Levels for Multiple Health Outcomes. *Sunlight, Vitamin D and Skin Cancer Advances in Experimental Medicine and Biology:55–71.*

Bolk, N, Visser, TJ, Nijman, J, et al. Effects of evening vs. morning levothyroxine intake: a randomized double-blind crossover trial. *Archives of Internal Medicine.* 2010;170(22):1996–2003.

Bugleweed: How It Works. University of Michigan Health System. 2015. http://www.uofmhealth.org/health-library/hn-2055003#hn-2055003-how-it-works.

Bunevicius, R, Kazanavicius, G, Zalinkevicius, R, et al. Effects of thyroxine as compared with thyroxine plus triiodothyronine in patients with hypothyroidism. *New England Journal of Medicine* 1999; 340:424–429.

Catargi, B, Parrot-Roulaud, F, Cochet, C, Ducassou, D, Roger, P, Tabarin, A. Homocysteine, Hypothyroidism, and Effect of Thyroid Hormone Replacement. *Thyroid.* 1999;9(12):1163–1166.

Cellini, M, Santaguida, MG, Gatto, I, Virili, C, Del Duca, SC, Brusca, N, Capriello, S, Gargano, L, Centanni, M. Systematic Appraisal of Lactose Intolerance as Cause of Increased Need for Oral Thyroxine. *National Center for Biotechnology Information.* U.S. National Library of Medicine, 2014. 99(8):E1454–458.

Clyde, PW, Harari, AE, Getka, EJ, et al. Combined levothyroxine plus liothyronine compared with levothyroxine alone in primary hypothyroidism: a randomized controlled trial. *Journal of the American Medical Association.* 2003; 290:2952–2958.

Cytomel—FDA prescribing information, side effects and uses. Drugs.com. 2014. http://www.drugs.com/pro/cytomel.html.

Doi, SA, Woodhouse, NJ, Thalib, L, Onitilo, A. Ablation of the Thyroid Remnant and I-131 Dose in Differentiated Thyroid Cancer: A Meta-Analysis Revisited. *Clinical Medicine and Research.* 2007;5(2):87–90.

Eiling, R, Weiland, V, Niestroj, M. Improvement of symptoms in mild hyperthyroidism with an extract of *Lycopus europaeus* (*Thyreogutt mono*). *Wiener Medizinische Wochenschrift.* 2013;163(3–4):95–101.

Fact Sheet: Guidelines for Patients Receiving Radioiodine I-131 Treatment. *Society of Nuclear Medicine and Molecular Imaging.* http://www.snmmi.org/about snmmi/content.aspx?itemnumber=5609.

Farhangi, MA, Keshavarz, SA, Eshraghian, M, Ostadrahimi, A, Saboor-Yaraghi, AA. The Effect of Vitamin A Supplementation on Thyroid Function in Premenopausal Women. *Journal of the American College of Nutrition.* 2012;31(4): 268–274.

Food and Agriculture Organization, World Health Organization. Iron. In *Human Vitamin and Mineral Requirements.* Rome: WHO; 2002.

Gaby, AR. Sub-laboratory hypothyroidism and the empirical use of Armour thyroid. *Alternative Medicine Review.* 2004;9:157–179.

Gharib, H, Papini, E, Garber, JR, et al. American Association of Clinical Endocrinologists, American College of Endocrinology, and Associazione Medici Endocrinologi Medical Guidelines for Clinical Practice for the Diagnosis and Management of Thyroid Nodules—2016 Update. *Endocrine Practice.* 2016; 22(5):622–639.

Grozinsky-Glasberg, S, Fraser, A, Nahshoni, E, et al. Thyroxine-triiodothyronine combination therapy versus thyroxine monotherapy for clinical hypothyroidism: meta-analysis of randomized controlled trials. *Journal of Clinical Endocrinology and Metabolism.* 2006; 91:2592–2599.

Goyal, N, Goldenberg, D. Thyroidectomy. *Medscape.* 2016. http://emedicine .medscape.com/article/1891109-overview.

Jabbar, A, Yawar, A, Waseem, S, et al. Vitamin B12 deficiency common in primary hypothyroidism. *Journal of the Pakistan Medical Association.* 2008;58(5): 258–261.

Jones, DS. *Textbook of Functional Medicine.* Gig Harbor, WA: Institute for Functional Medicine, 2010.

Lemon Balm. University of Maryland Medical Center. 2016. https://umm.edu/ health/medical/altmed/herb/lemon-balm.

Levothyroxine: MedlinePlus Drug Information. *Medline Plus.* https://www.nlm .nih.gov/medlineplus/druginfo/meds/a682461.html.

Liothyronine: MedlinePlus Drug Information. *Medline Plus.* 2010. https://www .nlm.nih.gov/medlineplus/druginfo/meds/a682462.html.

Look into Levoxyl. 2015. http://www.levoxyl.com/.

Low-Dose Naltrexone (LDN) Fact Sheet 2015. *Low-Dose Naltrexone (LDN) Fact Sheet 2015*. 2015. http://www.ldnresearchtrust.org/sites/default/files/ldn infor mation pack(1)_0.pdf.

Low-Dose Naltrexone. *Low-Dose Naltrexone*. http://www.lowdosenaltrexone .org/.

Mackawy, AMH, Al-Ayed, BM, Al-Rashidi, BM. Vitamin D Deficiency and Its Association with Thyroid Disease. *International Journal of Health Sciences*. 2013;7(3):267–275.

Mancini, A, Corbo, GM, Gaballo, A, et al. Relationships between plasma CoQ10 levels and thyroid hormones in chronic obstructive pulmonary disease. *Bio-Factors*. 2005;25(1–4):201–204.

Menke, T, Niklowitz, P, Reinehr, T, Sousa, GJD, Andler, W. Plasma Levels of Coenzyme Q10 in Children with Hyperthyroidism. *Hormone Research*. 2004;61(4):153–158.

Methimazole: MedlinePlus Drug Information. *Medline Plus*. 2010. https://www .nlm.nih.gov/medlineplus/druginfo/meds/a682464.html.

Morley, JE, Russell, RM, Reed, A, Carney, EA, Hershman, JM. The interrela-tionship of thyroid hormones with vitamin A and zinc nutritional status in patients with chronic hepatic and gastrointestinal disorders. *American Journal of Clinical Nutrition*. 1981;34(8):1489–1495.

Nedrebø, B, Ericsson, U-B, Nygård, O, et al. Plasma total homocysteine levels in hyperthyroid and hypothyroid patients. *Metabolism*. 1998;47(1):89–93.

Nygaard, B, Jensen, EW, Kvetny, J, et al. Effect of combination therapy with thy-roxine (T4) and 3,5,3'-triiodothyronin versus T4 monotherapy in patients with hypothyroidism, a double-blind, randomized cross-over study. *European Journal of Endocrinology*. 2009;161(6):895–902.

Oba, K, Kimura, S. Effects of vitamin A deficiency on thyroid function and serum thyroxine levels in the rat. *Journal of Nutritional Science and Vitaminology*. 1980;26(4):327–334.

Office of Dietary Supplements—Vitamin D. *Vitamin D—Health Professional Fact Sheet*. 2016. https://ods.od.nih.gov/factsheets/vitamind-healthprofessional/.

Owecki, M, Dorszewska, J, Sawicka-Gutaj, N, et al. Serum homocysteine levels are decreased in levothyroxine-treated women with autoimmune thyroiditis. *Endocrine Abstracts*. 2014.

Pandolfi, C, Ferrari, D, Stanic, I, Pellegrini, L. Circulating levels of CoQ10 in hypo- and hyperthyroidism. *Minerva Endocrinologica*. 1994;19(3):139–142.

Patient and Physician Hypothyroidism Information. Tirosint. 2015. http://www .tirosint.com/.

Propylthiouracil: MedlinePlus Drug Information. *Medline Plus*. 2011. https:// www.nlm.nih.gov/medlineplus/druginfo/meds/a682465.html.

Propylthiouracil oral: Uses, Side Effects, Interactions, Pictures, Warnings and Dos-ing. *WebMD*. http://www.webmd.com/drugs/2/drug-8883/propylthiouracil -oral/details.

Radioactive Iodine. *American Thyroid Association*. http://www.thyroid.org/ radioactive-iodine/.

Same, D. Effects of the Environment, Chemicals and Drugs on Thyroid Function.

www.thyroidmanager.org. 2010. http://www.ncbi.nlm.nih.gov/pubmed/25 905415.

Santini, F, Vitti, P, Ceccarini, G, et al. In vitro assay of thyroid disruptors affecting TSH-stimulated adenylate cyclase activity. *Journal of Endocrinological Investigation.* 2003;26(10):950–955.

Saravanan, P, Visser, TJ, Dayan, CM. Psychological well-being correlates with free thyroxine but not free 3,5,3'-triiodothyronine levels in patients on thyroid hormone replacement. *Journal of Clinical Endocrinology and Metabolism.* 2006;91(9):3389–3393.

Shikov, AN, Pozharitskaya, ON, Makarov, VG, Demchenko, DV, Shikh, EV. Effect of Leonurus cardiaca oil extract in patients with arterial hypertension accompanied by anxiety and sleep disorders. *Phytotherapy Research.* 2010;25(4): 540–543.

Silberstein, EB, Alavi, A, Balon, HR, Clarke, SE, Divgi, C, Gelfand, MJ, Goldsmith, SJ, Jadvar, H, Marcus, CS, Martin, WH, Parker, JA. The SNMMI practice guideline for therapy of thyroid disease with 131I 3.0. *Journal of Nuclear Medicine.* 2012 Oct 1;53(10):1633–1651.

Synthroid (levothyroxine sodium tablets, USP). https://www.synthroid.com/.

Thomson, CD. Assessment of requirements for selenium and adequacy of selenium status: a review. *European Journal of Clinical Nutrition.* 2004;58(3): 391–402.

Therapy That Works on Every Level. Unithroid. 2014. http://www.unithroid .com/.

Thyroid gland removal. *Medline Plus.* 2014. https://www.nlm.nih.gov/medline plus/ency/article/002933.htm.

Thyroid Hormone Treatment. *American Thyroid Association.* 2016. http://www .thyroid.org/thyroid-hormone-treatment/.

Thyroiditis. *University of Maryland Medical Center.* 2014. http://umm.edu/health/ medical-reference-guide/complementary-and-alternative-medicine-guide/ condition/thyroiditis.

Valizadeh, M, Seyyed-Majidi, MR, Hajibeigloo, H, et al. Efficacy of combined levothyroxine and liothyronine as compared with levothyroxine monotherapy in primary hypothyroidism: a randomized controlled trial. *Endocrine Research.* 2009;34(3):80–89.

Verdon, F. Iron supplementation for unexplained fatigue in non-anaemic women: double blind randomised placebo controlled trial. *British Medical Journal.* 2003;326(7399):1124.

Waldner, C, Campbell, J, Jim, GK, Guichon, PT, Booker, C. Comparison of 3 methods of selenium assessment in cattle. *Canadian Veterinary Journal.* 1998; 39(4):225–231.

Why Get Real. *GET REAL About Hyperthyroidism.* http://getrealthyroid.com/ why-get-real/.

Wojtyniak, K, Szymański, M, Matławska, I. Leonurus cardiaca L. (Motherwort): A Review of its Phytochemistry and Pharmacology. *Phytotherapy Research.* 2012;27(8):1115–1120.

Xue, H, Wang, W, Li, Y, et al. Selenium upregulates CD4 CD25 regulatory T cells in iodine-induced autoimmune thyroiditis model of NOD.H-2h4 mice. *Endocrine Journal.* 2010;57(7):595–601.

Yarnell, E, Abascal, K. Botanical Medicine for Thyroid Regulation. *Alternative and Complementary Therapies.* 2006;12(3):107–112.

Yokusoglu, M, Nevruz, O, Baysan, O, et al. The Altered Autonomic Nervous System Activity in Iron Deficiency Anemia. *Tohoku Journal of Experimental Medicine.* 2007;212(4):397–402.

Younger, J, Parkitny, L, Mclain, D. The use of low-dose naltrexone (LDN) as a novel anti-inflammatory treatment for chronic pain. *Clinical Rheumatology.* 2014;33(4):451–459.

Zeng, X, Yuan, Y, Wu, T, Yan, L, Su, H. Chinese herbal medicines for hyperthyroidism. *Protocols Cochrane Database of Systematic Reviews.* 2007.

Chapter 7. The Power of Food

Abraham, GE. The History of Iodine in Medicine Part III: Thyroid Fixation and Medical Iodophobia. *The Original Internist.* 2006;13:71–78.

Abraham, G, Brownstein, D. Validation of the orthoiodosupplementation program: A Rebuttal of Dr. Gaby's Editorial on iodine. http://www.optimox .com/pics/Iodine/IOD-12/IOD_12.htm.

Alissa, EM, Alshali, K, Ferns, GA. Iodine Deficiency Among Hypothyroid Patients Living in Jeddah. *Biological Trace Element Research.* 2009;130(3):193–203.

Allah, EA, Gomaa, A, Sayed, M. The effect of omega-3 on cognition in hypothyroid adult male rats. *Acta Physiologica Hungarica.* 2014;101(3):362–376.

Ballantyne, S. *The Paleo Approach: Reverse Autoimmune Disease and Heal Your Body.* Las Vegas: Victory Belt, 2013.

Benvenga, S, Vigo, MT, Metro, D, Granese, R, Vita, R, Donne, ML. Type of fish consumed and thyroid autoimmunity in pregnancy and postpartum. *Endocrine.* 2015;52(1):120–129.

Breese Mccoy, SJ. Coincidence of remission of postpartum Graves' disease and use of omega-3 fatty acid supplements. *Thyroid Research.* 2011;4(1):16.

Brown, T. Medscape Medical. "The 10 Most-Prescribed and Top-Selling Medications." *WebMD.* 2015.

Chandra, AK, Ghosh, D, Mukhopadhyay, S, Tripathy, S. Effect of bamboo shoot, Bambusa arundinacea (Retz.) Willd. on thyroid status under conditions of varying iodine intake in rats. *Indian Journal of Experimental Biology.* 2004;42(8): 781–786.

Chandra, AK, Mondal, C, Sinha, S, Chakraborty, A, Pearce, EN. Synergic actions of polyphenols and cyanogens of peanut seed coat (Arachis hypogaea) on cytological, biochemical and functional changes in thyroid. *Indian Journal of Experimental Biology* 2015;53(3):143–151.

Cinemre, H, Bilir, C, Gokosmanoglu, F, Bahcebasi, T. Hematologic effects of levothyroxine in iron-deficient subclinical hypothyroid patients: a randomized, double-blind, controlled study. *Journal of Clinical Endocrinology and Metabolism.*2009;94(1):151–156.

Danby, FW. Acne, Dairy, and Cancer. *Dermato-Endocrinology.* 2009;1(1):12–16.

Dietary Guidance 2011. National Agricultural Library, United States Department of Agriculture. http://fnic.nal.usda.gov/nal_display/index.php?info_center =4&tax_level=1&tax_subject=256.

Dillman, E, Gale, C, Green, W, Johnson, DG, Mackler, B, Finch, C. Hypothermia in iron deficiency due to altered triiodothyronine metabolism. *American Journal of Physiology—Regulatory, Integrative and Comparative Physiology.* 1980; 239(5):R377–R381.

Drutel, A, Archambeaud, F, Caron, P. "Selenium and the Thyroid Gland." *Clinical Endocrinology* 78.2 (2013):155–164.

Fisher, DA, Delange, F. Thyroid hormone and iodine requirements in man during brain development. In Stanbury, JB, et al., eds., *Iodine in Pregnancy.* New Delhi: Oxford University Press, 1998, 1–33.

Freed, DLJ. Do Dietary Lectins Cause Disease? *British Medical Journal* 1999; 318:1023.

Gaitan, E. Goitrogens. *Baillieres Clin Endocrinol Metab.* 1988;2(3):683–702.

Gärtner, R, Gasnier, BC, Dietrich, JW, Krebs, B, Angstwurm, MW. Selenium supplementation in patients with autoimmune thyroiditis decreases thyroid peroxidase antibodies concentrations. *Journal of Clinical Endocrinology and Metabolism.* 2002;87(4):1687–1691.

Goswami, R, Marwaha, RK, Gupta N, et al. Prevalence of vitamin D deficiency and its relationship with thyroid autoimmunity in Asian Indians: a community-based survey. *British Journal of Nutrition.* 2009;102(3):382–386.

Han, TS, Williams, GR, Vanderpump, MP. Benzofuran derivatives and the thyroid. Department of Endocrinology, Royal Free and University College Medical School, Royal Free Hospital, Hampstead, London.

Haq, MRU, Kapila, R, Sharma, R, Saliganti, V, Kapila, S. Comparative evaluation of cow β-casein variants (A1/A2) consumption on Th2-mediated inflammatory response in mouse gut. *European Journal of Nutrition.* 2013;53(4): 1039–1049.

Hinz, KM, Meyer, K, Kinne, A, Schülein, R, Köhrle, J, Krause, G. Structural Insights into Thyroid Hormone Transport Mechanisms of the L-Type Amino Acid Transporter 2. *Molecular Endocrinology.* 2015;29(6):933–942.

Ingenbleek, Y, McCully, KS. Vegetarianism Produces Subclinical Malnutrition, Hyperhomocysteinemia, and Atherogenesis. *Nutrition.* 2012;28(2):148–153.

Jönsson, T, Olsson, S, Ahrén, B, et al. Agrarian Diet and Diseases of Affluence—Do Evolutionary Novel Dietary Lectins Cause Leptin Resistance? *BMC Endocrine Disorders.* 2005;5:10.

Köhrle, J. The trace element selenium and the thyroid gland. *Biochimie.* 1999;81(5): 527–533.

Köhrle, J, Gärtner, R. Selenium and thyroid. *Best Practice and Research Clinical Endocrinology and Metabolism.* 2009;23(6):815–827.

König, F, Andersson, M, Hotz, K, Aeberli, I, Zimmermann, MB. Ten repeat collections for urinary iodine from spot samples or 24-hour samples are needed to reliably estimate individual iodine status in women. *Journal of Nutrition.* 2011;141(11):2049–2054.

Konno, N, Makita, H, Yuri, K, Iizuka, N, Kawasaki, K. Association between dietary iodine intake and prevalence of subclinical hypothyroidism in the coastal regions of Japan. *Journal of Clinical Endocrinology and Metabolism.* 1994;78(2):393–397.

Kralik, A, Eder, K, Kirchgessner, M. Influence of zinc and selenium deficiency on parameters relating to thyroid hormone metabolism. *Hormones and Metabolic Research.* 1996;28(5):223–226.

Kucharzewski, M, Braziewicz, J, Majewska, U, Góźdź, S. Concentration of selenium in the whole blood and the thyroid tissue of patients with various thyroid diseases. *Biological Trace Element Research.* 2002;88(1):25–30.

Lamberg, B-A. Endemic Goitre—Iodine Deficiency Disorders. *Annals of Medicine.* 1991;23(4):367–372.

Laney, N, Meza, J, Lyden, E, Erickson, J, Treude, K, Goldner, W. The Prevalence of Vitamin D Deficiency Is Similar Between Thyroid Nodule and Thyroid Cancer Patients. *International Journal of Endocrinology.* 2010;2010:805716.

Maret, W, Sandstead, HH. Zinc requirements and the risks and benefits of zinc supplementation. *Journal of Trace Elements in Medicine and Biology.* 2006;20(1): 3–18.

Mazokopakis, EE, Chatzipavlidou, V. Hashimoto's thyroiditis and the role of selenium. Current concepts. *Hellenic Journal of Nuclear Medicine.* 2007;10(1):6–8.

Mehran, S, Meilahn, E, Orchard, T, Foley et al. Prevalence of thyroid antibodies among healthy middle-aged women: Findings from the thyroid study in healthy women. *Annals of Epidemiology.* 1995; 5(3):229–233.

Melnik, BC. Evidence for Acne-Promoting Effects of Milk and Other Insulinotropic Dairy Products. *Nestlé Nutrition Institute Workshop Series: Pediatric Program.* 2001;67:131–145.

Nachbar, MS, Oppenheim, JD. Lectins in the United States Diet: A Survey of Lectins in Commonly Consumed Foods and a Review of the Literature. *American Journal of Clinical Nutrition.* 1980;33(11):2338–2245.

Neri, DF, Wiegmann, D, Stanny, RR, et al. The effects of tyrosine on cognitive performance during extended wakefulness. *Aviation, Space, and Environmental Medicine.* 1995; 66:313–319.

Nishiyama, S, Futagoishi-Suginohara, Y, Matsukura, M, et al. Zinc supplementation alters thyroid hormone metabolism in disabled patients with zinc deficiency. *Journal of the American College of Nutrition.* 1994;13(1):62–67.

Pal, A, Mohan, V, Modi, DR, et al. Iodine plus n-3 fatty acid supplementation augments rescue of postnatal neuronal abnormalities in iodine-deficient rat cerebellum. *British Journal of Nutrition.* 2013;110(04):659–670.

Pedersen, I, Knudsen, N, Jorgenson, H, et al. Large Differences in Incidences of Overt Hyper- and Hypothyroidism Associated with a Small Difference in Iodine Intake: A Prospective Comparative Register-Based Population Survey. *Journal of Clinical Endocrinology and Metabolism.* 2002; 87(10):4462–4469.

Pehowich, DJ. Thyroid hormone status and membrane n-3 fatty acid content influence mitochondrial proton leak. *Biochimica et Biophysica Acta (BBA)—Bioenergetics.* 1999;1411(1):192–200.

Perlmutter, D. *Grain Brain.* Boston: Little, Brown, 2013.

Rayman, MP. The importance of selenium to human health. *Lancet.* 2000; 356(9225):233–241.

Reinhardt, W, Luster, M, Rudorff, KH. Effect of small doses of iodine on thyroid function in patients with Hashimoto's thyroiditis residing in an area of mild iodine deficiency. *European Journal of Endocrinology*. 1998;139:23–28.

Ristic-Medic, D, Piskackova, Z, Hooper, L, et al. Methods of assessment of iodine status in humans: a systematic review. *American Journal of Clinical Nutrition*. 2009;89:2052S–2069S.

Roti, E, Vagenakis, G. Effect of excess iodide: clinical aspects. In Braverman, LE, Utiger, RD, eds. *The Thyroid: A Fundamental and Clinical Text*, 8th ed. Philadelphia: Lippincott, 2000, 316–329.

Sebastiano, V, Francesco, MD, Alessandro, V, Mattia, V. Environmental iodine deficiency: a challenge to the evolution of terrestrial life? *Thyroid*. 2000;10(8): 727–729.

Simonart, T. Acne and Whey Protein Supplementation Among Bodybuilders. *Dermatology*. 2012;225(3):256–258.

Souza, LL, Nunes, MO, Paula, GS, et al. Effects of dietary fish oil on thyroid hormone signaling in the liver. *Journal of Nutritional Biochemistry*. 2010;21(10): 935–940.

Teschemacher, H, Koch, G. Opioids in the Milk. *Endocrine Regulations*. 1991;25(3): 147–150.

Thilly, CH, Vanderpas, JB, Bebe, N, et al. Iodine deficiency, other trace elements, and goitrogenic factors in the etiopathogeny of iodine deficiency disorders (IDD). *Biological Trace Element Research*. 1992;32(1-3):229–243.

Tóth, G, Noszái, B. Thyroid hormones and their precursors. II. Species-specific properties. *Acta Pharm Hung*. 2014;84(1):21–37.

Toulis, KA, Anastasilakis, AD, Tzellos, TG, et al. Selenium supplementation in the treatment of Hashimoto's thyroiditis: a systematic review and a meta-analysis. *Thyroid*. 2010;20:1163–1173.

Toxicological Profile for Iodine. Agency for Toxic Substances and Disease Registry, http://www.atsdr.cdc.gov/toxprofiles/tp158.html.

Triggiani, V, Tafaro, E, Giagulli, VA, et al. Role of iodine, selenium and other micronutrients in thyroid function and disorders. *Endocrine, Metabolic, and Immune Disorders—Drug Targets*. 2009;(3):277–294.

Trumbo, P, Yates, A, Schlicker, S, Poos, M. Dietary reference intakes: Vitamin A, Vitamin K, arsenic, boron, chromium, copper, iodine, iron, manganese, molybdenum, nickel, silicon, vanadium, and zinc. *Journal of the American Dietetic Association*. 2001;101(3):294–301.

Urbano, G, López-Jurado, M, Aranda, P, et al. The Role of Phytic Acid in Legumes: Antinutrient or Beneficial Function? *Journal of Physiology and Biochemistry*. 2000;56(3):283–294.

Van Spronsen, FJ, van Rijn, M, Bekhof, J. Phenylketonuria: tyrosine supplementation in phenylalanine-restricted diets. *American Journal of Clinical Nutrition*. 2001;73:153–157.

Verdu, EF, Armstrong, D, Murray, JA. Between Celiac Disease and Irritable Bowel Syndrome: The "No Man's Land" of Gluten Sensitivity. *American Journal of Gastroenterology*. 2009;104:1587–1594.

Vojdani, A. The Characterization of the Repertoire of Wheat Antigens and

Peptides Involved in the Humoral Immune Responses in Patients with Gluten Sensitivity and Crohn's Disease. *ISRN Allergy.* 2011;1–12.

Vought, R, London, W, Brown, F, et al. Iodine Intake and Excretion in Healthy Nonhospitalized Subjects. *American Journal of Clinical Nutrition.* 1964;15: 124–132.

Zimmermann, MB. Interactions of Vitamin A and iodine deficiencies: effects on the pituitary-thyroid axis. *International Journal for Vitamin and Nutrition Research.* 2007;3:236–240.

Zimmermann, MB, Adou, P, Torresani, T, et al. Persistence of goitre despite oral iodine supplementation in goitrous children with iron deficiency anemia in Côte d'Ivoire. *American Journal of Clinical Nutrition.* 2000;71:88–93.

Zimmermann, MB, Köhrle, J. The impact of iron and selenium deficiencies on iodine and thyroid metabolism: biochemistry and relevance to public health. *Thyroid.* 2002;12(10):867–878.

Chapter 8. *Tame the Toxins*

Abdelouahab, N, Langlois, M-F, Lavoie, L, Corbin, F, Pasquier, J-C, Takser, L. Maternal and Cord-Blood Thyroid Hormone Levels and Exposure to Poly-brominated Diphenyl Ethers and Polychlorinated Biphenyls During Early Pregnancy. *American Journal of Epidemiology.* 2013;178(5):701–713.

Abdelouahab, N, Mergler, D, Takser, L, et al. Gender differences in the effects of organochlorines, mercury, and lead on thyroid hormone levels in lakeside communities of Quebec (Canada). *Environmental Research.* 2008;107(3): 380–392.

American Thoracic Society. HEPA Filters Reduce Cardiovascular Health Risks Associated with Air Pollution, Study Finds. *Science Daily.* 2011. www.science daily.com/releases/2011/01/110121144009.htm.

Antoniou, M, Robinson, C, Fagan, J. GMO Myths and Truths: An Evidence-Based Examination of the Claims Made for the Safety and Efficacy of Genetically Modified Crops and Foods. *Earth Open Source.* 2012. http://earthopensource .org/files/pdfs/GMO_Myths_and_Truths/GMO_Myths_and _Truths_1.3.pdf.

Bergmans, H, Logie, C, Maanen, KV, Hermsen, H, Meredyth, M, Vlugt, CVD. Identification of potentially hazardous human gene products in GMO risk assessment. *Environmental Biosafety Research.* 2008;7(1):1–9.

Biomonitoring Summary. National Biomonitoring Program. 2013. http://www .cdc.gov/biomonitoring/perchlorate_biomonitoringsummary.html.

Björkman, L, Lundekvam, BF, Lægreid, T, et al. Mercury in human brain, blood, muscle and toenails in relation to exposure: an autopsy study. *Environmental Health.* 2007;6(1):30.

Boas, M, Feldt-Rasmussen, U, Skakkebaek, NE, Main, KM. Environmental chemicals and thyroid function. *European Journal of Endocrinology.* 2006;154(5): 599–611. Review.

Boas, M, Main, KM, Feldt-Rasmussen, U. Environmental chemicals and thyroid function: an update. *Current Opinion in Endocrinology, Diabetes, and Obesity.* 2009;16(5):385–391. Review.

Burazor, I, Vojdani, A. Chronic Exposure to Oral Pathogens and Autoimmune Reactivity in Acute Coronary Atherothrombosis. *Autoimmune Diseases.* 2014;2014:1–8.

Carvalho, AN, Lim, JL, Nijland, PG, Witte, ME, Horssen, JV. Glutathione in multiple sclerosis: More than just an antioxidant? *Multiple Sclerosis Journal.* 2014;20(11):1425–1431.

Centers for Disease Control and Prevention. Community Water Fluoridation. www.cdc.gov/fluoridation/faqs/.

———. Fourth National Report on Human Exposure to Environmental Chemicals. 2009. www.cdc.gov/exposurereport/pdf/FourthReport.pdf. (The Fourth Report presents data for 212 chemicals and includes the findings from nationally representative samples for 1999–2004.)

———. Fourth National Report on Human Exposure to Environmental Chemicals. Updated Tables, July 2014. 2014. www.cdc.gov/exposurereport/pdf/FourthReport_UpdatedTables_Jul2014.pdf.

Chen, H-X, Ding, M-H, Liu, Q, Peng, K-L. Change of iodine load and thyroid homeostasis induced by ammonium perchlorate in rats. *Journal of Huazhong University of Science and Technology [Medical Sciences].* 2014;34(5):672–678.

Christensen, KLY. Metals in blood and urine, and thyroid function among adults in the United States 2007–2008. *International Journal of Hygiene and Environmental Health.* 2013;216(6):624–632.

Clauw, DJ. Fibromyalgia: A Clinical Review. *Journal of the American Medical Association.* 2014;311915):1547–1555.

Connett, P. 50 Reasons to Oppose Fluoridation. Fluoride Action Network. 2012. http://fluoridealert.org/articles/50-reasons/.

Corre, LL, Besnard, P, Chagnon, M-C. BPA, an Energy Balance Disruptor. *Critical Reviews in Food Science and Nutrition.* 2015;55(6):769–777.

Council on Environmental Health, Rogan, WJ, Paulson, JA, Baum, C, et al. Iodine Deficiency, Pollutant Chemicals, and the Thyroid: New Information on an Old Problem. *Pediatrics.* 2014;133(6):1163–1166.

Crinnion, W. *Clean, Green, and Lean.* New York: John Wiley and Sons, 2010.

———. Sauna as a Valuable Clinical Tool for Cardiovascular, Autoimmune, Toxicant-induced and other Chronic Health Problems. *Alternative Medicine Review: Environmental Medicine.* 16(3):215–225.

Darbre, PD, Harvey, PW. Paraben Esters: Review of Recent Studies of Endocrine Toxicity, Absorption, Esterase, and Human Exposure, and Discussion of Potential Human Health Risks. *Journal of Applied Toxicology.* 2008;28(5):561–578.

Desailloud, R, Wemeau, JL. Should we fear the perchlorate ion in the environment? *Presse Médicale.* 2016;45(1):107–116.

Diesendorf, M, Colquhoun, J, Spittle, B J, Everingham, DN, Clutterbuck, FW. New Evidence on Fluoridation. *Australia and New Zealand Journal of Public Health.* 1997;21(2):187–190.

Di Pietro, A, Baluce, B, Visalli, G, Maestra, SL, Micale, R, Izzotti, A. Ex vivo study for the assessment of behavioral factor and gene polymorphisms in individual susceptibility to oxidative DNA damage metals-induced. *International Journal of Hygiene and Environmental Health.* 2011;214(3):210–218.

Dr. Ben Lynch Network Sites. MTHFR.Net. http://MTHFR.net.

Ellingsen, DG, Efskind, J, Haug, E, Thomassen, Y, Martinsen, I, Gaarder, PI. Effects of low mercury vapour exposure on the thyroid function in chloralkali workers. *Journal of Applied Toxicology.* 2000;20(6):483–489.

Environmental Working Group and Commonweal. PFOA (Perfluorooctanoic Acid). Human Toxome Project. www.ewg.org/sites/humantoxome/chemicals/chemical.php?chemid=100307.

Environmental Working Group. EPA Proposes to Phase Out Fluoride Pesticide. 2011. www.ewg.org/news/testimony-official-correspondence/epa-proposes-phase-out-fluoride-pesticide.

———. EWG's 2014 Shopper's Guide to Pesticides in Produce. 2014. www.ewg.org/foodnews/.

———. EWG's Healthy Home Tips for Parents. 2008. http://static.ewg.org/reports/2008/EWGguide_goinggreen.pdf.

———. EWG's Skin Deep Cosmetics Database. www.ewg.org/skindeep/.

———. FDA Should Adopt EPA Tap Water Health Goals as Enforceable Limits for Bottled Water. 2008. www.ewg.org/news/testimony-official-correspondence/fda-should-adopt-epa-tap-water-health-goals-enforceable.

———. Is Your Bottled Water Worth It?: Bottle Vs. Tap—Double Standard. 2009. www.ewg.org/research/your-bottled-water-worth-it/bottle-vs-tap-double-standard.

———. Over 300 Pollutants in U.S. Tap Water. 2009. www.ewg.org/tapwater/.

———. Pollution in People: Cord Blood Contaminants in Minority Newborns. 2009. http://static.ewg.org/reports/2009/minority_cord_blood/2009-Minority-Cord-Blood-Report.pdf.

Erdemgil, Y, Gözet, T, Can, Ö, Ünsal, I, Özpınar, A. Perchlorate levels found in tap water collected from several cities in Turkey. *Environmental Monitoring and Assessment.* 2016;188(3).

Faber, S, Cluderay, T. 1,000 Chemicals. *EnviroBlog.* Environmental Working Group. 2014. www.ewg.org/enviroblog/2014/05/1000-chemicals.

Fujinami, RS, Herrath, MGV, Christen, U, Whitton, JL. Molecular Mimicry, Bystander Activation, or Viral Persistence: Infections and Autoimmune Disease. *Clinical Microbiology Reviews.* 2006;19(1):80–94.

Gallagher, CM, Meliker, JR. Mercury and thyroid autoantibodies in U.S. women, NHANES 2007–2008. *Environment International.* 2012;40:39–43.

Gasnier, C, Dumont, C, Benachour, N, Clair, E, Chagnon, MC, Séralini, GE. Glyphosate-Based Herbicides Are Toxic and Endocrine Disruptors in Human Cell Lines. *Toxicology.* 2009;262(3):184–191.

Geens, T, Dirtu, AC, Dirinck, E, et al. Daily intake of bisphenol A and triclosan and their association with anthropometric data, thyroid hormones and weight loss in overweight and obese individuals. *Environment International.* 2015; 76:98–105.

Genetics Home Reference. What Are Single Nucleotide Polymorphisms (SNPs)? http://ghr.nlm.nih.gov/handbook/genomicresearch/snp.

Ghosh, H, Bhattacharya, S. Thyrotoxicity of the chlorides of cadmium and mercury in rabbit. *Biomedical and Environmental Sciences.* 1992;5(3):236–240.

Gill, RF, McCabe MJ, Rosenspire, AJ. Elements of the B Cell Signalosome Are Differentially Affected by Mercury Intoxication. *Autoimmune Diseases.* 2014; 2014:1–10.

Guilford, FT, Hope, J. Deficient Glutathione in the Pathophysiology of Mycotoxin-Related Illness. *Toxins* [Basel]. 2014;6(2):608–623.

Horton, MK, Blount, BC, Valentin-Blasini, L, et al. Co-occurring exposure to perchlorate, nitrate and thiocyanate alters thyroid function in healthy pregnant women. *Environmental Research.* 2015;143:1–9.

Houlihan, J, Wiles, R, Thayer, K, Gray, S. Body Burden: The Pollution in People. Environmental Working Group. 2003.

Huggins, HA. *Uninformed Consent: The Hidden Dangers in Dental Care.* Newburyport, MA: Hampton Roads Publishing, 1999.

Hybenova, M, Hrda, P, Procházková, J, Stejskal, VD, Sterzl, I. The Role of Environmental Factors in Autoimmune Thyroiditis. *Neuro Endocrinology Letters.* 2010;31(3):283–289.

Institute for Functional Medicine. Advanced Practice Detoxification Modules. www.functionalmedicine.org/conference.aspx?id=2744&cid=35& section=t324.

Jain, RB, Choi, YS. Interacting effects of selected trace and toxic metals on thyroid function. *International Journal of Environmental Health Research.* 2016;26(1): 75–91.

Jiang, Y, Guo, X, Sun, Q, Shan, Z, Teng, W. Effects of Excess Fluoride and Iodide on Thyroid Function and Morphology. *Biological Trace Element Research.* 2016;170(2):382–389.

Jianjie, C, Wenjuan, X, Jinling, C, Jie, S, Ruhui, J, Meiyan, L. Fluoride caused thyroid endocrine disruption in male zebrafish (*Danio rerio*). *Aquatic Toxicology.* 2016;171:48–58.

Kaur, S, White, S, Bartold, PM. Periodontal Disease and Rheumatoid Arthritis: A Systematic Review. *Journal of Dental Research.* 2013;92(5):399–408.

Kharrazian, D. The Potential Roles of Bisphenol A (BPA) Pathogenesis in Autoimmunity. *Autoimmune Diseases.* 2014;2014:1–12.

Kinch, CD, Kurrasch, DM, Habibi, HR. Adverse morphological development in embryonic zebrafish exposed to environmental concentrations of contaminants individually and in mixture. *Aquatic Toxicology.* 2016;175:286–298.

Knott, KK, Schenk, P, Beyerlein, S, Boyd, D, Ylitalo, GM, O'Hara, TM. Blood-based biomarkers of selenium and thyroid status indicate possible adverse biological effects of mercury and polychlorinated biphenyls in Southern Beaufort Sea polar bears. *Environmental Research.* 2011;111(8):1124–1136.

Kumarathilaka, P, Oze, C, Indraratne, S, Vithanage, M. Perchlorate as an emerging contaminant in soil, water and food. *Chemosphere.* 2016;150:667–677.

Leung, AM, Pearce, EN, Braverman, LE. Environmental perchlorate exposure. *Current Opinion in Endocrinology and Diabetes and Obesity.* 2014;21(5):372–376.

Li, J, Liu, Y, Kong, D, Ren, S, Li, N. T-screen and yeast assay for the detection of the thyroid-disrupting activities of cadmium, mercury, and zinc. *Environmental Science and Pollution Research.* 2016;23(10):9843–9851.

Liang, S, Zhou, Y, Wang, H, Qian, Y, Ma, D, Tian, W, Persaud-Sharma, V, et al. The

Effect of Multiple Single Nucleotide Polymorphisms in the Folic Acid Pathway Genes on Homocysteine Metabolism. *BioMed Research International*. 2014;2014.

Liu, Q, Ding, MH, Zhang, R, Chen, HX, et al. Study on mechanism of thyroid cytotoxicity of ammonium perchlorate. *Zhonghua Lao Dong Wei Sheng Zhi Ye Bing Za Zhi*. 2013;31(6):418–421.

Llop, S, Lopez-Espinosa, M-J, Murcia, M, et al. Synergism between exposure to mercury and use of iodine supplements on thyroid hormones in pregnant women. *Environmental Research*. 2015;138:298–305.

Lunder, S. Flame Retardants Are Everywhere in Homes, New Studies Find. *EnviroBlog*. Environmental Working Group. 2012. www.ewg.org/enviro blog/2012/12/toxic-fire-retardants-are-everywhere-homes-new-studies -find.

Maffini, MV, Trasande, L, Neltner, TG. Perchlorate and Diet: Human Exposures, Risks, and Mitigation Strategies. *Current Environmental Health Reports*. 2016; 3(2):107–117.

Mervish, NA, Pajak, A, Teitelbaum, SL, et al. Thyroid Antagonists (Perchlorate, Thiocyanate, and Nitrate) and Childhood Growth in a Longitudinal Study of U.S. Girls. *EHP Environmental Health Perspectives*. 2015;124(4).

Mesnage, R, Gress, S, Defarge, N, Séralini, GE. Human Cell Toxicity of Pesticides Associated to Wide Scale Agricultural GMOs. *Theorie in der Ökologie*. 2013;17:118–120.

Meyer, E, Eagles-Smith, CA, Sparling, D, Blumenshine, S. Mercury Exposure Associated with Altered Plasma Thyroid Hormones in the Declining Western Pond Turtle (Emys marmorata) from California Mountain Streams. *Environmental Science and Technology*. 2014;48(5):2989–2996.

Minoia, C, Ronchi, A, Pigatto, P, Guzzi, G. Effects of mercury on the endocrine system. *Critical Reviews in Toxicology*. 2009;39(6):538–538.

Myers, A. Episode 11: Chemical-free and Gluten-free Skin Care with Bob Root. *The Myers Way*. 2013. http://www.amymyersmd.com/2013/07/tmw-episode -11-chemical-free-gluten-free-skin-care-with-bob-root/.

———. Episode 12: Biological Dentistry with Stuart Nunnally, DDS. *The Myers Way*. 2013. http://www.amymyersmd.com/2013/07/tmw-episode-12-bio logical-dentistry-with-stuart-nunnally-dds/.

———. Episode 17: Green Beauty With W3LL PEOPLE. The Myers Way. 2013. Available at http://www.amymyersmd.com/2013/08/tmw-episode-17-green -beauty-with-w3ll-people/.

Nakazawa, DJ. *The Autoimmune Epidemic: Bodies Gone Haywire in a World Out of Balance and the Cutting Edge Science That Promises Hope*. New York: Simon and Schuster, 2008.

Null, G. Fluoride: Killing Us Softly. *Global Research*. 2013. www.globalresearch .ca/fluoride-killing-us-softly/5360397.

Nuttall, SL, Martin, U, Sinclair, AJ, Kendall, MJ. Glutathione: In Sickness and in Health. *Lancet*. 1998;351(9103):645–646.

Ong, J, Erdei, E, Rubin, RL, Miller, C, Ducheneaux, C, O'Leary, M, Pacheco, B, et al. Mercury, Autoimmunity, and Environmental Factors on Cheyenne River Sioux Tribal Lands. *Autoimmune Diseases*. 2014. Article ID 325461.

Patrick, L. Thyroid disruption: mechanism and clinical implications in human health. *Alternative Medicine Review.* 2009 Dec;14(4):326–46. Review. Erratum in: *Alternative Medicine Review.* 2010;15(1):58.

Pinhel, MADS, Sado, CL, Longo, GDS, et al. Nullity of GSTT1/GSTM1 related to pesticides is associated with Parkinson's disease. *Arq Neuro-Psiquiatr Arquivos de Neuro-Psiquiatria.* 2013;71(8):527–532.

Porreca, I, Severino, LU, D'Angelo, F, et al. "Stockpile" of Slight Transcriptomic Changes Determines the Indirect Genotoxicity of Low-Dose BPA in Thyroid Cells. *PLoS ONE.* 2016;11(3).

Procházková, J, Sterzl, I, Kucerova, H, Bartova, J, Stejskal, VD. The Beneficial Effect of Amalgam Replacement on Health in Patients with Autoimmunity. *Neuro Endocrinology Letters.* 2004;25(3):211–218.

Reisman, RE, Mauriello, PM, Davis, GB, Georgitis, JW, DeMasi, JM. A Double-Blind Study of the Effectiveness of a High-Efficiency Particulate Air (HEPA) Filter in the Treatment of Patients with Perennial Allergic Rhinitis and Asthma. *Journal of Allergy and Clinical Immunology.* 1990;85(6):1050–1057.

Richard, S, Moslemi, S, Sipahutar, H, Benachour, N, Seralini, GE. Differential Effects of Glyphosate and Roundup on Human Placental Cells and Aromatase. *Environmental Health Perspectives.* 2005;113(6):716–720.

Rogers, JA, Metz, L, Yong, VW. Review: Endocrine Disrupting Chemicals and Immune Responses: A Focus on Bisphenol-A and Its Potential Mechanisms. *Molecular Immunology.* 2013;53(4):421–430.

Romano, ME, Webster, GM, Vuong, AM, et al. Gestational urinary bisphenol A and maternal and newborn thyroid hormone concentrations: The HOME Study. *Environmental Research.* 2015;138:453–460.

Root, B. *Chemical-Free Skin Health.* M42 Publishing, 2010.

Samsel, A, Seneff, S. Glyphosate, Pathways to Modern Diseases II: Celiac Sprue and Gluten Intolerance. *Interdisciplinary Toxicology.* 2013;6(4):159–184.

———. Glyphosate's Suppression of Cytochrome P450 Enzymes and Amino Acid Biosynthesis by the Gut Microbiome: Pathways to Modern Diseases. *Entropy.* 2013;15:1416–1463.

Sarkar, C, Pal, S. Ameliorative Effect of Resveratrol Against Fluoride-Induced Alteration of Thyroid Function in Male Wistar Rats. *Biological Trace Element Research.* 2014;162(1–3):278–287.

Schaller, J. *Mold Illness and Mold Remediation Made Simple: Removing Mold Toxins from Bodies and Sick Buildings.* Tampa, FL: Hope Academic Press, 2005.

Schell, LM, Gallo, MV. Relationships of putative endocrine disruptors to human sexual maturation and thyroid activity in youth. *Physiology and Behavior.* 2010;99(2):246–253.

Schell, LM, Gallo, MV, Denham, M, Ravenscroft, J, Decaprio, AP, Carpenter, DO. Relationship of Thyroid Hormone Levels to Levels of Polychlorinated Biphenyls, Lead, p,p'-DDE, and Other Toxicants in Akwesasne Mohawk Youth. *Environmental Health Perspectives.* 2008;116(6):806–813.

Seymour, GJ, Ford, J, Cullinan, MP, Leishman, S, Yamazaki, K. Relationship Between Periodontal Infections and Systemic Disease. *Clinical Microbiology and Infection.* 2007;13(4):3–10.

Shoemaker, RC. *Mold Warriors: Fighting America's Hidden Health Threat.* Baltimore: Gateway Press, 2005.

———. *Surviving Mold: Life in the Era of Dangerous Buildings.* Baltimore: Otter Bay Books, 2010.

Sigurdson, T, Fellow, S. Exposing the Cosmetics Cover-Up: True Horror Stories of Cosmetic Dangers. Environmental Working Group. 2013. www.ewg.org/research/exposing-cosmetics-cover/true-horror-stories-of-cosmetic-dangers.

Singh, N, Verma, K, Verma, P, Sidhu, G, Sachdeva, S. A comparative study of fluoride ingestion levels, serum thyroid hormone and TSH level derangements, dental fluorosis status among school children from endemic and non-endemic fluorosis areas. *SpringerPlus.* 2014;3(1):7.

Sirota, M, Schaub, MA, Batzoglou, S, Robinson, WH, Butte, AJ. Autoimmune Disease Classification by Inverse Association with SNP Alleles. *PLoS Genetics.* 2009;5(12): e1000792.

Smith, JM. Genetically Engineered Foods May Cause Rising Food Allergies—Genetically Engineered Corn. In the Institute for Responsible Technology newsletter *Spilling the Beans.* 2007.

Smith, JM, Institute for Responsible Technology. *Genetic Roulette.* Institute for Responsible Technology; 2012. http://geneticroulettemovie.com.

Song, GG, Bae, SC, Lee, YH. Association of the MTHFR C677T and A1298C Polymorphisms with Methotrexate Toxicity in Rheumatoid Arthritis: A Meta-Analysis. *Clinical Rheumatology.* 2014.

Steinmaus, CM. Perchlorate in Water Supplies: Sources, Exposures, and Health Effects. *Current Environmental Health Reports.* 2016;3(2):136–143.

Steinmaus, C, Pearl, M, Kharrazi, M, et al. Thyroid Hormones and Moderate Exposure to Perchlorate during Pregnancy in Women in Southern California. *EHP Environmental Health Perspectives.* 2015.

Stejskal, J, Stejskal, VD. The Role of Metals in Autoimmunity and the Link to Neuroendocrinology. *Neuro Endocrinology Letters.* 1999;20(6):351–364.

Surviving Mold website. www.survivingmold.com.

Tan, SW, Meiller, JC, Mahaffey, KR. The endocrine effects of mercury in humans and wildlife. *Critical Reviews in Toxicology.* 2009;39(3):228–269.

Teens Turning Green. Sustainable Food Resources: Dirty Thirty. http://www.teensturninggreen.org/wordpress/wp-content/uploads/2013/03/dirtythirty-10-11-10.pdf.

Tiwari, V, Bhattacharya, L. Adverse effects of mercuric chloride on thyroid of mice, *Musculus albinus,* and pattern of recovery of the damaged activity. *Journal of Environmental Biology.* 2004;25(1):109–111.

U.S. Environmental Protection Agency. Ground Water and Drinking Water. http://water.epa.gov/drink/.

———. Indoor Air Quality (IAQ). www.epa.gov/iaq/.

———. Perfluorooctanoic Acid (PFOA) and Fluorinated Telomers. www.epa.gov/oppt/pfoa/pubs/pfoainfo.html.

———. Targeting Indoor Air Pollutants: EPA's Approach and Progress. March 1993. http://nepis.epa.gov

————. TSCA Chemical Substance Inventory. www.epa.gov/oppt/existingchem icals/pubs/tscainventory/basic.html.

Wada, H, Cristol, DA, Mcnabb, FA, Hopkins, WA. Suppressed Adrenocortical Responses and Thyroid Hormone Levels in Birds near a Mercury-Contaminated River. *Environmental Science and Technology.* 2009;43(15):6031–6038.

Wang, N, Zhou, Y, Fu, C, et al. Influence of Bisphenol A on Thyroid Volume and Structure Independent of Iodine in School Children. *PLoS ONE.* 2015;10(10).

Williams, RH, Jaffe, H, Taylor, JA. Effect of Halides, Thiocyanate and Propyl-thiouracil upon the Distribution of Radioiodine in the Thyroid Gland, Blood and Urine. *American Journal of the Medical Sciences.* 1950;219(1):7–15.

Wu, Y, Beland, FA, Fang, J-L. Effect of triclosan, triclocarban, 2,2',4,4' -tetrabromodiphenyl ether, and bisphenol A on the iodide uptake, thyroid peroxidase activity, and expression of genes involved in thyroid hormone syn-thesis. *Toxicology in Vitro.* 2016;32:310–319.

Yang, H, Xing, R, Liu, S, Yu, H, Li, P. γ-Aminobutyric acid ameliorates fluoride-induced hypothyroidism in male Kunming mice. *Life Sciences.* 2016;146:1–7.

Yang, J, Chan, KM. Evaluation of the toxic effects of brominated compounds (BDE-47, 99, 209, TBBPA) and bisphenol A (BPA) using a zebrafish liver cell line, ZFL. *Aquatic Toxicology.* 2015;159:138–147.

Zeng, Q, Cui, YS, Zhang, L, et al. Studies of fluoride on the thyroid cell apoptosis and mechanism. *Zhonghua Yu Fang Yi Xue Za Zhi.* 2012;46(3):233–236.

Zhao, H, Chai, L, Wang, H. Effects of fluoride on metamorphosis, thyroid and skeletal development in Bufo gargarizans tadpoles. *Ecotoxicology.* 2013;22(7): 1123–1132.

Zoeller, RT. Environmental chemicals impacting the thyroid: targets and conse-quences. *Thyroid.* 2007;17(9):811–817.

————. Environmental chemicals targeting thyroid. *Hormones (Athens).* 2010; 9(1):28–40.

Zoeller, RT, Rovet, J. Timing of thyroid hormone action in the developing brain: clinical observations and experimental findings. *Journal of Neuroendocrinology.* 2004;16(10):809–818.

Chapter 9. The Infection Connection

Alam, J, Kim, YC, Choi, Y. Potential Role of Bacterial Infection in Autoimmune Diseases: A New Aspect of Molecular Mimicry. *Immune Network.* 2014;14(1): 7–13.

Allen, K, Shykoff, BE, Izzo Jr., JL. Pet Ownership, but Not ACE Inhibitor Ther-apy, Blunts Home Blood Pressure Responses to Mental Stress. *Hypertension.* 2001;38:815–820.

American College of Rheumatology. Study Provides Greater Understanding of Lyme Disease-Causing Bacteria. Press release. 2009.

Bach, J-F. The Effect of Infections on Susceptibility to Autoimmune and Allergic Diseases. *New England Journal of Medicine.* 2002;347:911–920.

Brady, DM. Molecular Mimicry, the Hygiene Hypothesis, Stealth Infections, and Other Examples of Disconnect Between Medical Research and the Practice of

Clinical Medicine in Autoimmune Disease. *Open Journal of Rheumatology and Autoimmune Diseases*. 2013;3:33–39.

Broccolo, F, Fusetti, L, Ceccherini-Nelli, L. Possible Role of Human Herpesvirus 6 as a Trigger of Autoimmune Disease. *Scientific World Journal*. 2013;2013:1–7.

Brucker-Davis, F, Hiéronimus, S, Fénichel, P. Thyroid and the environment. *Presse Médicale*. 2016;45(1):78–87.

Casiraghi, C, Horwitz, MS. Epstein–Barr virus and autoimmunity: the role of a latent viral infection in multiple sclerosis and systemic lupus erythematosus pathogenesis. *Future Virology*. 2013;8(2):173–182.

Chastain, EML, Miller, SD. Molecular Mimicry as an Inducing Trigger for CNS Autoimmune Demyelinating Disease. *Immunological Reviews*. 2012;245(1): 227–238.

Collingwood, J. The Power of Music to Reduce Stress. *Psych Central*. http://psych central.com/lib/the-power-of-music-to-reduce-stress/000930?all=1.

Cusick, MF, Libbey, JE, Fujinami, RS. Molecular Mimicry as a Mechanism of Autoimmune Disease. *Clinical Reviews in Allergy and Immunology;* 2012;42(1): 102–111.

Davis, SL. Environmental Modulation of the Immune System via the Endocrine System. *Domestic Animal Endocrinology;* 1998;15(5):283–289.

Delogu, LG, Deidda, S, Delitala, G, Manetti, R. Infectious Diseases and Autoimmunity. *Journal of Infection in Developing Countries*. 2001;5(10):679–687.

Desailloud, R, Hober, D. Viruses and thyroiditis: an update. *Virology Journal*. 2009;6(1):5.

Draborg, AH, Duus, K, Houen, G. Epstein-Barr Virus in Systemic Autoimmune Diseases. *Clinical and Developmental Immunology*. 2013;2013:1–9.

Ercolini, AM, Miller, SD. The Role of Infections in Autoimmune Disease. *Clinical and Experimental Immunology*. 2009;155(1):1–15.

Getts, DR, Chastain, EML, Terry, RL, Miller, SD. Virus Infection, Antiviral Immunity, and Autoimmunity. *Immunological Reviews*. 2013;255(1):197–209.

Institute for Functional Medicine. The Challenge of Emerging Infections in the 21st Century: Terrain, Tolerance, and Susceptibility. *Annual International Conference,* Bellevue, Wash., 2011.

Janegova, A, Janega, P, Rychly, B, Kuracinova, K, Babal, P. The role of Epstein-Barr virus infection in the development of autoimmune thyroid diseases. *Endokrynologia Polska*. 2015;66(2):132–136.

Kaňková, Š, Procházková, L, Flegr, J, Calda, P, Springer, D, Potluková, E. Effects of Latent Toxoplasmosis on Autoimmune Thyroid Diseases in Pregnancy. *PLoS ONE*. 2014;9(10).

Patil, AD. Link between Hypothyroidism and Small Intestinal Bacterial Overgrowth. *Indian Journal of Endocrinology and Metabolism*. 2014;18(3):307–309.

Pender, MP. CD8+ T-Cell Deficiency, Epstein-Barr Virus Infection, Vitamin D Deficiency, and Steps to Autoimmunity: A Unifying Hypothesis. *Autoimmune Diseases*. 2012;2012:1–16.

Rajič, B, Arapović, J, Raguž, K, Babić, SM, Maslać, S. Eradication of Blastocystis Hominis Prevents the Development of Symptomatic Hashimoto's Thyroiditis: A Case Report. *National Center for Biotechnology Information*. U.S. National Library of Medicine. 2015;9(7):788–791.

Rashid, T, Ebringer, A. Autoimmunity in Rheumatic Diseases Is Induced by Microbial Infections via Crossreactivity or Molecular Mimicry. *Autoimmune Diseases*. 2012:1–9.

Sfriso, P, Ghirardello, A, Botsios, C, et al. Infections and autoimmunity: the multifaceted relationship. *Journal of Leukocyte Biology*. 2009;87(3):385–395.

Shapira, Y, Agmon-Levin, N, Selmi, C, et al. Prevalence of anti-toxoplasma antibodies in patients with autoimmune diseases. *Journal of Autoimmunity*. 2012; 39(1–2):112–116.

Smolders, J. Vitamin D and Multiple Sclerosis: Correlation, Causality, and Controversy. *Autoimmune Diseases*. 2011;2011:1–3.

Szymula, A, Rosenthal, J, Szczerba, BM, Bagavant, H, Fu, SM, Deshmukh, US. T cell epitope mimicry between Sjögren's syndrome Antigen A (SSA)/Ro60 and oral, gut, skin and vaginal bacteria. *Clinical Immunology*. 2014;152(1–2):1–9.

Tomer, Y, Davies, TF. Infection, Thyroid Disease, and Autoimmunity. *National Center for Biotechnology Information*. U.S. National Library of Medicine. 1993;14(1):107–120.

Tozzoli, R, Barzilai, O, Ram, M, et al. Infections and autoimmune thyroid diseases: Parallel detection of antibodies against pathogens with proteomic technology. *Autoimmunity Reviews*. 2008;8(2):112–115.

Uchakin, PN, Parish, DC, Dane, FC, et al. Fatigue in Medical Residents Leads to Reactivation of Herpes Virus Latency. *Interdisciplinary Perspectives on Infectious Diseases*. 2011;2011:1–7.

Vojdani, A. A Potential Link Between Environmental Triggers and Autoimmunity. *Autoimmune Diseases*. 2014;2014:1–18.

Wasserman, EE, Nelson, K, Rose, NR, et al. Infection and thyroid autoimmunity: A seroepidemiologic study of TPOaAb. *Autoimmunity*. 2009;42(5): 439–446.

Wucherpfennig, KW. Mechanisms for the Induction of Autoimmunity by Infectious Agents. *Journal of Clinical Investigation*. 2001;108(8):1097–1104.

———. Structural Basis of Molecular Mimicry. *Journal of Autoimmunity*. 2001; 16(3):293–302.

Yang, CY, Leung, PS, Adamopoulos, IE, Gershwin, ME. The Implication of Vitamin D and Autoimmunity: A Comprehensive Review. *Clinical Reviews in Allergy and Immunology*. 2013;45(2):217–226.

Chapter 10. The Stress Solution

Adrenal Fatigue website. www.adrenalfatigue.org.

Al-Massadi, O, Trujillo, M, Señaris, R, et al. The vagus nerve as a regulator of growth hormone secretion. *Regulatory Peptides*. 2011;166(1-3):3–8.

Assaf, AM. Stress-Induced Immune-Related Diseases and Health Outcomes of Pharmacy Students: A Pilot Study. *Saudi Pharmaceutical Journal*. 2013;21(1): 35–44.

Attia, AMM, Ibrahim, FAA, El-Latif, NAA, et al. Therapeutic antioxidant and anti-inflammatory effects of laser acupuncture on patients with rheumatoid arthritis. *Lasers in Surgery and Medicine*. 2016.

Blase, KL, van Dijke, A, Cluitmans, PJ, Vermetten, E. Efficacy of HRV-biofeedback as additional treatment of depression and PTSD. *Tijdschr Psychiatr*. 2016;58(4):292–300.

Burkhart, K, Phelps, JR. Amber Lenses to Block Blue Light and Improve Sleep: A Randomized Trial. *Chronobiology International*. 2009;26(8):1602–1612.

Canadian Agency for Drugs and Technologies in Health. Neurofeedback and Biofeedback for Mood and Anxiety Disorders: A Review of the Clinical Evidence and Guidelines—An Update [Internet]. CADTH Rapid Response Reports. 2014. www.ncbi.nlm.nih.gov/pubmed/25411662.

Cheon, E-J, Koo, B-H, Choi, J-H. The Efficacy of Neurofeedback in Patients with Major Depressive Disorder: An Open Labeled Prospective Study. *Applied Psychophysiology and Biofeedback*. 2015;41(1):103–110.

Fan, S. Floating Away: The Science of Sensory Deprivation Therapy. *The Crux*. 2014. http://blogs.discovermagazine.com/crux/2014/04/04/floating-away-the-science-of-sensory-deprivation-therapy/#.vz58c2qriff.

Ghosh, T, Jahan, M, Singh, A. The efficacy of electroencephalogram neurofeedback training in cognition, anxiety, and depression in alcohol dependence syndrome: A case study. *Industrial Psychiatry Journal*. 2014;23(2):166.

Godbout, JP, Glaser, R. Stress-Induced Immune Dysregulation: Implications for Wound Healing, Infectious Disease, and Cancer. *Journal of Neuroimmune Pharmacology*. 2006;1(4):421–427.

Gomez-Merino, D, Drogou, C, Chennaoui, M, Tiollier, E, Mathieu, J, Guezennec, CY. Effects of Combined Stress during Intense Training on Cellular Immunity, Hormones and Respiratory Infections. *Neuroimmunomodulation*. 2005;12(3):164–172.

Grossman, P, Niemann, L, Schmidt, S, Walach, H. Mindfulness-Based Stress Reduction and Health Benefits: A Meta-Analysis. *Journal of Psychosomatic Research*. 2004;57(1):35–43.

Huang, WQ, Zhou, QZ, Liu, XG, et al. Effects of Acupuncture Intervention on Levels of T Lymphocyte Subsets in Plasma and Thymus in Stress-induced Anxiety Rats. *Zhen Ci Yan Jiu*. 2015;40(4):265–269.

Innes, KE, Selfe, TK, Khalsa, DS, Kandati, S. Effects of Meditation versus Music Listening on Perceived Stress, Mood, Sleep, and Quality of Life in Adults with Early Memory Loss: A Pilot Randomized Controlled Trial. *Journal of Alzheimer's Disease*. 2016.

Irwin, M, Daniels, M, Risch, SC, Bloom, E, Weiner, H. Plasma cortisol and natural killer cell activity during bereavement. *Biological Psychiatry*. 1988;24(2):173–178.

Kabat-Zinn, J, Massion, AO, Kristeller, J, Peterson, LG, Fletcher, KE, Pbert, L, Lenderking, WR, et al. Effectiveness of a Meditation-Based Stress Reduction Program in the Treatment of Anxiety Disorders. *American Journal of Psychiatry*. 1992;149(7):936–943.

Khansari, DN, Murgo, AJ, Faith, RE. Effects of Stress on the Immune System. *Immunology Today*. 1990;11:170–175.

Kjellgren, A, Sundequist, U, et al. Effects of flotation-REST on muscle tension pain. *Pain Research and Management.* 2001;6(4):181–189.

Kobayashi, I, Lavela, J, Bell, K, Mellman, TA. The Impact of Posttraumatic Stress Disorder Versus Resilience on Nocturnal Autonomic Nervous System Activity as Functions of Sleep Stage and Time of Sleep. *Physiology and Behavior.* 2016.

Kok, BE, Coffey, KA, Cohn, MA, et al. How Positive Emotions Build Physical Health: Perceived Positive Social Connections Account for the Upward Spiral Between Positive Emotions and Vagal Tone. *Psychological Science.* 2013;24(7): 1123–1132.

Labrique-Walusis, F, Keister, KJ, Russell, AC. Massage Therapy for Stress Management: Implications for Nursing Practice. *Orthopedic Nursing.* 2010;29(4): 254–257.

Lampert, R, Tuit, K, Hong, K-I, Donovan, T, Lee, F, Sinha, R. Cumulative stress and autonomic dysregulation in a community sample. *Stress.* 2016:1–11.

Le Scouarnec, RP, Poirier, RM, Owens, JE, Gauthier, J, Taylor, AG, Foresman, PA. Use of binaural beat tapes for treatment of anxiety: a pilot study of tape preference and outcomes. *Alternative Therapies in Health and Medicine.* 2001;7(1):58–63.

Liu, Y, Wheaton, AG, Chapman, DP, Croft, JB. Sleep Duration and Chronic Diseases among US Adults Age 45 Years and Older: Evidence from the 2010 Behavioral Risk Factor Surveillance System. *Sleep.* 2013;36(10):1421–1427.

Lutz, B. An Institutional Case Study: Emotion Regulation with HeartMath at Santa Cruz County Children's Mental Health. *Global Advances in Health and Medicine.* 2014;3(2):68–71.

Masuda, A, Kihara, T, Fukudome, T, Shinsato, T, Minagoe, S, Tei, C. The effects of repeated thermal therapy for two patients with chronic fatigue syndrome. *Journal of Psychosomatic Research.* 2005;58(4):383–387.

Masuda, A, Miyata, M, Kihara, T, Minagoe, S, Tei, C. Repeated Sauna Therapy Reduces Urinary 8-Epi-Prostaglandin F 2α. *Japanese Heart Journal.* 2004; 45(2):297–303.

Masuda, A, Nakazato, M, Kihara, T, Minagoe, S, Tei, C. Repeated Thermal Therapy Diminishes Appetite Loss and Subjective Complaints in Mildly Depressed Patients. *Psychosomatic Medicine.* 2005;67(4):643–647.

Mccraty, R, Atkinson, M, Lipsenthal, L, Arguelles, L. New Hope for Correctional Officers: An Innovative Program for Reducing Stress and Health Risks. *Applied Psychophysiology and Biofeedback.* 2009;34(4):251–272.

Mccraty, R, Zayas, MA. Cardiac coherence, self-regulation, autonomic stability, and psychosocial well-being. *Frontiers in Psychology.* 2014;5.

———. Intuitive Intelligence, Self-regulation, and Lifting Consciousness. *Global Advances in Health and Medicine.* 2014;3(2):56–65.

Moncayo, R, Moncayo, H. The WOMED model of benign thyroid disease: Acquired magnesium deficiency due to physical and psychological stressors relates to dysfunction of oxidative phosphorylation. *BBA Clinical.* 2015;3: 44–64.

Mooventhan, A, Shetty, G, Anagha, N. Effect of electro-acupuncture, massage, mud, and sauna therapies in patient with rheumatoid arthritis. *Journal of Ayurveda and Integrative Medicine.* 2015;6(4):295–299.

Myers, A. Episode 10: Sleep Expert Dan Pardi. *The Myers Way.* 2013. http://www .amymyersmd.com/2013/06/tmw-episode-10-sleep-expert-dan-pardi/.

Nasirinejad, F, Hoomayoonfar, H. Study on the Effects of Vagus Nerve in Controlling of Testosterone Secretion. *Razi Journal of Medical Sciences.* 1999;6(1):58–65.

O'Keane, V, Dinan, TG, Scott, L, Corcoran, C. Changes in Hypothalamic– Pituitary–Adrenal Axis Measures After Vagus Nerve Stimulation Therapy in Chronic Depression. *Biological Psychiatry.* 2005;58(12):963–968.

Padmanabhan, R, Hildreth, AJ, Laws, D. A prospective, randomised, controlled study examining binaural beat audio and pre-operative anxiety in patients undergoing general anaesthesia for day case surgery. *Anaesthesia.* 2005;60(9): 874–877.

Panossian, A, Wikman, G. Evidence-based efficacy of adaptogens in fatigue, and molecular mechanisms related to their stress-protective activity. *Current Clinical Pharmacology.* 2009 Sep;4(3):19–219.

Panossian, A, Wikman, G, Kaur, P, Asea, A. Adaptogens exert a stress-protective effect by modulation of expression of molecular chaperones. *Phytomedicine.* 2009 Jun;16(6–7):617–622.

Prasad, R, Kowalczyk, JC, Meimaridou, E, Storr, HL, Metherell, LA. Oxidative Stress and Adrenocortical Insufficiency. *Journal of Endocrinology.* 2014;221(3): R63–R73.

Ravalier, JM, Wegrzynek, P, Lawton, S. Systematic review: complementary therapies and employee well-being. *Occupational Medicine (Lond).* 2016.

Reyna-Garfias, R, Barbosa-Cabrera, E, Drago-Serrano, ME. Stress Modulates Intestinal Secretory Immunoglobulin A. *Frontiers in Integrative Neuroscience.* 2013;7:86.

Ruotsalainen, JH, Verbeek, JH, Mariné, A, Serra, C. Preventing occupational stress in healthcare workers. *Sao Paulo Medical Journal.* 2016;134(1):92.

Sapolsky, R. *Why Zebras Don't Get Ulcers.* New York: Holt, 2004.

Schoenberg, PLA, David, AS. Biofeedback for Psychiatric Disorders: A Systematic Review. *Applied Psychophysiology and Biofeedback.* 2014;39(2):109–135.

Segerstrom, SC, Miller, GE. Psychological Stress and the Human Immune System: A Meta-Analytic Study of 30 Years of Inquiry. *Psychological Bulletin.* 2004;130(4):601–630.

Shaffer, F, Mccraty, R, Zerr, CL. A healthy heart is not a metronome: an integrative review of the heart's anatomy and heart rate variability. *Frontiers in Psychology.* 2014;5.

Sripongngam, T, Eungpinichpong, W, Sirivongs, D, Kanpittaya, J, Tangvoraphonkchai, K, Chanaboon, S. Immediate Effects of Traditional Thai Massage on Psychological Stress as Indicated by Salivary Alpha-Amylase Levels in Healthy Persons. *Medical Science Monitor Basic Research.* 2015;21:216–221.

Summa, KC, Turek, FW. Chronobiology and Obesity: Interactions between Circadian Rhythms and Energy Regulation. *Advances in Nutrition: An International Review Journal.* 2014;5(3).

Talley, G. About Floating Guide. Float Tank Solutions. http://www.floattank solutions.com/product/free-guide-float-tanks-20-page-primer/.

Verkuil, B, Brosschot, JF, Tollenaar, MS, Lane, RD, Thayer, JF. Prolonged Non-metabolic Heart Rate Variability Reduction as a Physiological Marker of Psychological Stress in Daily Life. *Annals of Behavioral Medicine*. 2016.

Wahbeh, H, Calabrese, C, Zwickey, H. Binaural Beat Technology in Humans: A Pilot Study to Assess Psychologic and Physiologic Effects. *Journal of Alternative and Complementary Medicine*. 2007;13(1):25–32.

Wang, Y, Kondo, T, Suzukamo, Y, Oouchida, Y, Izumi, S-I. Vagal Nerve Regulation Is Essential for the Increase in Gastric Motility in Response to Mild Exercise. *Tohoku Journal of Experimental Medicine*. 2010;222(2):155–163.

Weiland, TJ, Jelinek, GA, Macarow, KE, et al. Original sound compositions reduce anxiety in emergency department patients: a randomised controlled trial. *Medical Journal of Australia*. 2011;195(11):694–698.

Wilson, J, Wright, JV. *Adrenal Fatigue: The 21st Century Stress Syndrome*. Smart Publications, 2001.

Zubeldia, JM, Nabi, HA, Del Río, MJ, Genovese, J. Exploring new applications for Rhodiola rosea: can we improve the quality of life of patients with short-term hypothyroidism induced by hormone withdrawal? *Journal of Medicinal Food*. 2010 Dec;13(6):1287–1292.

Chapter 11: *The Myers Way Thyroid Connection Plan*

Cordain, L, SB, Eaton, A, Sebastian, N, Mann, S, Lindeberg, BA, Watkins, O'Keefe, JH, et al. Origins and Evolution of the Western Diet: Health Implications for the 21st Century. *American Journal of Clinical Nutrition*. 2005;81(2): 341–354.

García-Niño, WR, Pedraza-Chaverrí, J. Protective Effect of Curcumin Against Heavy Metals-Induced Liver Damage. *Food and Chemical Toxicology*. 2014; 69C:182–201.

Gleeson, M. Nutritional Support to Maintain Proper Immune Status During Intense Training. *Nestlé Nutrition Institute Workshop Series*. 2013;75:85–97.

Harris, E, Macpherson, H, Pipingas, A. Improved Blood Biomarkers but No Cognitive Effects from 16 Weeks of Multivitamin Supplementation in Healthy Older Adults. *Nutrients*. 2015;7(5):3796–3812.

Institute for Functional Medicine. *Clinical Nutrition: A Functional Approach Textbook*. 2nd ed. 2004.

———. Functional Perspectives on Food and Nutrition: The Ultimate Upstream Medicine. Annual International Conference, San Francisco, CA, May 29–31, 2014. www.functionalmedicine.org/conference.aspx?id=2711&cid=35&section=t281.

———. *Textbook of Functional Medicine*. September 2010. www.functionalmedicine.org/listing_detail.aspx?id=2415&cid=34.

Kazi, YF, Saleem, S, Kazi, N. Investigation of Vaginal Microbiota in Sexually Active Women Using Hormonal Contraceptives in Pakistan. *BMC Urology*. 2012;18(12):22.

Krause, R, Schwab, E, Bachhiesl, D, Daxböck, F, Wenisch, C, Krejs, GJ, Reisinger, EC. Role of Candida in Antibiotic-Associated Diarrhea. *Journal of Infectious Diseases*. 2001;184(8):1065–1069.

Lieberman, S, Enig, MG, Preuss, HG. A Review of Monolaurin and Lauric Acid: Natural Virucidal and Bactericidal Agents. *Alternative and Complementary Therapies.* 2006;12(6):310–314.

Ludvigsson, JF, Neovius, M, Hammarström, L. Association Between IgA Deficiency and Other Autoimmune Conditions: A Population-Based Matched Cohort Study. *Journal of Clinical Immunology.* 2014;34(4):444–451.

Naglik, JR, Moyes, DL, Wächtler, B, Hube, B. *Candida albicans* Interactions with Epithelial Cells and Mucosal Immunity. *Microbes and Infection.* 2011;13 (12–13):963–976.

Nicholson, JK, Holmes, E, Kinross, J, Burcelin, R, Gibson, G, Jia, W, Pettersson, S. Host-Gut Microbiota Metabolic Interactions. *Science.* 2012;336(6086): 1262–1267.

Ogbolu, DO, Oni, AA, Daini, OA, Oloko, AP. In Vitro Antimicrobial Properties of Coconut Oil on Candida Species in Ibadan, Nigeria. *Journal of Medicinal Food.* 2007;10(2):384–387.

Özdemir, Ö. Any Role for Probiotics in the Therapy or Prevention of Autoimmune Diseases? Up-to-Date Review. *Journal of Complementary and Integrative Medicine.* 2013;10.

Patavino, T, Brady, DM. Natural Medicine and Nutritional Therapy as an Alternative Treatment in Systemic Lupus Erythematosus. *Alternative Medicine Review.* 2001;6(5):460–471.

Scrimgeour, AG, Condlin, ML. Zinc and Micronutrient Combinations to Combat Gastrointestinal Inflammation. *Current Opinion in Clinical Nutrition and Metabolic Care.* 2009;12(6):653–660.

Spampinato, C, Leonardi, D. Candida Infections, Causes, Targets, and Resistance Mechanisms: Traditional and Alternative Antifungal Agents. *BioMed Research International.* 2013. Article ID 204237.

Truss, CO. Metabolic Abnormalities in Patients with Chronic Candidiasis: The Acetaldehyde Hypothesis. *Journal of Orthomolecular Psychiatry.* 1984;13(2):66–93.

Van de Wijgert, JH, Verwijs, MC, Turner, AN, Morrison, CS. Hormonal Contraception Decreases Bacterial Vaginosis but Oral Contraception May Increase Candidiasis: Implications for HIV Transmission. *AIDS.* 2013;27(13):2141–2153.

Vojdani, A, Rahimian, P, Kalhor, H, Mordechai, E. Immunological Cross-Reactivity Between Candida albicans and Human Tissue. *Journal of Clinical and Laboratory Immunology.* 1996;48(1):1–15.

Wang, G, Wang, J, Ma, H, Ansari, G, Khan, MF. N-Acetylcysteine protects against trichloroethene-mediated autoimmunity by attenuating oxidative stress. *Toxicology and Applied Pharmacology.* 2013;273(1):189–195.

Wilhelm, SM, Rjater, RG, Kale-Pradhan, PB. Perils and Pitfalls of Long-Term Effects of Proton Pump Inhibitors. *Expert Review of Clinical Pharmacology.* 2013;6(4):443–451.

Wright, J, Lenard, L. *Why Stomach Acid Is Good for You: Natural Relief from Heartburn, Indigestion, Reflux, and GERD.* New York: M. Evans, 2001.

Zakout, YM, Salih, MM, Ahmed, HG. Frequency of Candida Species in Papanicolaou Smears Taken from Sudanese Oral Hormonal Contraceptives Users. *Biotech and Histochemistry.* 2012;87(2):95–97.

Index

Note: Italic page numbers refer to illustrations.

My Story

Helping people is my passion.

It's why I joined the Peace Corps, why I became a physician, why I did not stop searching, challenging, learning, and growing until I found what I believe to be the best way to heal people. My passion is to reach as many people, in as many places, in as many ways as possible, not just those people who are at the end of their rope or have the ability to see me.

Why? Because conventional medicine is a one-size-fits-all model. My belief is that health shouldn't be viewed as a cookie-cutter solution; it's more complex than that. Functional medicine is personalized medicine. I understand that no two people are alike. Each of us is unique in our genetic makeup and physiology. What ultimately causes illness in one person is not the same for another, and treatment for each will therefore be different. I know this from personal experience.

Every detail of your health history is interconnected like a web; everything is a clue to your present state of health and I want to absorb it all. With each patient, I seek to find the common link and solve problems from the root cause — not simply treat the symptoms.

For those who cannot see me in person, I share all that I can through my books, website, blog, podcasts, online courses, eBooks, and phone consultations. I've done the hard work as well and I practice what I preach. I've seen incredible health changes with my patients in my clinic. Now let's see what I can help you discover.